# A More Excellent Way

## Dr. Henry W. Wright

WHITAKER
HOUSE

# What Doctors and Others Are Saying...

As a physician, *A More Excellent Way*™ has changed my practice; as a believer, it has changed my life. It will change yours also.
—**Dr. Frans J. Cronje, MBChB, MSc**

In my 20+ years of dental practice, I have seen a direct connection between an individual's personal history and his overall health condition. Unless people are unusually strong spiritually, the more life trauma they experience, the more "sickly" they become. Henry Wright is not a simple "healer," but a man of faith who has used modern scientific methods to research and document the actual spiritual causes of specific diseases. Once the spiritual roots are dealt with, the body will heal itself.
—**Robert G. Wiese, DDS, Cosmetic & Laser Dentistry, Garland, TX**

Henry Wright gives a very unique biblical insight into the healing ministry, along with medical footnotes that point out the spiritual roots and causes of disease. Every pastor, evangelist, teacher and Christian layperson ought to have this manual as a follow-up to their healing ministry. The principles of the book *A More Excellent Way*™ brought clarity and understanding in my moments of personal tragedy.
—**Jimmie McDonald, author of the book *The Kathryn Kuhlman I Knew***
    **Ordained Elder in the African Methodist Episcopal Church**

It is a privilege to add my recommendation to this life-changing book. I have been a practicing physician for more than 20 years and when I first heard of *A More Excellent Way*™, I had significant skepticism and reservations. I have not only seen the transformed lives and physical healings, but have also experienced a personal transformation in my life and in my family. I feel I finally have an answer to so many of my patients' needs.
    My prayer for anyone reading this for the first time is that you will let the Word of God bring the transforming power it was always meant to.
—**Robert Wayne Inzer, MD, FACOG**

I found this book to be very informative, both spiritually and in the natural realm. You will be surprised to see how our spirit man and our spiritual condition affect our physical well-being. This is one great book, and I certainly recommend it for anyone suffering with disease or just wanting to maintain good health in their body. Packed full of "whys"; packed full of "how to correct"; packed full of encouragement for hurting souls. A real eye-opener!
—**Shirley Johnson, Senior Reviewer, Midwest Book Review**

# What Doctors and Others Are Saying…

This book is one of the most important books you will ever read. Definitely worth your time and may be hard to put down once you've started reading it! Be ready to be transformed in your thinking about disease.
**—Amazon.com Review**

In the monthly report of the Top 100 Books, *A More Excellent Way*™ has been as high as #3 in the Top 100 Christian Books and #1 in the category of Health/Fitness.
**—*Christian Retailing*, A Strang Publication**

All Scripture quotations are taken from the King James Version of the Holy Bible.

*Note:* This book is not intended to provide medical advice or to take the place of medical advice and treatment from your personal physician. Neither the publisher, nor the author, nor the author's ministry takes any responsibility for any possible consequences from any action taken by any person reading or following the information in this book. If readers are taking prescription medications, they should consult with their physicians and not take themselves off prescribed medicines without the proper supervision of a physician. Always consult your physician or other qualified health-care professional before undertaking any change in your physical regimen, whether fasting, diet, medications, or exercise.

## A More Excellent Way
### *commemorative trade paperback edition*

ISBN: 978-1-60374-101-9
eBook ISBN: 978-1-60374-202-3
Printed in the United States of America
© 1999, 2005, 2009 by Be in Health™, Inc. All rights reserved.

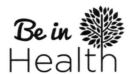

If you wish to contact Dr. Henry W. Wright or Be in Health™:
4178 Crest Highway
Thomaston, GA 30286
phone: 706.646.2074 • 800.453.5775
fax: 706.646.2864
info@beinhealth.com
www.beinhealth.com

Whitaker House
1030 Hunt Valley Circle
New Kensington, PA 15068
www.whitakerhouse.com

**Library of Congress Cataloging-in-Publication Data**

Wright, Henry (Henry W.)
 A more excellent way / by Henry W. Wright. — Commemorative ed.
  p. cm.
 Rev. ed. of: A more excellent way (1 Corinthians 12:31).
 Summary: "Presents the case that the roots of psychological and biological diseases are spiritual, and provides advice on how to eradicate disease instead of treating symptoms"—Provided by publisher.
 Includes bibliographical references (p.    ) and index.
 ISBN 978-1-60374-102-6 (trade hardcover : alk. paper) — ISBN 978-1-60374-101-9 (trade pbk. : alk. paper) 1. Spiritual healing—Christianity. 2. Diseases—Religious aspects—Christianity. 3. Spiritual life—Christianity. I. Wright, Henry (Henry W.). More excellent way, 1 Corinthians 12:31. II. Title.
 BT732.5.W755 2009
 234'.131—dc22
                      2008052913

7  8  9  10  11  12  13  14  **ʊʃ**  21  20  19  18  17  16

## *What you're about to read is dangerous!*

This book is one of the most thought-provoking and challenging works you may ever read. Satan, the enemy of God, hates this book because people read it and many are radically changed and even healed of their diseases.

Have you ever met Christians who believe in God but are miserable? Where's the victory? Is God the problem or are we? Could it be we are ignorant in some areas and that lack of understanding is costing us our joy?

This book will give you knowledge and discernment to help you recover yourself from the things that are interfering with your life. The text was taken from a live conference, so it's very conversational, and disease topics are sown throughout. If you have an illness, syndrome, or disease, you'll be very tempted to go to the index and look up every reference. Don't stop there. The healing you're looking for is woven into the *entire message*. We hope you can overcome and read the whole book!

In addition to the testimonies you'll find at the back, you can go to **iamchanged.com** and watch amazing videos of healing. Sign up there to connect with us through social media and receive our weekly emails. We hope you'll also consider attending our weeklong program of teaching and ministry in Thomaston, Georgia, called **For My Life**®.

You have so much to gain by reading this book. We hope you'll open your heart to this message from God's Word and dive right in!

With love,

The Be in Health Team

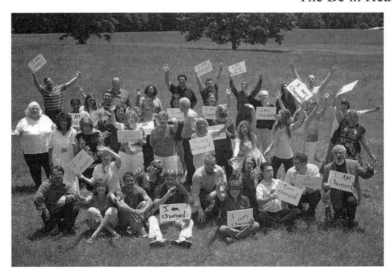

# Contents

# Meet Dr. Wright

Dr. Henry W. Wright is the Senior Pastor of Hope of the Generations Church in Thomaston, Georgia, and President/Founder of Be in Health®. He conducts conferences all over the world and has developed several ministry programs, including **For My Life**®. Dr. Wright grew up knowing that God heals disease. His mother was dying from a tumor that had wrapped itself around her jugular vein. At church one Sunday, she repented for bitterness and cried out to God. Instantly, the tumor was gone and she lived another 33 years! Her prayer was that her son would one day serve God, too.

Dr. Wright has dedicated his life to God and helping others find the spiritual roots to disease so they can live in wholeness. He holds a doctorate of Christian Therapeutic Counseling from Chesapeake Bible College in Ridgely, MD. In the past 25 years, he and his team have touched the lives of one million people, helping them overcome disease and find their place in God.

# Dedication

This book is dedicated to my mother, Norma Anne Wilson Wright, who went to be with the LORD on Thanksgiving Day, 1977. When I was in her womb, she was dying with fibrosarcoma cancer, fast-growing and fatal. This cancer was wrapped around her jugular vein and had spread to large areas in her neck and up into the base of her brain. In this condition, paralyzed, wasting away and dying, she was present at a church service in Hatfield Point, New Brunswick, Canada, about two months after I was born. At this service, God touched her and she was instantly healed. Her doctors were unable to find any trace of the masses of cancer that they had observed previously. The cancer was gone. No medical treatment had been given. She lived for 33 more years and was probably the only place of peace I ever had growing up. Her faith and her example and the testimony of her life continue to set an example for me and not only for me but for others whom I can touch because of her steadfast faith in God. Her healing set a standard within me against the enemy. In truth, God is no respecter of persons and what He has done for one, He will do for another.

# Foreword

When one goes to a physician, he expects to be given something to counteract what is wrong in his body. For example, if the blood pressure is high, one is given a chemical (medicine) that lowers blood pressure. A prescription medicine "pushes" one's body chemistry to a more "normal" state, alleviating discomfort and sometimes slowing the destruction of the body caused by disease. Nevertheless, many chronic diseases such as diabetes mellitus, heart disease and arthritis continue to get worse despite the administration of more and more medicines. At its best, medical care appears to help the suffering person to live with his or her disease more comfortably and perhaps a little longer than otherwise might be the case.

This book outlines a simple approach to the prevention and elimination of chronic disease. Its approach is not about living a better life with a chronic disease, but living free of disease. Originally, the word disease meant "lack of ease" or "LACK OF PEACE." When a person is not at peace, this is not a medical issue but a spiritual issue that has many facets, each of which God has a specific, individualized solution for. This book does not have all the answers; yet, this book can direct the thoughtful reader onto a path, a highway of discovery that is life changing and where the root causes of disease can be addressed and eliminated. Jesus said, "Peace I leave with you, my peace I give unto you: not as the world giveth, give I unto you. Let not your heart be troubled, neither let it be afraid" (John 14:27). This book is not against medicine, but goes beyond what medical care offers because it addresses the connection between the human spirit and the human chemistry that a doctor understands. Reader, you have been fearfully and wonderfully made; many of you have also been unmade by spiritual forces that have stolen your peace. It is not too late—don't leave your doctor. But take God's hand and allow Him to lead you as you read this book—then there may come a time when your doctor says to you, "we can stop this medicine; it is not needed any more."

—*William Gottlob Berlinger III, MD*
Internal Medicine and Geriatrics
Philadelphia, Pennsylvania

# Disclaimer

We do not seek to be in conflict with any medical or psychiatric practices, any church or its religious doctrines, beliefs or practices. We are not part of medicine or psychology; we are working to make them more effective, believing many human problems are fundamentally spiritual with associated physiological and psychological manifestations. This information is intended for your general knowledge only, to give insight into disease, its problems, and possible solutions. It is not a substitute for medical advice or treatment from specific medical conditions or disorders. We do not diagnose or treat disease.

You should seek prompt medical care for any specific health issues. Treatment modalities around your specific health issues are between you and your physician. We are not responsible for a person's disease or their healing. We are administering the Scriptures and what they say about this subject, along with what the medical and scientific communities have observed in line with this insight. There is no guarantee any person will be healed or any disease prevented. The fruits of this teaching will come forth out of the application of the principles and the relationship between each person and God. Be in Health is patterned after 2 Corinthians 5:18–20; 1 Corinthians 12; Ephesians 4; and Mark 16:15–20.

# What We Believe

The Holy Bible—and only the Bible—is 100% the Word of God. 2 Timothy 3:16; 2 Peter 1:20–21. Our foundation is the Authorized King James Version of the Bible, translated from Hebrew as the Masoretic Text and from Greek as the Majority Text. The eternal Godhead is revealed in the Hebrew Masoretic Text (OT) and the Greek Majority Text (NT). Deut. 6:4; Gen. 1:26; Is. 48:16; Matt. 28:19; 1 Cor. 10:1–11. All the purposes of God are now a finished work through Jesus Christ by faith; by which He created all things, by whom He saved and restored all things and whom He has made the head of all things, forever. Is. 48; John 1:1–36; Col. 1:12–29; Heb. 1.

**Jesus Christ is the LORD God**; God the Word. He came in the flesh and is the only begotten Son of God. He was conceived by God the Holy Ghost in the womb of Mary, the Virgin, and lived a sinless life as a human being. Jesus was anointed by God with the Holy Ghost to destroy the works of the devil and to show us the ministry of believer/priest to preach the good news, call for men everywhere to repent and turn to God, heal the sick and do cures in His name, and cast out devils. He died for our sins and for the sins of all who believe on His name. He is the sacrificial Lamb; by His shed blood we have remission of sins. He reconciled us to God by faith and indwells us by the Holy Spirit. His body lay in the grave three days and three nights and on the third day God raised Him from the dead. After that He walked on this earth for 40 days and was seen by up to 500 people at one time.

He ascended into heaven and sat down on the right hand of God. He is coming again, first in the "First Resurrection." Seven years later in the "Day of the Lord" He will come and all the saints with Him to defeat the antichrist and set up Christ's millennial reign as the Messiah, Zechariah 14:1-5. As the fullness of the Godhead rested bodily on Jesus as a work of the Holy Spirit, this fullness of the Godhead should rest on the body of Christ (the Church) in the earth today. 1 Corinthians 12

**The Doctrines of Christ - Hebrews 6:1–2 -** are repentance from dead works, faith towards God, the doctrine of baptisms, laying on of hands, resurrection of the dead, and eternal judgment. **The Sacraments of the Church** include the LORD's Supper (Communion), water baptism, footwashing. **The Great Commission** is a world vision for the body of Christ (the Church.) We are the salt of the earth, the light of the world, called to show the love of God by the love we have one for another, called to a fast of service as servants, called to be a gift to mankind. **Healing and Miracles** are part of the atonement , valid for today (Jesus Christ the same, yesterday, today and forever.) Ps. 103:3; 1 Thes. 5:23; 3 John 2; 1 Cor. 12.

# Preface

This book is designed to sow seeds of knowledge into your hearts about a big problem. The problem is spiritual, psychological and biological disease and what can we do about it and where is God in it today.

I ask for much grace and mercy in the reading because this teaching is not designed to be a theological dissertation, but is designed to be an insight into a problem and its solution: disease prevention and eradication. You will find this material to be scripturally accurate as well as medically and scientifically observable.

I find myself on the cutting edge of a problem and its solution. I do not have all the answers and I am still learning more every day. I reserve the right to revise this information as God increases the depth of my understanding.

One of my desires is to better equip the Church with respect to defeating spiritual, psychological and biological diseases. Also, one of my goals is to take away the mystery of disease and to be able to show, from God's perspective, why mankind has disease.

Over the years, God has shown me many insights into why mankind has disease. It is not that God cannot heal or that He doesn't want to; the problem is that man doesn't understand disease. We have gone into captivity and are perishing because of either lack of knowledge or just no knowledge at all. My investigation over the years, from the Scriptures and by practical discernment, has unearthed many spiritual roots and blocks to healing. In fact, the basic principles that, when applied, will move the hand of God to heal, are the same that, when applied, will prevent disease.

God's perfect will is not to heal you; His perfect will is that you do not get sick. Today, this church/ministry and I stand 100 percent for disease eradication and prevention, not disease management, on a regular basis, if at all possible. To this end, this church and I are dedicated.

I do not want this book to become a method or a science or a formula or a quick fix to take the place of relationship with God. One of the main themes of this book is the connection between sin and disease. Another theme in the book is the consequence of separation from God, His Word, His love, separation from ourselves and separation from others.

One of the things that concerns me for those who will use this book to try to help others is that they will make it into a science or, at worst, use the knowledge in a legalistic manner to condemn others. A heart of compassion is the key to ministry. This current edition adds testimonies and guides to ministering in *A More Excellent Way*™.

The Authorized King James Version of the Bible is the foundation for this teaching. Please do not change the King James Version as a scriptural foundation because this teaching will lose the integrity and intent of its meaning.

—*Dr. Henry W. Wright*

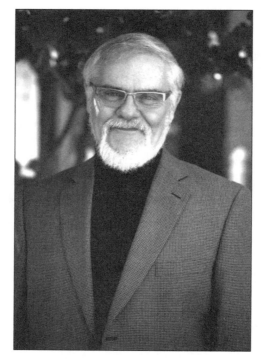

Dr. Henry W. Wright, DCTC, MCM

# Chapter One
# My Purpose and Insight

## Introduction

When I began in ministry in the early 1980s, I was part of a church that believed God did get involved in people's lives and there was something happening between conversion and heaven. But even in that church of over 1500 people, coming week after week, the elders anointing them with oil, praying the prayer of faith, fasting and praying and standing on the Word, people were not getting well from incurable diseases.

As I crossed America, I observed that regardless of denomination, regardless of the church, less than 5 percent of all of God's people (forget about the world) were getting healed of their diseases. It is even worse than that today. I do not know if you have ever been prayed for because of a disease and didn't get well. If you went before God and believed Him, believed He loved you and He would heal you, yet it didn't happen, that is a staggering attack on your faith and your trust in the living God.

Scripture tells us God loves us and He came and died for us in the person of the Lord Jesus. He healed the people of their diseases and cast out their evil spirits. The disciples did it, the 70 did it and the early Church did it. Then we entered into a dark age of time from which I do not think we have ever recovered.

When I began in ministry, I wanted to know why God said He not only forgives us of all our iniquities, but He heals us of all our diseases.

> **Who forgiveth all thine iniquities; who healeth all thy diseases; Psalm 103:3**

In the Old Testament, people were raised from the dead, people were healed and many other miracles were done. In the New Testament I found we had a new and better covenant. In 3 John it says,

> **Beloved, I wish above all things that thou mayest prosper and be in health, even as thy soul prospereth. 3 John 1:2**

In 1 Thessalonians, Paul says, May the God of Peace sanctify you **wholly** in **spirit**, in **soul** and in **body**.

> **And the very God of peace sanctify you wholly; and I pray God your whole spirit and soul and body be preserved blameless unto the coming of our Lord Jesus Christ. 1 Thessalonians 5:23**

Well, I didn't see much sanctification of the body. I didn't see much sanctification of the soul and I found a need for sanctification of God's people in holiness. I have found God's people struggle with the things of life. Paul did in Romans.

> **¹⁴For we know that the law is spiritual: but I am carnal, sold under sin. ¹⁵For that which I do I allow not: for what I would, that do I not; but what I hate, that do I. ¹⁶If then I do that which I would not, I consent unto the law that *it is* good. ¹⁷Now then it is no more I that do it, but sin that dwelleth in me. Romans 7:14–17**

Paul had a major struggle with his own spirituality. In fact, he said he had a **sin that dwelt within him**.

When I began to become involved with people in their lives, I prayed for them and believed God would heal them, but less than 5 percent of everyone I prayed was healed. I preached a gospel, helped people be saved and go to heaven, but left them stranded between conversion and heaven. Would that be the gospel I would preach? Would I come up with a doctrine that would establish it? It would be easy to say, "Sorry, no help for you, no hope for you." But in my heart, the Scriptures I read seemed to indicate differently.

I went to God one day and said, "You had better talk to me, Boss, because if You have called me to represent You to Your people and to those yet unsaved, You had better show me a little more fruit. If it's not happening, You had better tell me why or else I am going to go back into sales and marketing. I'll go to church, I'll love you, I'll be a good Christian, I might even be a deacon, but you can forget about me speaking. I am not speaking for You if my words are not being honored, because that is fraud."

The Bible says if any man lack wisdom, let him ask of God and God will give it to him liberally and upbraid him not because he has the audacity to ask God for a little information!

> **If any of you lack wisdom, let him ask of God, that giveth to all *men* liberally, and upbraideth not; and it shall be given him. James 1:5**

I went before God in the early 1980s and He began to show me His truth about disease from the Scriptures. It wasn't that He *could not* heal. It was that we had to become sanctified in certain areas of our lives before He *would* heal.

### *Diseases in our lives can be the result of a separation from Him and His Word in specific areas of our lives.*

God would have to become double minded, would have to become evil in condoning evil, in order to bless us in our sins. Except for those times when He will have mercy on whom He will have mercy, disease is an issue that has to do with circumcision of the heart.

> And he said, I will make all my goodness pass before thee, and I will proclaim the name of the LORD before thee; and will be gracious to whom I will be gracious, and will shew mercy on whom I will shew mercy. **Exodus 33:19**

> For he saith to Moses, I will have mercy on whom I will have mercy, and I will have compassion on whom I will have compassion. **Romans 9:15**

A lot of people struggle with the supposed "gaps" between the Gospels, the book of Acts and the Epistles. After Acts, there is very little discussion about healing and deliverance. Thus, some have said, "Well, it passed away because you do not find it," or "Healing was only for Christ or the disciples and not for us." I struggled with that. I'll be honest with you.

One day, my eyes were opened and I saw something. I have never looked back from the ministry God set before me.

The Lord came and He demonstrated the love of God and power over the devil and disease in spite of sin. He demonstrated it in Matthew, Mark, Luke and John. His disciples and the early Church also demonstrated it in Acts. Then from Romans all the way through Jude you will find the Scriptures teaching us about sanctification.

You cannot have Matthew, Mark, Luke, John and Acts until you have dealt with Romans to Jude. You cannot expect God to bless you if you are separated from Him in an area that needs to be dealt with.

### *We have been taught so much about God's promises and not much about His Spirit of discernment and the consequence of sin.*

If someone came to me with simple arthritis and asked me to pray for them, I would say, "No, I'm not going to do it."

If they said, "But the Word says to come before the elders and be anointed with oil and be prayed for," I would respond, "No, I've been there, done that!"

Do you know how many times I have prayed for people with arthritis in the past? None of them were healed. I quit praying for them; it was a waste of my time. But one day God opened my heart. I was ministering in 1985, when five ladies came up to me. Each of them had arthritis. Two of the ladies had gnarly disfiguration. I said to them, "You know, there is sometimes a responsibility to God for healing."

I want to tell you that healing and things you receive from God, to a degree, are conditional to your obedience. I am not into legalism. I am into grace and mercy. **But I want to tell you that with freedom comes a degree of responsibility.**

As you study through this teaching, I am going to touch the very fabric of your lives. If you're interested in your life and your family's lives, this is a good time to listen. I am going to sow seed. Just as the rain comes down and waters the crops and returns to the clouds, the Bible says the Word does not return void.

> **So shall my word be that goeth forth out of my mouth: it shall not return unto me void, but it shall accomplish that which I please, and it shall prosper *in the thing* whereto I sent it. Isaiah 55:11**

I am going to seed (plant) **knowledge** into your life.

The knowledge I have is not only accurate scripturally, but it is also accurate medically. Coast-to-coast in America, I deal with disease. Even doctors have contacted me regarding their own lives. There are doctors in America who call and discuss with me the implications of their patient's disease. I have doctors who refer their patients to me to discuss the spiritual roots of disease.

I sense the tide shifting across broad denominational lines. Our ministry is a nondenominational ministry. What is a nondenominational ministry? It is one that believes that, in spite of denominations, God is still on the throne. The Lord Jesus is still the Word Who came in the flesh and the Holy Spirit is still on the earth today—One Faith, One Lord and One Baptism until we come into the unity of faith.

> **One Lord, one faith, one baptism, Ephesians 4:5**

> **Till we all come in the unity of the faith, and of the knowledge of the Son of God, unto a perfect man, unto the measure of the stature of the fulness of Christ: Ephesians 4:13**

If I stumble over your sacred cows of theology, I am sorry. It is not in my heart to do that even unintentionally. I ask you to listen thoughtfully to what I have to say. You will find what I have to say may bear witness and answer a lot of your questions.

I told the five ladies with arthritis *there would be a condition to their healing*. I asked them to think about the people who had injured each of them in their lifetime, either through word or deed—someone who didn't treat them right, victimized them, lied about them, abused them, either emotionally, physically, verbally or maybe even sexually.

I asked them, "When you think of their name, or their face, whether they're living or dead, what do you feel? Do any of you have that high-octane ping going off inside?"

They all said, "Yes, there is somebody I have not had resolution with." There was bitterness and unforgiveness. I told them that in exchange for their healing, they would have to get that right with God, right then, or else we were wasting our time. They were going to have to forgive that person. The Scriptures say:

> But if ye forgive not men their trespasses, neither will your Father forgive your trespasses. Matthew 6:15

Have you ever read that Scripture? Do you think it is there just for fun? Do you think it is a situational Scripture that only applies to some and not to all?

People ask me, "Does God forgive all manner of sin?" Yes and no. He wants to; that is His nature. He said He does:

> If we confess our sins, he is faithful and just to forgive us *our* sins, and to cleanse us from all unrighteousness. 1 John 1:9

But after conversion, there is an absolute requirement and responsibility to forgive others. How do you resolve this Scripture in 1 John with the one in Matthew that says, "If you from your heart do not forgive your brother his trespass, your Father which is in heaven will not forgive you yours"?

> [14]For if ye forgive men their trespasses, your heavenly Father will also forgive you: [15]But if ye forgive not men their trespasses, neither will your Father forgive your trespasses. Matthew 6:14–15

When you take a good look at these Scriptures, you will find you can go to heaven with sin because it is by faith we are saved, not by works.

> [8]For by grace are ye saved through faith; and that not of yourselves: *it is* the gift of God: [9]Not of works, lest any man should boast. Ephesians 2:8–9

But the consequences of unforgiveness may bind you to a disease resulting from this sin of bitterness and unforgiveness. Christians, for the most part, believe we are saved by grace and by faith. But just because you are born again and your spirit has become alive in God, it does not mean you have resolved the consequences of the sin issue in your life. Otherwise, we would not need sanctification, would we?

I told the five ladies an exchange would happen for their obedience. I said, "If you, from your heart, will sincerely forgive that person of their trespasses whether you feel like it or not, I am going to ask God to heal you. If you just do it because you want the healing for selfish reasons and you are using this kind of like a mechanism, or a system or a mantra, then we are still wasting our time."

The Bible says that if you forgive from your heart…

> So likewise shall my heavenly Father do also unto you, if ye from your hearts forgive not every one his brother their trespasses. Matthew 18:35

Your head might still be pitching a fit about what they did to you because it is in your memory. The Bible says,

**For as many as are led by the Spirit of God, they are the sons of God. Romans 8:14**

Are you being led by your psychology (soul) or is the Spirit of God leading you? Who lives within your human spirit and makes you sons and daughters of God? Are you being led by the Spirit of God or by the intellect and other thoughts? I ask because it is an important question.

I led them into a prayer of repentance and forgiveness. I am here to tell you that when I finished the prayer, I looked up to them and said, "How's your arthritis doing?" All of a sudden it dawned on them: they had no more pain. Fingers had straightened. The pain was gone. All five ladies stood there totally freed from crippling arthritis and its pain. *I had never ministered healing one time.*

When they met the conditions of *God's* nature, He was there to heal. So I am not too impressed (I say this carefully) by healing crusades not taking into account that a disease may be the result of sin not dealt with.

I do not know if you are aware of this, but fear is a sin. Fear is a sin. Fear is the  number one plague of America and it is the number one plague of the world—fear of tomorrow, fear of death, fear of man, fear of dying, fear of disease, fear of mothers-in-law, fear of your neighbor and fear of yourself.

We are a people of God who are in bondage. We are paying an incredibly high price. God's people are being sent back into the world for help when the answer to setting them free is waiting in His Word. I am more interested in getting you into a better life, not just getting you into heaven.

The Lord's prayer says,

**⁹...Our Father which art in heaven, Hallowed be thy name. ¹⁰Thy kingdom come. Thy will be done in earth, as *it is* in heaven. Matthew 6:9–10**

When I read 3 John 2, it was over for me.

**Beloved, I wish above all things that thou mayest prosper and be in health, even as thy soul prospereth. 3 John 2**

*God's perfect will is not to heal you.*
*God's perfect will in the Word is that you do not get sick.*

In Exodus 15 and Deuteronomy 28, God promised if we are obedient to Him, none of the diseases of Egypt will fall upon us.

And said, If thou wilt diligently hearken to the voice of the LORD thy God, and wilt do that which is right in his sight, and wilt give ear to his commandments, and keep all his statutes, I will put none of these diseases upon thee, which I have brought upon the Egyptians: for I *am* the LORD that healeth thee. Exodus 15:26

And it shall come to pass, if thou shalt hearken diligently unto the voice of the LORD thy God, to observe *and* to do all his commandments which I command thee this day, that the LORD thy God will set thee on high above all nations of the earth: Deuteronomy 28:1

Deuteronomy also makes mention of the diseases of Egypt coming upon us because of disobedience.

Moreover he will bring upon thee all the diseases of Egypt, which thou wast afraid of; and they shall cleave unto thee. Deuteronomy 28:60

*Newsweek* magazine, in a 1990 article called "The Power to Heal," said: "The fate of the spirit is relegated to religious specialists who have little to say about their followers' physical well being."

Many pastors in America today do not understand diseases and they do not understand psychological problems. They know how to help you become born again. They know how to balance a budget. They know how to visit hospitals, marry people and bury the dead, but they do not know what to do with disease. So they will send you out into the street to an unregenerated, unrenewed specialist in a disease and maybe even call them the anointed of God.

In the Old Testament, if someone had leprosy and later said they were clean, to whom were they sent to determine if they were healed? The priest! The New Testament says, if there be any sick among you, call who? The elders of the Church.

Is any sick among you? let him call for the elders of the church; and let them pray over him, anointing him with oil in the name of the Lord: James 5:14

*If I have anything to do with it in my lifetime,*
*I intend to bring the pastoral ministry*
*back to where God wanted it from the beginning.*

This happens when God honors what ministers are teaching by healing diseases as the Word is applied to the lives of the people.

In 1996, I taught in a church in Texas where a member was healed of multiple chemical sensitivity (MCS/EI). She had not been able to go to church for over 20 years. She was isolated. She could only eat two to four foods, suffered from electromagnetic sensitivity, chronic fatigue syndrome and multiple allergies. God healed her. He healed all the peripheral diseases around MCS/EI.

That church is really rocking because she is back singing in the choir every Sunday. They asked me to come and teach on roots of disease, so I went there and taught. I came back again that evening and taught for another 2½ hours on the spiritual roots of disease and the consequences of sin.

The next morning, they brought a lady to me privately who had cancer of the lung and cancer of the bone. She had been to all the doctors and had all the bone scans and x-rays. She was the mother of two children.

Because I knew the spiritual root of her disease, I just kind of laid it out. This is your disease; this is what I see. It took about three seconds and she was bawling like a baby. I had touched her pain. I had touched her spiritual dynamics. God opened her up with discernment and I put my hand right on that thing that had been festering for years, causing eventual destruction of the two sentries of her immune system (called anti-oncogenes) that protect us from cancer. When those enzymes are destroyed in our bodies, the cell is compromised and cancer cell mitosis can begin at any time.

I told her, "I do not know what God's going to do, but I do know you are going to have to get right with God in this area of your life."

She said, "I've known that all the time, but I just couldn't get there. I just couldn't get over it."

I said, "Would you like to go there and get over it?"

She said, "Yes." I led her into a place before the Lord and before the Father, a place of soul searching, a place of repentance and of getting right with God. I took authority over the spirit of death and the cancer.

Thirty days later, I got a phone call. She had been back to the doctor and had bone scans and X-rays. There was no evidence of lung cancer or bone cancer. Her pastor has already sent me two letters, asking me to train his deacons and his teams. He and the members of his congregation were ready to start learning how to care for the sheep in *a more excellent way*™. He said, "Thank you for coming and allowing the Lord to speak through you about the connection between sin and disease."

We think of sin as robbing banks. We think of sin as maybe prostitution, lying and stealing. Would you consider fear to be sin? Would you consider bitterness to be sin? Would you consider self-hatred to be sin? Would you consider these things to be sin? The Word says they are. I think certain sins have become socially acceptable. We are paying too high a price for these areas of unrecognized sin in the area of disease.

About 30 percent of all cancers have a spiritually rooted component. I specialize in cancer to some degree, but I do not have all the answers. We are somewhat familiar with uterine, ovarian, breast and prostate cancer. We have insight into how these cancers develop. In the section on the spiritual roots of disease, I'll go into this in detail.

About 80 percent of all diseases have a spiritual root with various psychological and biological manifestations. I am not a doctor or psychologist. I do not mix psychology with ministry. I am a servant of the Father and the Lord Jesus Christ. No man has taught me, but He has taught me.

## Disease Prevention, Not Disease Management, Is My Goal

My parents were ministers. I am a third generation spiritual leader. I grew up with the knowledge that God heals because of my mother's miraculous healing.

My mother was dying with fibrosarcoma cancer, fast-growing and fatal, which had wrapped around her jugular vein. Just two months after my birth, she was dying. She was paralyzed. Masses of cancer had grown around her jugular vein and up into the base of her brain—up and down her whole neck area. She repented of bitterness and made a Hannah-type covenant that if God would heal her, she would raise me, Henry, in the knowledge of God.

In this private moment of prayer while others were praying for her, God healed her instantly. When the doctors checked, they were amazed to find no evidence of cancer. No medical treatment had been given, yet the masses of cancer were gone, evaporated. Even more remarkable, *her healing broke a pattern*, a genetic curse from her past. You see, her mother had died of cancer within two months of giving birth to her. With this curse defeated, my mother lived another 33 years.

In my later years—you noticed I said, "later years…"—I dedicated my life to God and the study of the Scriptures. The Bible says to teach a child in the way he should go and when he is old, he shall not depart from it.

> **Train up a child in the way he should go: and when he is old, he will not depart from it. Proverbs 22:6**

The Scriptures seem to indicate the Lord wants to heal *all* of our diseases.

> **Who forgiveth all thine iniquities; who healeth all thy diseases; Psalm 103:3**

Yet I observed that only a small percentage of people have ever defeated incurable diseases, including those who looked to churches for their healing.

I understood the frustration of Carl Jung as he observed his minister father preach a gospel that offered no solutions for the diseases of the soul and the body. Today's psychology is in part the fruit of that frustration as an attempt to manage the diseases of the soul through therapy and drugs.

I observed the Church, religions, alternative medicine, spiritual groups, allopathic medicine, chiropractic and eastern mysticism trying to decrease the effects of disease through various methods. **In the end, all I really ever saw was disease management.**

I want to say something to you: the best you have going for you in American medicine is HMOs. The insurance industry recognizes disease is on the increase, so they are going to cut their costs, cut their risk for the benefit of the stockholders and you are going to pay the price. They are going to pay what they want to pay for your medical care and no more. I suggest that there is *a more excellent way™*.

I did a seminar in New York City in an off-Broadway theater that was donated to our ministry for two days. In my audience was a doctor from New York. At the end of two days, he came up to me and said,

> I am a member of the medical community here in New York City. I have been here listening to you for two days. When you say that disease management is the best that the medical community can offer, you have been very generous to our industry. *The best we could only hope to achieve is disease management.* It would be good if we could do that.

Recent national statistics show with all modalities of treatment for cancer, including surgery, chemotherapy, vitamins, supplements and all the various types of therapies, the average life extension was only one year. That one year of prolonged life came at great expense and with tremendous pain and suffering.

Psalm 103:3 says the Lord not only forgives us of all our iniquities, but He heals us of all our diseases. It doesn't say, "He helps us manage all our diseases."

> **Who forgiveth all thine iniquities; who healeth all thy diseases;**
> **Psalm 103:3**

Let me say something to you: I couldn't heal a fly with a toothache. I do not have any powers; I am just a sheepherder. I am not a healer; I am just a guy. I know Him Who is God and I know His Word. As a minister, I cannot teach a gospel that makes God less than *omnipotent*; I have to hold out for that. I also have to hold out that God is *omniscient*. He knows everything: past, present and future. I also have to hold out that He is *omnipresent*. He is available worldwide, all the time, everywhere.

The fourth area that I have to hold out for is something you have probably not heard a lot about; **God is also omnificent**, all creative, ever able to fix that which needs to be fixed. *Being omnificent makes Him* *magnificent*—King of kings and LORD of all lords. He is God of all gods. He is the Creator of all flesh. He is the Sustainer of all mankind. He is in love with you and I am in love with Him. I hope you are too!

Over the years, God has shown me many insights into why mankind has disease.

> *It is not that God cannot heal you, or that He doesn't want to.*
> *The problem is that man does not understand disease.*

We have gone into captivity and are perishing either because of lack of knowledge or just no knowledge at all.

God said to the prophet Isaiah, "My people are gone into captivity, because they have no knowledge...." Hell hath enlarged herself and swallowed them up and all of their fame into the depths of hell.

> **13Therefore my people are gone into captivity, because *they have* no knowledge: and their honourable men *are* famished, and their multitude dried up with thirst. 14Therefore hell hath enlarged herself, and opened her mouth without measure: and their glory, and their multitude, and their pomp, and he that rejoiceth, shall descend into it. Isaiah 5:13–14**

He is not talking about unsaved Gentiles; He's talking about *My people*, called by My Name, set aside by My covenant. My people in the earth are going into captivity because they have no knowledge.

Hosea says God's people perish because of lack of knowledge.

> **My people are destroyed for lack of knowledge: because thou hast rejected knowledge, I will also reject thee, that thou shalt be no priest to me: seeing thou hast forgotten the law of thy God, I will also forget thy children. Hosea 4:6**

So whether it's lack of knowledge or no knowledge,

> **All we like sheep have gone astray; we have turned every one to his own way... Isaiah 53:6**

I would like to make sure we change that, if we can.

My investigation over the years from the Scriptures, practical discernment and review of scientific and medical evidence, has unearthed many spiritual roots and blocks to healing.

> *In fact, the basic principles that, when applied,*
> *will move the hand of God to heal,*
> *are the same principles that, when applied,*
> *will prevent disease.*

The very same principles that you can apply in your life to move the hand of God to sustain you, to heal you and to deliver you—if you start applying them now in your life even if you do not have a disease—may keep you from getting that disease in your lifetime.

Deuteronomy 28 and Exodus 15 say because of our obedience to God and His Word and our fellowship with Him in the covenant, He will put none of the diseases of Egypt upon us.

> **And said, If thou wilt diligently hearken to the voice of the LORD thy God, and wilt do that which is right in his sight, and wilt give ear to his commandments, and keep all his statutes, I will put none of these diseases upon thee, which I have brought upon the Egyptians: for I *am* the LORD that healeth thee. Exodus 15:26**

*That is a valid promise even today. So either we are going to continue in promise or we are going to teach bondage.*

### God's Perfect Will is Not to Heal You; His Perfect Will is That You Do Not Get Sick.

Today, I stand 100 percent not for disease management, but for disease eradication and prevention on a regular basis, if at all possible.

> **[14]Turn, O backsliding children, saith the LORD; for I am married unto you: and I will take you one of a city, and two of a family, and I will bring you to Zion: [15]And I will give you pastors according to mine heart, which shall feed you with knowledge and understanding. Jeremiah 3:14–15**

It is my prayer that you will and can receive this. I consider this to be my ministry and a gift to you. I desire to feed you with knowledge and understanding. Paul instructed Timothy,

> **[24]And the servant of the Lord must not strive; but be gentle unto all *men,* apt to teach, patient, [25]In meekness instructing those that oppose themselves; if God peradventure will give them repentance to the acknowledging of the truth; [26]And *that* they may recover themselves out of the snare of the devil, who are taken captive by him at his [the devil's] will. 2 Timothy 2:24–26**

In this teaching, I can give you enough information and enough knowledge so you will be able to come before God and so the work of sanctification, healing and deliverance can begin for you and your loved ones—your friends and your families. Remember, I told you that my purpose is to sow seed—to leave behind a foundation for God, by His Spirit, according to the Word of God and according to knowledge that is available both from the scientific and medical communities and from the Word. My purpose is to bring you to a place where you may recover yourself from the snare of the devil.

One day, someone said, "I believe God gave me my disease. I am closer to Him because of it."

I had someone else say, "Well, I just believe my disease is from God—it just teaches me how to be humble. It's my thorn in the flesh, but His grace is sufficient for me."

Could be, but I asked him if he was going to a doctor.

He said, "Oh, yes."

I asked, "Why are you going to a doctor?"

He said, "So I can get well."

I said, "You hypocrite! How dare you interfere with God's will in your life by going to a doctor?"

I was ministering in a Church of Christ in southern Maine many years ago and the head deacon came up to me after the service. It had been a powerful service that lasted 3½ hours. This deacon had injured himself. He was moaning, groaning and complaining, so I said, "Would you mind if I pray for you? Maybe God would heal you of that pain."

He said, "Oh no, brother, I do not want any prayer; this pain reminds me of the sufferings of Christ and what He did for me on the cross. It is a constant reminder of what He did for me."

I looked at him and said, "Suffer on, brother!"

I think that sometimes we create theologies based on our lack of knowledge.

> *The beginning of all healing of spiritually rooted diseases*
> *begins when you make your peace with God,*
> *and accept His love once and for all,*
> *accepting yourself and accepting others.*

In Deuteronomy 6:5, it says, Thou shalt love the LORD thy God with all thine heart and with all thy soul and with all thy might.

**And thou shalt love the LORD thy God with all thine heart, and with all thy soul, and with all thy might. Deuteronomy 6:5**

Leviticus says, Thou shalt love thy neighbor as thyself: I am the LORD.

**Thou shalt not avenge, nor bear any grudge against the children of thy people, but thou shalt love thy neighbour as thyself: I *am* the LORD. Leviticus 19:18**

And then again it says in Matthew 22:37–40:

> ³⁷Jesus said unto him, Thou shalt love the Lord thy God with all thy heart, and with all thy soul, and with all thy mind. ³⁸This is the first and great commandment. ³⁹And the second *is* like unto it, Thou shalt love thy neighbour as thyself. ⁴⁰On these two commandments hang all the law and the prophets. Matthew 22:37–40

*If you do not love yourself, you cannot love your neighbor.*
*You may pretend you do.*
*If you do not love yourself, then you cannot love your neighbor,*
*because you are unable to receive their love.*

The inability to give and receive love today is a tragedy. If someone were to come up to you, give you a big hug, give you a million dollars and say you were the best thing since peanut butter, could you receive that? Could you receive it without feeling guilty?

We have been so tragically victimized in the family that it is amazing we are even here today. **The failure in all family problems begins with the man.** The salvation of the whole family should begin with the salvation of the father and husband of the home. God did not create woman to be the spiritual leader of the home, He created the man to be. The Bible says the head of the woman is the man. The head of the man is Christ and the head of Christ is the Father.

> ²²Wives, submit yourselves unto your own husbands, as unto the Lord. ²³For the husband is the head of the wife, even as Christ is the head of the church: and he is the saviour of the body. ²⁴Therefore as the church is subject unto Christ, so *let* the wives *be* to their own husbands in every thing. Ephesians 5:22–24

Many women today are having real problems; 85 to 90 percent of all those we minister to nationally are female. God has used me to heal more females than you can imagine. God's first ministry is to the fatherless and the widows, not to how many Scriptures you can read in your Bible (even though it is important to be in the Word to build your faith). James says:

> Pure religion and undefiled before God and the Father is this, To visit the fatherless and widows in their affliction, *and* to keep himself unspotted from the world. James 1:27

That is sanctification. Pure religion is when you begin taking care of the fatherless, taking care of the widows and keeping yourself unspotted from the world.

I deal with many people whose fathers are still alive but they are fatherless. I deal with many women whose husbands or ex-husbands are still alive yet they are spiritual widows. The fallout and the diseases coming upon us because of these sins are of great magnitude.

I think the world will come to a well church faster than it will come to a sick church. There is more to salvation than being saved from hell. The gospel message includes day by day blessings. I believe it is God's will to bless people.

## Faith vs. Fear

Many people struggle with faith. Maybe you are sick with a disease and have been told you do not have enough faith. Maybe you have been listening to some of these people who teach you need to do something to get more faith.

The Bible says every man and woman has been given a measure of faith.

> …through the grace given unto me, to every man that is among you…but to think soberly, according as God hath dealt to every man the measure of faith. Romans 12:3

You have enough faith. You could always pray, "Lord, increase my faith"; however, you have enough if you only believe. You are going to have to determine the difference as to whether you are following God from your head or your heart.

If we follow God out of our head, we are all in trouble. My poor head pitches a fit most of the time. If I did not have the Word of God down in my spirit, mixed with faith by the Holy Spirit who lives within me, my life would be a wasteland. My poor head sometimes pitches a fit with the Word of God.

We need to be continually renewed by the washing of the water of the Word.

> That he might sanctify and cleanse it with the washing of water by the word, Ephesians 5:26

> And be renewed in the spirit of your mind; Ephesians 4:23

> For which cause we faint not; but though our outward man perish, yet the inward man is renewed day by day. 2 Corinthians 4:16

> And have put on the new man, which is renewed in knowledge after the image of him that created him: Colossians 3:10

Romans says faith comes by hearing and hearing by the Word of God.

> So then faith *cometh* by hearing, and hearing by the word of God. Romans 10:17

In Hebrews, we are told faith is the substance of things hoped for, the evidence of things not yet seen.

> Now faith is the substance of things hoped for, the evidence of things not seen. Hebrews 11:1

Do you have hopes or are you hopeless? Do you have something burning on the inside that represents hope about something in your life, about you or someone else? Do you? Then you have faith, because faith is the substance of things hoped for, the evidence of things not yet seen. If it has already come to pass, do you need hope? Do you need faith?

I was hungry this morning; I am no longer hungry. I ate. I no longer need hope or faith regarding my lunch. I am dreaming about dinner.

*Fear* is the substance of things *not* hoped for, the evidence *not* yet seen. Do you know how many of God's people are in "fear faith," not real faith? You may be in fear faith and think it is real faith, but if you were in real faith, you would not have the problem unless you did not understand why you had the problem. I deal with fears such as phobias, paranoia, delusions, projections, anxiety, panic, panic attacks, phobic realities, agoraphobia, claustrophobia and mother-in-law phobia.

**Fear projects into the future.** Faith also projects into the future, does it not? Fear involves projection, number one, and then displacement, which is avoidance. God has taught you in the Word from the Old Testament all the way through the New Testament, you do *not* run from an enemy. When you study the warfare garments in Ephesians 6:11–20, you do not find anything for your backside!

You do not run from an enemy in your life and you do not hide from your mother-in-law. You do not hide from your enemy. You do not hide from fear of disease. You do not hide from your disease. You do not go and disappear down inside.

It is time for you to come up and take your place in the land of the living once and for all. What is the worst that can happen to you, anyway? You can die and go to heaven, so what is your problem? What are you afraid of?

In the Church, we sometimes attack each other. That is an autoimmune disease! The sign out in front of your church, the one you see as you walk in the front door, says, "Hallelujah, Love One Another." You will know them because of the love they have one for another.

> **Wherefore by their fruits ye shall know them. Matthew 7:20**

> **[34]A new commandment I give unto you, That ye love one another; as I have loved you, that ye also love one another. [35]By this shall all *men* know that ye are my disciples, if ye have love one to another. John 13:34–35**

Isaiah 58 says the people of God were saying, "Hallelujah, LORD, we love You. You are our Father and You have redeemed us from Egypt." Yet they were destroying each other and God would not protect them or hear them.

> **[58:1]Cry aloud, spare not, lift up thy voice like a trumpet, and shew my people their transgression, and the house of Jacob their sins. [2]Yet they seek me daily, and delight to know my ways, as a nation that did**

**righteousness, and forsook not the ordinance of their God: they ask of me the ordinances of justice; they take delight in approaching to God. ³Wherefore have we fasted, *say they,* and thou seest not? *wherefore* have we afflicted our soul, and thou takest no knowledge? Behold, in the day of your fast ye find pleasure, and exact all your labours. ⁴Behold, ye fast for strife and debate, and to smite with the fist of wickedness: ye shall not fast as *ye do this* day, to make your voice to be heard on high. Isaiah 58:1–4**

Yes, we come and we worship You with the songs of David, and we come before You, and yes, You are our LORD, our God, and we love to come, we love to pray, we love to fast, we love the law, we love, love, love— but, why haven't You healed us?

That is the question of God's people in Isaiah 58. Do you know what God said? "Yes, I've watched you fasting and praying, but you pray for strife and eat each other alive. I have caused My ears to become deaf to you."

What is Isaiah saying? God is saying: you want My blessings but you do not want My friends; you do not want My sons and daughters.

I was talking with someone the other day who was kind of chewing about someone…you know, gossiping. I looked at them and I said, "How dare you say that about a friend of Jesus? Do you realize that person is a friend of Jesus? What do you think Jesus thinks about you talking that way about His friend?"

Do you think Jesus is our friend? Do you think I have a Scripture to stand on? He said, "I no longer call you servants, I call you friends" (John 15:15, among many others).

**Henceforth I call you not servants; for the servant knoweth not what his lord doeth: but I have called you friends; for all things that I have heard of my Father I have made known unto you. John 15:15**

Friends do not talk about each other. Friends build each other up. Friends cover with love—perfect love covers a multitude of sins.

**And above all things have fervent charity among yourselves: for charity shall cover the multitude of sins. 1 Peter 4:8**

In Galatians 6, we are told if a brother be overtaken in a fault, those of you who consider yourselves spiritual, restore such a one—not stone him by sundown. Restore such a one in a spirit of meekness and consider yourself also, lest you be tempted in like manner and fall away in the same type of bondage. Then, we are told to bear one another's burdens and thus fulfill the law of Christ.

**¹Brethren, if a man be overtaken in a fault, ye which are spiritual, restore such an one in the spirit of meekness; considering thyself, lest thou also be tempted. ²Bear ye one another's burdens, and so fulfil the law of Christ. Galatians 6:1–2**

My purpose is to sow seed into your hearts. Whether God gives the increase or not, I do not know. I do not know you. I do not live inside your body; you do. I do not know if you are going to get lost in the desert between Egypt and the Promised Land or not. I am sure going to lay some stuff on you—I am going to bring you some insight and I am going to bring you some discernment.

I promise you I have the fruit to prove, nationally, that God has honored this teaching. Many times I know disease. Even when I do not know the person and do not know the circumstances, I know what is behind the disease spiritually. I was able last evening to tell a person the secret parts of their heart. Why? So they could recover themselves into right standing with God and be healed. That is the fruit of this ministry.

When people are in captivity by the devil, they do not know it. They do not understand. Why? No one has told them. Read 2 Timothy 2:23 to the end of the chapter in the Majority Text (otherwise known as the King James):

> [23]**But foolish and unlearned questions avoid, knowing that they do gender strifes. [24]And the servant of the Lord must not strive; but be gentle unto all men, apt to teach, patient, [25]In meekness instructing those that oppose themselves; if God peradventure will give them repentance to the acknowledging of the truth; [26]And that they may recover themselves out of the snare of the devil, who are taken captive by him at his [the devil's] will. 2 Timothy 2:23–26**

## Promise without Discernment is Still Bondage

Jeremiah says:

> [14]**Turn, O backsliding children, saith the LORD; for I am married unto you: and I will take you one of a city, and two of a family, and I will bring you to Zion: [15]And I will give you pastors according to mine heart, which shall feed you with knowledge and understanding. Jeremiah 3:14–15**

He gave them pastors according to His own heart to teach them with knowledge and understanding. What am I doing with you? Giving you knowledge and understanding and discernment. Say this with me:

*"Promise without discernment is still bondage."*

The last verse of Hebrews 5 says one who is able to handle strong meat is one who, by reason of exercise of his senses, is able to *discern both good and evil.*

> **But strong meat belongeth to them that are of full age, *even* those who by reason of use have their senses exercised to discern both good and evil. Hebrews 5:14**

I think, ladies and gentlemen, that we have been so God-conscious that we have forgotten discernment concerning evil. A sign of maturity is not just knowing good, but knowing evil as well, so you know what is of God and what is not. That is a sign of maturity.

I am not into sin consciousness. That produces condemnation. I am into conviction, and that requires discernment. *All condemnation is of the devil. All conviction is of God.* They both say the same thing, but there is a wrong spirit behind one and a right spirit behind the other. If you are under condemnation, you are trying to hide from the problem. If you are under conviction, you are running to face the problem. Have you been there? Have you done that?

## Communion

In dealing with autoimmune disease, 1 Corinthians 11:29–31 is an example of a block, not a root, but a block to healing:

> **²⁹For he that eateth and drinketh unworthily, eateth and drinketh damnation to himself, not discerning the Lord's body. ³⁰For this cause many *are* weak and sickly among you, and many sleep. ³¹For if we would judge ourselves, we should not be judged. 1 Corinthians 11:29–31**

Many of God's people were weak. Could that be like Chronic Fatigue Syndrome? A little exhaustion?

When we get into the fear, anxiety and stress teaching, I'll show you where exhaustion comes from in the human body, other than from a hard day's work. We'll talk about potassium depletion and what the medical community knows about exhaustion tied to Multiple Chemical Sensitivity/Environmental Illness and also Chronic Fatigue Syndrome.

Some people are sick; some are sickly. Does the word "sickly" mean "sick" to you? What about "and many sleep"? It does not mean they sleep in church; it means they die premature deaths. Why? Because they do not rightly discern the Lord's body.

There are two realities of the Lord's Supper or Communion. The first is that people are sick and weak and die premature deaths because we have eliminated one-half of communion. I may bump into some of your theology but, if I do, I sure do love you and I hope you love me, too!

It splits right down the middle—those who believe God heals today and those who do not believe God heals today. It is a dispensational issue.

**Communion, or the Lord's Supper, represents two realities:** the shed blood which is the cup and the bread which is His broken body. *Christ's* *broken body is not for forgiveness of sin.* The Bible says without the shedding of blood, there is no forgiveness of sins.

> **And almost all things are by the law purged with blood; and without shedding of blood is no remission. Hebrews 9:22**

> **For the life of the flesh is in the blood: and I have given it to you upon the altar to make an atonement for your souls: for it is the blood that maketh an atonement for the soul. Leviticus 17:11**

So His shed blood makes forgiveness of sin possible because He was the sacrificial Lamb that allows us to appropriate forgiveness from God our Father. It is by His shed blood we have the penalty paid for sin.

Many people are appropriating the blood for the curse. However, it is Jesus' broken body that paid the penalty for the curse to fulfill the law that says, cursed is he that hangeth on a tree.

> **His body shall not remain all night upon the tree, but thou shalt in any wise bury him that day; (for he that is hanged *is* accursed of God;) that thy land be not defiled, which the LORD thy God giveth thee *for* an inheritance. Deuteronomy 21:23**

> **Christ hath redeemed us from the curse of the law, being made a curse for us: for it is written, Cursed *is* every one that hangeth on a tree: Galatians 3:13**

It is by His stripes we were healed and we appropriate that today to our lives.

> **But he *was* wounded for our transgressions, *he was* bruised for our iniquities: the chastisement of our peace *was* upon him; and with his stripes we are healed. Isaiah 53:5**

> **Who his own self bare our sins in his own body on the tree, that we, being dead to sins, should live unto righteousness: by whose stripes ye were healed. 1 Peter 2:24**

If we come to a Communion service and partake of the cup and the bread, but we deny healing and deliverance as part of the atonement today, we eliminate the provision of God in our lives as human beings apart from salvation and eternal life in that day. For that reason, because we eliminate the broken body but celebrate it and do not believe it, we cannot partake. For that reason, many of us are filled with disease and insanity today, because we have said in our hearts that healing passed away two thousand years ago; yet we still participate in the sacrament of Communion, which represents its reality for today. If you do not believe it, you do not have to worry about it happening. But be careful—ignorance is a form of knowledge and so is unbelief.

*If you do not believe God heals today, do not worry about it; He won't.*

*If you do not believe that God heals today, then He will not.* According to your faith be it unto you!

> **Then touched he their eyes, saying, According to your faith be it unto you. Matthew 9:29**

Let every man be fully persuaded in his own mind.

> **⁵One man esteemeth one day above another: another esteemeth every day *alike*. Let every man be fully persuaded in his own mind. Romans 14:5**

I have taken this position: many times we have disease among God's people *because we have eliminated one-half of the provision of the Communion and the sacrament of Communion (the Lord's Supper).*

Now, the other aspect of 1 Corinthians 11:29–31 has to do with us eating each other alive. This is "not discerning the Lord's body." Who was the Lord's body apart from what He did at the cross? Who else, if not the Lord's body in the earth today: the Church? We are the body of Christ. When we go to Isaiah, we read:

> **Cry aloud, spare not, lift up thy voice like a trumpet, and shew my people their transgression, and the house of Jacob their sins. Isaiah 58:1**

This has to do with God's people, the Old Testament Church. He is not talking about the heathen; he is not talking about Gentiles. He is talking about God's people and, ladies and gentlemen, God's people blow it and sin. We fall short of the glory of God continually in some areas of our lives. Hebrews says,

> **Looking diligently lest any man fail of the grace of God; lest any root of bitterness springing up trouble *you*, and thereby many be defiled; Hebrews 12:15**

When you are around someone who falls short of the glory of God, it means they have spiritually dumped all over you. They have defiled you, they have violated you and they have demonstrated part of their old nature.

What are you going to do with it? Eye for eye, tooth for tooth? That passed away! Jesus did away with eye for eye and tooth for tooth when He said, "You're going to love them."

> **³⁸Ye have heard that it hath been said, An eye for an eye, and a tooth for a tooth: ³⁹But I say unto you, That ye resist not evil: but whosoever shall smite thee on thy right cheek, turn to him the other also...⁴⁴But I say unto you, Love your enemies, bless them that curse you, do good to them that hate you, and pray for them which despitefully use you, and persecute you; Matthew 5:38–44**

If we have bitterness, if we have rejection, if we have unloving spirits, if we have hatred, it is ping-pong time and then slam-dunk, right? Many times our lives are like a massive ping-pong game: I am going to get you before you get me. That root of bitterness will keep you from the blessings of God.

God, speaking by the prophet Isaiah, says:

> ²Yet they seek me daily, and delight to know my ways, as a nation that did righteousness, and forsook not the ordinance of their God: they ask of me the ordinances of justice; they take delight in approaching to God. ³Wherefore have we fasted, *say they,* and thou seest not? *wherefore* have we afflicted our soul, and thou takest no knowledge? Behold, in the day of your fast ye find pleasure, and exact all your labours. Isaiah 58:2–3

This is a conversation from God's people to Him: "We have been fasting and praying. We need some help. Help, God! It looks like the heavens are brass. You're not listening. You're not listening; You are not answering our prayers. We have been fasting, we have afflicted our soul and *You do not even pay attention.* You take no knowledge."

> Behold, ye fast for strife and debate, and to smite with the fist of wickedness: ye shall not fast as *ye do this* day, to make your voice to be heard on high. Isaiah 58:4

God goes on and talks about the fast He's called us to—it is not absence of food and water. Many people quote verse 6 out of context to try to prove fasting and prayer will move God's hand to heal and deliver you.

> *Is* not this the fast that I have chosen? to loose the bands of wickedness, to undo the heavy burdens, and to let the oppressed go free, and that ye break every yoke? Isaiah 58:6

I do not find it in the Scriptures. I do not find it there; quite the opposite. In fact, in verses 7–12 of Isaiah 58, the fast that God has called us to is that of service to others in love.

Could it be we have mixed up *fellowship* with *petition*? Could it be we misunderstand that God is not just interested in being our Provider, He's interested in being our Father? The Lord is interested in being our Savior, our spiritual Husband forever. That is why we are called the bride of Christ. There is a marriage supper; do you all teach that in your church?

## Medication Insight

I have my *PDR (Physician's Desk Reference)* manual on drugs. In any seminar where I am dealing with disease, almost everyone is on a wide variety of drugs. That is what you have going for you in today's world and with every drug you are taking there is a component called "side effects."

One of the things I do in ministry is, before you receive ministry, my staff does a general intake and a medical intake. In the medical intake, we want to know all the medicine and drugs you are taking. Each of those drugs has side effects. You may be struggling with what seems to be a disease, but instead it may be the side effect of a drug.

I tell you, *I cannot minister to side effects.* I tried years ago and found out I was wasting my time. We are very careful in determining in a person's life what they are dealing with, which is actually the root problem of disease and not the side effects from a drug they are taking. Do you know how many pastors are trying to help people get free of diseases and are, in effect, ministering to the side effects of drugs and wondering why God is not healing the problem? There is no healing for the side effects of a drug.

*USA Today* (April 24, 1998) contained an article about deadly drugs: "Why Are So Many Drugs Killing So Many Patients?" "Adverse reactions to prescription drugs are the fourth-largest cause of death nationally." It is a Pandora's Box of hell. We will teach you about *pharmakeia* and sorcery.

Now, if you are taking prescription drugs, do not let me condemn you. If that's where you're at, that's where you're at.

## Depression, Anxiety Attacks and the Use of Prozac and Other Drugs

The side effects of these drugs are incredible. They are serotonin enhancers. When serotonin is released off the dendrite ends in the body, the drugs block the return, thus prolonging the effectiveness of it. It is out there longer, which gives the person a sense of well being.

The key issue that we need to deal with is: Why do we have a serotonin deficiency?

A serotonin deficiency will cause depression. *Depression,* by clinical definition, is the result of a chemical imbalance in the body through the introduction of drugs, uppers and downers, over- or under-production (hyper-/hypo-) of normal neurotransmitters, which are manufactured by the body.

One of the things I deal with in this ministry is the over- (hyper-) or under- (hypo-) secretion of neurotransmitters. For example, *manic depression* may be associated with an underproduction of serotonin caused by a genetic defect producing a wide range of highs and lows from manic to depressive. Migraines, binge eating, weight problems, or obsessive/compulsive behavior (OCD) may also indicate an under-secretion of serotonin. It is non-genetic and it is not the same as an anxiety disorder.

*Prozac* and other drugs used to treat depression are designed to increase your self-esteem. *A lack of self-esteem is the root problem.*

*Lack of self-esteem, self-rejection, self-hatred and guilt are very damaging to the human spirit and are many times caused by a father, although in some cases it can be the mother. Somewhere, there has been a lack of nurturing in childhood. Sometimes it can be inherited because the lack of nurturing has not been there from generation to generation.*

*Prozac* is the drug of choice today. It sometimes is being prescribed by doctors without any thought of the consequences or who do not have any understanding as to what it even involves. The problem with *Prozac* is this: Prozac is sometimes given to people who have anxiety. Yet one of the primary side effects of *Prozac* is anxiety and a secondary side effect is reduction of libido. That creates a double problem.

Females taking *Prozac* may lose their libido and that has a negative effect on their sexual relationship with their husbands. Do you know what loss of libido is? Loss of sex drive. Males can lose their sex drive with their wives. The guy is depressed and anxious and now his wife wonders why he has lost all interest and he is not chasing her. That is going to create another problem: more anxiety, more guilt, more rejection and more conflict. This may result in a further decrease in serotonin levels and now we have a bigger problem: a deeper depression. Galatians 5:20 in the Majority Text (King James Version) calls it witchcraft. (We'll study what Paul has to say about that subject later.) The only way to unravel this thing is to take a look at what may be causing this serotonin deficiency and that is a *spiritual problem.*

## Would You Be Interested in *A More Excellent Way*™?

Through this ministry, there are many people in America today who no longer need drugs of any type and who are living normal lives. Would you consider that to be a viable option for your life? We are on the "cutting edge" of medicine in America and it is awesome to be involved as a pastor. Isn't the "cutting edge of medicine" a funny place for a pastor to be?

The April 24, 1998, article in *USA Today* about deadly drugs continues: the number one killer in America is heart disease. Number two is cancer, number three is strokes, number four is adverse drug reactions to prescription drugs, number five is pulmonary disease and number six is accidents of all classes. Is that a sobering statistic?

Updated statistics in *USA Today*, November 30, 1999, quote the number eight killer as the medical profession. The number three killer is now quoted as death from properly prescribed and administered FDA-approved drugs with side effects.

A well-known talk show host, out of concern for the rapidly increasing death rate from FDA-approved drugs, made this statement: "The number of people actually dying from properly prescribed FDA-approved drugs is equal to the number of people dying when a jumbo 747 jet crashes and all the people aboard lose their lives...every single day of the year. That is how many people are actually dying every day. That does not include the two million people damaged by medically prescribed drugs."

Death from illegal drug use in America does not even make the top 10 in causes of death in America. Yet death by properly prescribed drugs and medical mistakes are listed on the top 10 killers list by *USA Today* and *Time Magazine* (April 27, 1998). I think it is time to stop and rethink what in the world are we doing and why are we doing it. Could it be that we have such a fear of death and disease that we have lost our spiritual sanity? It is amazing to me how many Christians have the same problems as the unchurched. There has to be *a more excellent way*™.

I operate in various gifts of the Holy Spirit. I do not make a big deal of it. It is there when it needs to be there. I do not know if you believe in the gifts of the Holy Spirit found in 1 Corinthians 12 or not. They are there and they are there for a reason. If I did not believe in them, I would not be teaching about spiritual healing. I would not be teaching about disease. I would not have any basis for doing it. To teach about disease and teach about healing and have no one healed is kind of ridiculous.

I am reminded of the Scriptures: You say you have faith; I'll show you my faith by my works (James 2:18). Faith without works is dead (James 2:17). There is another Scripture that is a little tougher. It says, They who say, "Yea Lord" but deny the power thereof, from such turn away (2 Timothy 3:5). When the Lord comes, will He find faith in the earth? (Luke 18:8).

> Yea, a man may say, Thou hast faith, and I have works: shew me thy faith without thy works, and I will shew thee my faith by my works. James 2:18

> Even so faith, if it hath not works, is dead, being alone. James 2:17

> Having a form of godliness, but denying the power thereof: from such turn away. 2 Timothy 3:5

> I tell you that he will avenge them speedily. Nevertheless when the Son of man cometh, shall he find faith on the earth? Luke 18:8

In Hebrews 4, we learn that the children of Israel did not enter into the land of promise because they did not mix faith with the gospel they had heard and received.

> [19]So we see that they could not enter in because of unbelief. [4:1]Let us therefore fear, lest, a promise being left *us* of entering into his rest, any of you should seem to come short of it. [2]For unto us was the gospel preached, as well as unto them: but the word preached did not profit them, not being mixed with faith in them that heard *it.* Hebrews 3:19–4:2

This is the first reason; the second reason is they did not enter into their rest (as God entered into His rest in creation; He rested on the seventh day) and they did not cease from their own labors.

> **⁹There remaineth therefore a rest to the people of God. ¹⁰For he that is entered into his rest, he also hath ceased from his own works, as God *did* from his. Hebrews 4:9–10**

Do you know when you start truly believing God, you cease to perform as if you were God? Do you also know there are so many people trying to be a god to themselves *that they truly are the author and finisher of their own life?*

Do you know how many people I deal with who are driven to succeed, to leave a million dollars for their children even when they know their children are going to blow it on nothing?

> **¹⁸Yea, I hated all my labour which I had taken under the sun: because I should leave it unto the man that shall be after me. ¹⁹And who knoweth whether he shall be a wise *man* or a fool? yet shall he have rule over all my labour wherein I have laboured, and wherein I have shewed myself wise under the sun. This *is* also vanity. Ecclesiastes 2:18–19**

So, can this be called vanity? Do you know how many people are driven?

Have you not heard the verse in the "book of whoever" that says as many as are *driven* by the Spirit of God are the sons of God? Does it say that? In the "book of whoever" it does. But it does not say it in the Word of God, does it? What does the Scripture say? For as many as are *led* by the Spirit of God, they are the sons of God.

> **For as many as are led by the Spirit of God, they are the sons of God. Romans 8:14**

*The devil drives and God leads.* That is why the Lord is called the Shepherd Who leads us into green pastures.

> **A Psalm of David. The LORD *is* my shepherd; I shall not want. ²He maketh me to lie down in green pastures: he leadeth me beside the still waters. Psalm 23:1–2**

## We Cannot Bypass the Penalty of Sin in Our Lives

I would say that probably 70 to 80 percent of all disease in America and in the world, with the name *syndrome* or *incurable* attached to it, has a spiritual root.

I am not against nutritionists; in fact, we have two nutritionists who are part of our ministry. I believe in a well-balanced diet; I believe you have to take care of the temple. I believe that when you get your rest, drink enough water, eat the proper foods and so on, you will have overall good health on that basis. *However, good nutrition, rest and water in themselves do not heal the defects that come because of separation from God and His Word, or deal with sanctification and sin and the resultant diseases.*

I want to say something to you. *Nutrition does not replace repentance.* I am reminded of the Lord when He was ministering; He had just healed someone and He made this incredible statement: Go your way and sin no more, lest a worse thing come upon you.

> **Afterward Jesus findeth him in the temple, and said unto him, Behold, thou art made whole: sin no more, lest a worse thing come unto thee. John 5:14**

Why did He say that? Because the Lord Himself, your Savior, my Savior, my Boss, directly tied the lack of sanctification to disease.

There are many people today trying to bypass the penalty of the curse of disobedience with various modalities and they are getting nowhere. Allopathic medicine has its place. We need doctors. We need people who understand the human body and the human soul, but there aren't many practitioners for the human spirit. That is our next topic.

## God Wants to Heal Us

In my investigation, in getting involved in people's lives, I have found God wanted to heal us. He said that He forgives us of all our iniquities and heals us of all our diseases.

> **Who forgiveth all thine iniquities; who healeth all thy diseases; Psalm 103:3**

I also found it in 3 John 2: Beloved, I wish above all things that thou mayest prosper and be in health, even as thy soul prospereth.

> **Beloved, I wish above all things that thou mayest prosper and be in health, even as thy soul prospereth. 3 John 1:2**

I read in 1 Thessalonians 5:23, May the God of peace sanctify you **wholly** in spirit, in soul and in body.

> **And the very God of peace sanctify you wholly; and *I pray God* your whole spirit and soul and body be preserved blameless unto the coming of our Lord Jesus Christ. 1 Thessalonians 5:23**

I believe God wants to work with us. I believe He is a loving Father. I also believe we have become separated from God in our understanding of disease. We would like to take a shot at correcting that.

In understanding disease—spiritual, psychological and biological—we will find the Bible has a lot to say about the subject. I am privileged to be on the "cutting edge" of medicine from coast-to-coast because of this biblical understanding of disease. There are doctors as well as therapists, psychologists, pastors and individuals across America who consult with me.

It is a funny thing to minister on the "cutting edge" of medicine. It is an enigma to the medical community. As one doctor said, "What is a pastor from Georgia doing messing around with disease?" Well, I am messing around with it because my Boss is the Great Physician. I am messing around in it because the Creator of all flesh is the One who knows what is wrong with us. I am messing around with it because God ordained it. I'll show you in Scripture that the pastor is to be responsible for all the affairs of God's people.

I think, and I say this very carefully, God is ticked off at the psychologists being the pastors of America. If there are any psychologists reading this, I love you man, I love you woman. But I do think you have taken some things away from the pastors that are rightfully theirs to deal with. Under Old Testament law, if anyone had leprosy, in order to be considered cured, to whom did they go show themselves? The priest. In the New Testament, it goes a little further. James says:

> **¹⁴Is any sick among you? let him call for the elders of the church; and let them pray over him, anointing him with oil in the name of the Lord: ¹⁵And the prayer of faith shall save the sick, and the Lord shall raise him up; and if he have committed sins, they shall be forgiven him. James 5:14–15**

So, in these verses, we see the lack of sanctification in a believer's life and the consequence, which shows us the relationship of sin to disease.

When I began to serve God in ministry, I believed God could heal. I saw it in the Word and I saw it in life. As I mentioned before, I would pray for people, but less than 5 percent ever got well. The same thing happened in the church I was in and in other churches across America. In my prayer time, I went to God and asked Him about this dilemma. I saw just as many Christians in doctors' offices as non-believers. I saw the same number of people in psychiatrists' offices, saints or sinners. Both were there with psychological and biological problems. I did not see any difference between saint and sinner when it came to any other of the pathologies of mankind: drug use, divorce, alcohol, etc.

I said, "God, my name is Henry. I feel Your call on my life and if You want me to help mankind, You had better solve this dilemma of what happens between salvation and heaven." I began to search the Scriptures and give my heart to God. The Bible says, If any of you lack wisdom, let him ask of God, that giveth to all men liberally and upbraideth not [because he had the audacity to ask God something]; and it shall be given him (James 1:5).

> If any of you lack wisdom, let him ask of God, that giveth to all *men* liberally, and upbraideth not; and it shall be given him. James 1:5

Then I ran across another Scripture: you have not, because you ask not.

> Ye lust, and have not: ye kill, and desire to have, and cannot obtain: ye fight and war, yet ye have not, because ye ask not. James 4:2

> And if we know that he hear us, whatsoever we ask, we know that we have the petitions that we desired of him. 1 John 5:15

I just figured I would ask. Gradually and surely I began to understand.

> *It wasn't that God could not heal;*
> *it was that He could not without denying His own holiness*
> *and giving us a leavened gospel that would say*
> *we could keep our sin and receive His blessings.*

## The Doctrine of Balaam

I bumped into the reality of the doctrine of Balaam (Numbers 22–24, 31; 2 Peter 2:15; Jude 11; Revelation 2:14). I really believe the doctrine of Balaam is in the Church today. This is not an indictment; it is an observation. What is the doctrine of Balaam? Do you know who Balaam and Balak were? Balaam was the seer; Balak was the heathen king. Balak wanted the children of Israel destroyed. He didn't like them—they were in his country and he wanted them out. But they were blessed.

He called for Balaam the seer to find a way to curse God's people. The first thing Balaam should have done was stay home, but he didn't. The Bible says Balaam taught Balak how to get God's people cursed. Here is the deal. Balak came to Balaam and said, "I want them cursed."

Balaam said, "I can't do it. They are a blessed people. God is their Father. He's bringing them out of Egypt. They are in covenant; they have the law. I cannot curse them for they are blessed."

Balak had this incredible thought: What would happen if I could get them to sin? He came up with the idea of tempting the girls of Israel with the boys from his country and tempting the boys with the girls in his country. He tempted them to worship the pagan idols. The first thing you know, Israel was sinning. Guess what came? *The curse came, there was no longer any provision for safety and 24,000 Israelites died in the plague that came as the result of their sin.*

I think the Church has come to a place where they have overplayed grace and mercy to the point of saying, "Because you are in covenant, you can sin like the devil and there are no consequences." I disagree!

I'll tell you why I disagree. I have had to get sanctified and still am under the pressure of the Holy Spirit every single day. I used to be so afraid that I would shake like a leaf when someone came to the door. If I talked to you, I would never look you in the eye. I would look at your nose, your toes, or the ceiling. Now people wish I would stop looking them in the eye!

I used to be a walking hypochondriac. I was in the doctor's office six months out of the year. I had strep throat four or five times a year and missed from two to three months of work because of massive infections. God healed me of all of it. My immune system was healed. How and why was I healed? I had to confess sin in my life. I had to get sanctified. I am working out my own salvation every single day now with fear and trembling. I do not mind repenting to God.

I heard someone teaching, "You never have to repent again once you are saved." I disagree! If I blow it, if I sin against you, I am going to repent to you. If I sin against you and I injure you knowingly or unknowingly and I am aware of it, I'll repent to you and ask you to forgive me. I'll do that with every single person I have known, do know, or ever will know.

The Bible says if you have anything against your brother, go to your brother alone.

> **[22]But I say unto you, That whosoever is angry with his brother without a cause shall be in danger of the judgment: and whosoever shall say to his brother, Raca, shall be in danger of the council: but whosoever shall say, Thou fool, shall be in danger of hell fire. [23]Therefore if thou bring thy gift to the altar, and there rememberest that thy brother hath ought against thee; [24]Leave there thy gift before the altar, and go thy way; first be reconciled to thy brother, and then come and offer thy gift. Matthew 5:22–24**

If this is the condition between us and another person, *how much more should it be with us and our heavenly Father?* But if we walk in the light, as He is in the light, we have fellowship one with another.

> **But if we walk in the light, as he is in the light, we have fellowship one with another... 1 John 1:7a**

And if we do not, the blood of Jesus Christ His Son cleanseth us from all unrighteousness.

> **...and the blood of Jesus Christ his Son cleanseth us from all sin. 1 John 1:7b**

Scripture tells us *we must ask* for forgiveness.

> [9]**If we confess our sins, he is faithful and just to forgive us** *our* **sins, and to cleanse us from all unrighteousness.** [10]**If we say that we have not sinned, we make him a liar, and his word is not in us. 1 John 1:9–10**

These Scriptures are addressed to the Church, not to the unchurched!

Second Corinthians says, Beloved, let us cleanse ourselves from all filthiness of the flesh and spirit.

> **Having therefore these promises, dearly beloved, let us cleanse ourselves from all filthiness of the flesh and spirit, perfecting holiness in the fear of God. 2 Corinthians 7:1**

He is speaking to the saints, not to the heathen!

I want to tell you something: The principles you apply to your life that will move the hand of God to heal you in covenant are the same principles that will, if you apply them to your life, prevent disease in your life.

## The Spirit of Fear

Second Timothy 1:7 says, "For God hath not given us the spirit of fear; but of power and of love and of a sound mind."

All three members of the Godhead are present in this Scripture:

- Power—Who is the power of God? God the Holy Spirit.

- Love—Who is the Love factor? God the Father.

John 3:16 says,

> **For God so loved the world, that he gave his only begotten Son, that whosoever believeth in him should not perish, but have everlasting life. John 3:16**

1 John 4 says God is love.

> **…for God is love. 1 John 4:8**

Talking about the Father, Psalm 68:19–20 says He (the Father) daily loadeth us with benefits, even the Elohiym of our salvation, who is the Lord Jesus. The Father is Love and is also our Provider.

> [19]**Blessed** *be* **the Lord,** *who* **daily loadeth us** *with benefits, even* **the God of our salvation. Selah.** [20]*He that is* **our God** *is* **the God of salvation; and unto God the Lord** *belong* **the issues from death. Psalm 68:19–20**

In Ezekiel 18, the last verse says "Adonay Yehovih" (the Father)—it is not the Father's will any man should perish but all should be saved.

> **For I have no pleasure in the death of him that dieth, saith the Lord GOD: wherefore turn** *yourselves,* **and live ye. Ezekiel 18:32**

That is what it says in the Old Testament in the Hebrew. In the New Testament, the Greek says the same thing in harmony with the Old. The Father's intention is to save and to preserve because of love.

- A sound mind—Who is the Word? Jesus is the Word.

How do we get a sound mind? Our mind is renewed by the washing of the water of the Word. John 1:1 tells us:

> **In the beginning was the Word, and the Word was with God, and the Word was God. John 1:1**

In verse 14, we learn that the Word became flesh.

> **And the Word was made flesh, and dwelt among us, (and we beheld his glory, the glory as of the only begotten of the Father,) full of grace and truth. John 1:14**

Revelation 19:11–14 says one comes on the white horse and the saints with Him and His name is the Word of God. Jesus Christ is the Living Word.

> **[11]And I saw heaven opened, and behold a white horse; and he that sat upon him *was* called Faithful and True, and in righteousness he doth judge and make war. [12]His eyes *were* as a flame of fire, and on his head *were* many crowns; and he had a name written, that no man knew, but he himself. [13]And he *was* clothed with a vesture dipped in blood: and his name is called The Word of God. [14]And the armies *which were* in heaven followed him upon white horses, clothed in fine linen, white and clean. Revelation 19:11–14**

What is the antidote to fear? A relationship with the whole Godhead: fellowship with the Father, fellowship with Jesus Who is the Word and fellowship with the Holy Spirit as He indwells you. You will not have any fear then. You will be hanging out with God.

The people coming out of Egypt under Moses did not enter into their promise first because of *unbelief* and second because they *did not cease from their own labors.*

> **[19]So we see that they could not enter in because of unbelief. [4:1]Let us therefore fear, lest, a promise being left *us* of entering into his rest, any of you should seem to come short of it. [2]For unto us was the gospel preached, as well as unto them: but the word preached did not profit them, not being mixed with faith in them that heard *it*.... [9]There remaineth therefore a rest to the people of God. [10]For he that is entered into his rest, he also hath ceased from his own works, as God *did* from his. [11]Let us labour therefore to enter into that rest, lest any man fall after the same example of unbelief. Hebrews 3:19–4:2, 9–11**

Do you know man is trying to become his own healer? How much money have you spent trying to heal yourself and how much money have you spent on physicians? I know of one person with Multiple Chemical Sensitivities/ Environmental Illness who spent over $500,000 trying to get well.

The Lord and I did not charge her one cent! The father of another person who was healed of MCS/EI had spent $400,000. She is well today and it did not cost her a cent.

### DON'T YOU THINK THAT IS *A MORE EXCELLENT WAY*™?

It is free—a free gift. Just like salvation is a free gift, God's love and His knowledge and His understanding are free gifts. The Bible says in Proverbs 25:2 it is the glory of God to conceal a thing, but the honor of kings is to search out a matter.

> *It is* the glory of God to conceal a thing: but the honour of kings *is* to search out a matter. Proverbs 25:2

When we minister to someone and they are not healed, what do you think we ought to do? Make up a theology saying God does not heal today? Make up a theology that someone did not have enough faith? What do you think we ought to do?

I'll tell you what I do: I go to work. I go back to God and say, "Why not? You had better talk to me, Boss. Why weren't they healed?" Do you know what? Many times *there is a reason* healing didn't happen.

Paul said to Timothy:

> [24]And the servant of the Lord must not strive; but be gentle unto all men, apt to teach, patient, [25]In meekness *instructing those that oppose themselves*; if God peradventure will give them repentance to the acknowledging of the truth; [26]And that they may recover themselves out of the snare of the devil, who are taken captive by him at his [the devil's] will. 2 Timothy 2:24–26

Now what are we doing when we give God the glory for disease and it was the devil who put it on us to begin with? I said this the other day to someone and they said, "I believe God gave me this disease. It is from Him. It is my thorn and His grace is sufficient for me. I believe this disease is God working me over. It is His chastening."

It is amazing to me to hear people giving God the glory for a disease and then go to a doctor trying to get healed. If that is the case, if disease is from God, then Jesus Christ of Nazareth was the biggest rebel against His Father I have ever seen. The Bible says He healed everyone that came to Him and cast out all their devils. Not one time did He say, "This disease is from God, so enjoy it."

> How God anointed Jesus of Nazareth with the Holy Ghost and with power: who went about doing good, and healing all that were oppressed of the devil; for God was with him. **Acts 10:38**

> …For this purpose the Son of God was manifested, that he might destroy the works of the devil. **1 John 3:8**

Now, I do not know whose Lord you follow, but that is the Lord I see; that is my Boss. That is the gospel I preach. If someone is not healed, there is a spiritual root and there is a block that has to be dealt with. There is a root problem that gives the devil a right to your life. Go before God and just lay it out. When you get the root figured out, we will check and see if any blocks to healing exist.

I have documented from Scripture over 30 blocks that will prevent God from healing you. You know, this is why we get so disillusioned when people go to healing seminars, listen to television evangelists or go to church healing services. They sincerely pray for God to heal them. What happens when they do not get healed? What do you do then?

I'll tell you what I do: I go and find out why they are not being healed. We are finding the reasons every day.

Do you think fear is sin? I deal with allergies, simple and multiple. I tell people with allergies this: "When the spies came into the promised land, what was the land filled with? Dairy products, sugar and wheat."

> And they told him, and said, We came unto the land whither thou sentest us, and surely it floweth with milk and honey; and this *is* the fruit of it. **Numbers 13:27**

It is time to take back your dairy products, your sugar and your wheat (grains). The Word of God tells us there is nothing evil in itself (including food), but all things taken with thanksgiving are sanctified with prayer and the Word of God. There is nothing evil in itself.

> [1]Now the Spirit speaketh expressly, that in the latter times some shall depart from the faith, giving heed to seducing spirits, and doctrines of devils; [2]Speaking lies in hypocrisy; having their conscience seared with a hot iron; [3]Forbidding to marry, *and commanding* to abstain from meats, which God hath created to be received with thanksgiving of them which believe and know the truth. [4]For every creature of God *is* good, and nothing to be refused, if it be received with thanksgiving: [5]For it is sanctified by the word of God and prayer. **1 Timothy 4:1–5**

> I know, and am persuaded by the Lord Jesus, that *there is* nothing unclean of itself: but to him that esteemeth any thing to be unclean, to him *it is* unclean. **Romans 14:14**

When I read Genesis 1:31, it said God created all things. He did not say His creation was "good." He said it was "very good."

> And God saw every thing that he had made, and, behold, *it was* very good…. Genesis 1:31

Do you think I am going to tell my Father in heaven and the Lord Jesus what they created in food was bad?

There are many people who were allergic to food but are eating it normally today, without any reactions or problems and who are now living normal lives. **Would that be *a more excellent way™*?**

Proverbs says:

> A merry heart doeth good *like* a medicine…. Proverbs 17:22

Our success rate with MCS/EI in America today is phenomenal after many years of ministry for this one disease. Our success rate with Chronic Fatigue Syndrome is equally incredible. Our success rate in certain diseases is so phenomenal it defies imagination. I get calls and letters frequently from people who have listened to my tapes. The lights go on. Remember 2 Timothy 2: God meets them and heals them. They walk out of diseases.

When we do not get a healing, what do we do? Will we go into unbelief, go into doubt, make a new doctrine, rewrite the Bible, go hide and become atheists? No! We will go back to God and ask Him why the devil still holds us captive at his will. That is what 2 Timothy seems to indicate. We need to find the strongholds in our lives keeping us from receiving God's healing.

Isaiah says,

> But this *is* a people robbed and spoiled; *they are* all of them snared in holes, and they are hid in prison houses: they are for a prey, and none delivereth; for a spoil, and none saith, Restore. Isaiah 42:22

### *I say restore!*

I stand boldly before God and all men and I say, restore those who are in prison houses and are a prey to the beast of the field. I take a stand; I put my foot down and say, let's go for the win.

God is still on the throne. He still answers prayer. He still talks to His people and gives them knowledge and understanding and He shows Himself strong. His eyes still rove to and fro throughout the earth. His ears are still open to their cries and He is looking to see if there are any who do seek after Him so that He may show Himself on their behalf.

> For the eyes of the LORD run to and fro throughout the whole earth, to shew himself strong in the behalf of *them* whose heart *is* perfect toward him… 2 Chronicles 16:9

*I believe that!*

Jeremiah said that the priests didn't ask, "Where is the LORD?"

> The priests said not, Where *is* the LORD? and they that handle the law knew me not: the pastors also transgressed against me, and the prophets prophesied by Baal, and walked after *things that* do not profit. Jeremiah 2:8

In the case of diseases in God's people in the Christian Church, not many pastors are saying today, "Where is the Lord?"

We taught earlier from 1 Corinthians 11 about communion, the Lord's Supper. Scripture tells us many are sick, many are weak and many die premature deaths. They did not rightly discern the body of Christ. Do you think this is an indictment or do you think it is a challenging statement of discernment?

In Jeremiah 2:8, it is very clear the priests did not say, "Where is the LORD?" They who handled the law did not know God, the pastors also transgressed against God and the prophets prophesied by Baal and walked after things that did not profit.

Look at Jeremiah 6:13–14 concerning the spiritual condition of the Old Testament Church and its leadership:

> <sup>13</sup>For from the least of them even unto the greatest of them every one *is* given to covetousness; and from the prophet even unto the priest every one dealeth falsely. <sup>14</sup>They have healed also the hurt *of the daughter* of my people slightly, saying, Peace, peace; when *there is* no peace. Jeremiah 6:13–14

Today, there are many sermons about God being our peace and Jesus being made peace unto us. But the evidence of this is missing. There is little peace. There are as many believers on Prozac as there are unbelievers on Prozac. I know because I talk to them every week. Prozac is a cheap substitute for the Holy Spirit, who is called the Comforter by the Lord.

Later on in chapter 8, Jeremiah again picked up the theme by saying the same thing all over again. Jeremiah said, Turn, oh backsliding children, saith the LORD, for I am married unto you.

> <sup>14</sup>Turn, O backsliding children, saith the LORD; for I am married unto you: and I will take you one of a city, and two of a family, and I will bring you to Zion: <sup>15</sup>And I will give you pastors according to mine heart, which shall feed you with knowledge and understanding. Jeremiah 3:14–15

> For thy Maker *is* thine husband; the LORD of hosts *is* his name; and thy Redeemer the Holy One of Israel; The God of the whole earth shall he be called. Isaiah 54:5

The Lord is your *spiritual* Husband. You men have a Husband, too, not in the carnal, human standpoint, but in the mystical standpoint of His being our Master forever. The Lord is my Husband and I want to be a good helpmate. We are going to have a marriage supper of the Lamb.

> **Let us be glad and rejoice, and give honour to him: for the marriage of the Lamb is come, and his wife hath made herself ready. Revelation 19:7**

> **And the Spirit and the bride say, Come. And let him that heareth say, Come. And let him that is athirst come. And whosoever will, let him take the water of life freely. Revelation 22:17**

We are all called the bride of Christ. Do you believe this? I believe it. Where the Lamb goes, I go. Where He has been, I am going. What He has done, I want to do. What He has said, I want to say. Because He said, "I only do and say the things I heard My Father saying" (John 14:9–10; 5:19; 8:28).

> **⁹Jesus saith unto him, Have I been so long time with you, and yet hast thou not known me, Philip? he that hath seen me hath seen the Father; and how sayest thou *then,* Shew us the Father? ¹⁰Believest thou not that I am in the Father, and the Father in me? the words that I speak unto you I speak not of myself: but the Father that dwelleth in me, he doeth the works. John 14:9–10**

If it pleased Jesus to do and say the things the Father said, then I ought to be obedient and follow Him and my Father, and say the same things, think the same things and do the same things. We would be a better Church.

There are always some who claim to have a new special revelation and are seeking followers. When you have mastered Genesis to Revelation, we will talk about new revelations. "Turn away, oh backsliding children, saith the LORD, for I am married unto you…" (Jeremiah 3:14). If you are ever struggling with your identity problem, you ought to take this Scripture and stick it in the face of the enemy and say, "My husband is the Lord; I am married to Him."

Take this lack of self-esteem, this self-hatred, this guilt and tell it to hit the road! "I am the Lord's and He loves me; He has called me and the Father has given me to the Lord forever.

You are no accident in God's heart. "I will take you one of a city and two of a family and I'll bring you to Zion. I will give you pastors according to my heart which shall feed you with knowledge and understanding."

> **¹⁴Turn, O backsliding children, saith the LORD; for I am married unto you: and I will take you one of a city, and two of a family, and I will bring you to Zion: ¹⁵And I will give you pastors according to mine heart, which shall feed you with knowledge and understanding. Jeremiah 3:14–15**

I won't say "peace, peace" when there isn't any. Nor am I going to send you to Prozac. We are going to come before God, find where the bondage is, where the roots are, where the blocks are and get right before God, so the Scriptures can be fulfilled.

Christ said, Peace I leave with you, my peace I give unto you: not as the world giveth, give I unto you.

> **Peace I leave with you, my peace I give unto you: not as the world giveth, give I unto you. Let not your heart be troubled, neither let it be afraid. John 14:27**

Would you be interested in this kind of peace, the peace that passeth all understanding? Do you believe this is a rare commodity or can it be reclaimed? I am here to tell you we are reclaiming it all over the globe with God's help. Jesus also said, Come unto Me all you who are heavy laden and I will give you rest.

> **Come unto me, all *ye* that labour and are heavy laden, and I will give you rest. Matthew 11:28**

I was asked to sit down with the leadership of a large denomination in America for a spiritual think-tank workshop. They staggered under the revelation of what I taught. People in their churches all over the country are now being healed. Their hearts are now open to *a more excellent way*™ with the Lord's blessing and grace as they deal with sanctification and the healing coming into their people. I have been asked to present ideas that will lead this denomination into healing and deliverance as a way of life. I think it is about time.

Whether it be Lutheran, Baptist, Nazarene, Episcopal, Independent Baptist, Free Will Baptist, whatever the denomination is from coast-to-coast, the truth of God's Word is true for each one.

> **Knowing this first, that no prophecy of the scripture is of any private interpretation. 2 Peter 1:20**

I had another wonderful opportunity of sitting down with the head of a Christian denomination in America. Many of their pastors and their people are in contact with our ministry and their hearts are open to *a more excellent way*™. I told the leader the worst thing that can happen to them is to become another dead church. Do not go there! Let me challenge you: do not throw the baby out with the bath water. Love the people, hate the sin, but separate the people from their sin so the love of God might possibly flow into them through you regardless of denomination or theological positioning.

> **[13]Therefore my people are gone into captivity, because *they have* no knowledge: and their honourable men *are* famished, and their multitude dried up with thirst. [14]Therefore hell hath enlarged herself, and opened her mouth without measure: and their glory, and their multitude, and their pomp, and he that rejoiceth, shall descend into it. Isaiah 5:13–14**

> **My people are destroyed for lack of knowledge: because thou hast rejected knowledge, I will also reject thee, that thou shalt be no priest to**

me: seeing thou hast forgotten the law of thy God, I will also forget thy children. Hosea 4:6

*Ignorance is a form of knowledge but it can be dangerous to our health.*

God loves people even when they are in error. Were you ever in error? Have you ever been ignorant? Were you ever lost in your sins? Have you ever had to change your theology? I have had to change mine. Do you think it is possible to change your thinking? God said, I'll give you pastors according to My own heart.

> And I will give you pastors according to mine heart, which shall feed you with knowledge and understanding. Jeremiah 3:15

Go to Jeremiah 32:17–18:

> [17]Ah Lord GOD! behold, thou hast made the heaven and the earth by thy great power and stretched out arm, and there is nothing too hard for thee: [18]Thou shewest lovingkindness unto thousands, and recompensest the iniquity of the fathers into the bosom of their children after them... Jeremiah 32:17–18

## Why Are Some Not Healed?

Sometimes you can have two people with the same sin and the same identical disease, yet **one is healed and the other is not. Why?** God does not necessarily judge you in your sin immediately; *He judges you for your heart toward it*. It is hard to teach this because if you are not careful, you will make sin abound again.

King David was called a man after God's own heart. Yet David had a man killed, he was an adulterer, etc. What made David different from Saul, his predecessor? Saul never repented. Psalm 51 tells us David did. *The difference is in our attitude toward sin*. Your heart toward God concerning sin is what moves Him. Isaiah said:

> For thus saith the high and lofty One that inhabiteth eternity, whose name *is* Holy; I dwell in the high and holy *place,* with him also *that is* of a contrite and humble spirit, to revive the spirit of the humble, and to revive the heart of the contrite ones. Isaiah 57:15

What is the predicator for moving the hand of God? Your sinlessness or your heart toward sin? I'll be very honest with you; historically and scripturally, it seems that even if you are still in your sin, if you have a hatred for sin, God judges you according to the righteousness of your heart toward Him. Out of the perfect hatred for sin, God starts to deal with you so you are better able to resist the sin and thus remove the torment and the struggle and eventually produce your freedom from sin.

There are other people who, when confronted with sin, harden their hearts and are not convicted. They do not have a perfect hatred for it. In fact, they either condone it or ignore it. God is going to judge you after the intent of your heart, not to the degree of your sanctification first. In Romans 7 we saw the apostle Paul, who also struggled with the issue of sin in his life.

I did a teaching some years ago called the 7 Steps to Sin (James 1:12–16). (See Teaching Unit 4 for "7 Steps to Sin.") Temptation is not sin. Having evil thoughts is not sin. If this were the case, we are all deep in sin. Thoughts come and go. The evil one in his kingdom is always out there tempting you. Temptation is not sin. Jesus was tempted in all points such as we are, yet was without sin.

> **For we have not an high priest which cannot be touched with the feeling of our infirmities; but was in all points tempted like as *we are, yet* without sin. Hebrews 4:15**

Many people, because they are tempted, feel they have sinned. You only have sin when the action of the sin is fulfilled. This is when it becomes your sin. I know what the Word says about a man lusting in his heart after a woman.

> **But I say unto you, That whosoever looketh on a woman to lust after her hath committed adultery with her already in his heart. Matthew 5:28**

There is a difference between temptation concerning women and fantasy lust. Fantasy lust is a sin because you are committing the act in your mind, not just being tempted with the act. Many men and women fall because of being ignorant at this level. They say, "Well, I'll just go ahead and do it because I have already thought about it." *This is Satan's snare: convincing you the temptation equals the act.*

The seven steps to sin are found in James 1:12–16:

> **[12]Blessed *is* the man that endureth temptation: for when he is tried, he shall receive the crown of life, which the Lord hath promised to them that love him. [13]Let no man say when he is tempted, I am tempted of God: for God cannot be tempted with evil, neither tempteth he any man: [14]But every man is tempted, when he is drawn away of his own lust, and enticed. [15]Then when lust hath conceived, it bringeth forth sin: and sin, when it is finished, bringeth forth death. [16]Do not err, my beloved brethren. James 1:12–16**

*Temptation is not sin.*

## How Do We Correct a Wrong When the Person is Dead?

Many people are bound by disease because of unresolved issues concerning people who have died. Do you know how many people have bitterness against dead people? How can you make it right with a dead person? You cannot. The same is true if you do not know where the person is.

I'll tell you how God judges it. *He judges it by your heart.* If you have something from your past and it is not possible for you to make it right with the person, then you make it right with God and it is taken care of. You do not have to carry the guilt any longer.

*If someone is holding a sin against you, it is their problem, not yours. They have to get it right before God just like you do. Whether they do or they do not really doesn't have anything to do with you because you are standing alone before God in the integrity of your heart.*

You need to stay in freedom and not in guilt. There may be something in your life such as a breach with someone and they won't even talk to you. They won't make peace with you. Your ability to be free of the situation does not mean you have to resolve it personally with this person. You can come before God. He will work with your heart, but you do not have to have it resolved with anyone in order to be free. You have to have it resolved before God. Your heart has to make the paradigm shift concerning this issue.

## Conflict Resolution

Let me tell you something with great authority: *you do not have to resolve one issue with someone who has victimized you in order for God to heal you,* providing you have resolved the issue between you and God concerning them.

If you are waiting for resolution between the other person and you before you can be well, you have bought the biggest lie you have ever bought. This would be tying you back to the tragedy, back to the victimization, back to the breakdown.

You stand alone before God and alone you shall be in your salvation, in your healing, in your deliverance and in your judgment. All of us shall stand before God one day and we cannot take a bunch of people with us and say, "They made me do it. They made me do it." You will stand alone.

Remember, God has not given us the spirit of fear, but of power and of love and of a sound mind.

> **For God hath not given us the spirit of fear; but of power, and of love, and of a sound mind. 2 Timothy 1:7**

*The antidote to fear is the Godhead.* The antidote to fear is trusting the Godhead. All three members of the eternal Godhead are found in this Scripture as follows: power is the Holy Ghost; love is God the Father and a sound mind is God the Word. John says, For God so loved the world that He gave His only begotten Son. Who gave the only begotten Son? The Father.

**For God so loved the world, that he gave his only begotten Son...**
**John 3:16**

Jesus said, You've seen Me, so you've seen the Father. I only do the things I see My Father doing, I only say the things I hear My Father saying.

**Jesus saith unto him, Have I been so long time with you, and yet hast thou not known me, Philip? he that hath seen me hath seen the Father; and how sayest thou *then*, Shew us the Father? John 14:9**

**Then answered Jesus and said unto them, Verily, verily, I say unto you, The Son can do nothing of himself, but what he seeth the Father do: for what things soever he doeth, these also doeth the Son likewise. John 5:19**

**Then said Jesus unto them, When ye have lifted up the Son of man, then shall ye know that I am *he,* and *that* I do nothing of myself; but as my Father hath taught me, I speak these things. John 8:28**

**I speak that which I have seen with my Father: and ye do that which ye have seen with your father. John 8:38**

**I can of mine own self do nothing: as I hear, I judge: and my judgment is just; because I seek not mine own will, but the will of the Father which hath sent me. John 5:30**

The Father is Love, but the sound mind comes from which other member of the Godhead? *Jesus, Who is God the Word.*

You have God the Father, God the Word, who came in the flesh and God the Holy Spirit. The eternal Godhead. God in three Persons. Deuteronomy 6:4 says, "Hear, O Israel, the LORD our God is one LORD." The word "one" is the Hebrew word *echad*, which translated means *plural unity*. Right there in the Torah (in Deuteronomy), you find the Godhead. You also find it other places, such as Genesis 1:26 and Isaiah 48:16–17.

**And God said, Let us make man in our image, after our likeness: and let them have dominion over the fish of the sea, and over the fowl of the air, and over the cattle, and over all the earth, and over every creeping thing that creepeth upon the earth. Genesis 1:26**

**[16]Come ye near unto me, hear ye this; I have not spoken in secret from the beginning; from the time that it was, there *am* I: and now the Lord GOD, and his Spirit, hath sent me. [17]Thus saith the LORD, thy Redeemer, the Holy One of Israel; I *am* the LORD thy God which teacheth thee to profit, which leadeth thee by the way *that* thou shouldest go. Isaiah 48:16–17**

From this standpoint, the antidote to fear is fellowship with the Godhead. I will tell you what I think: if I threw a $1,000,000 bill out here, you would be scrambling for it because it would be your prize. I think we have lost our first love. *I think it is time to get hot for God again.* I think it is time to fall in love with Who He is, all over again.

## Victimization

How do you honor your parents, or husband, or wife, (or children,) when they constantly "beat you up" in some manner? There are many people condemned by the Scripture, you are to honor your mother and your father.

> **Honour thy father and *thy* mother... Matthew 19:19**

You only have to honor your mother or father or anyone to the degree they honor God. If you have a mother and father who are evil before God, you do not have to honor them in their evil. But, you cannot touch them either. You do not have to go along with their sin. Some people tell me: "I just do not want to talk about what my mother did to me or my father did to me because it is not honoring them."

No, this is not about honoring them, it is just defining the evil. You do not have to honor the evil in parents. We cannot afford to preach a gospel that produces a codependency with evil. My definition of codependency is calling evil good in the name of love.

However, the first thing you must be able to do is separate them from their sin. You must always have a perfect hatred for evil.

> **Ye that love the LORD, hate evil... Psalm 97:10**

The Bible says you are to have a perfect hatred for evil, but you must love the person. This is hard to do.

What happens to us because someone behaves in an evil manner against us? We believe them to be evil. God looked down from heaven when I was evil. He separated me in His mind and in His heart from my sins and from my evil and He loved me. He looked past my sins and loved me anyway.

Pure religion and undefiled is to visit the fatherless, take care of the widows in their afflictions and keep yourself undefiled from the world.

> **Pure religion and undefiled before God and the Father is this, To visit the fatherless and widows in their affliction, *and* to keep himself unspotted from the world. James 1:27**

If you leave mother and father, brother and sister, houses and lands for the gospel and what God stands for, God will give to you, in this life, a hundredfold—mothers and fathers, brothers and sisters, houses and lands, and in the world to come eternal life.

> **29And Jesus answered and said, Verily I say unto you, There is no man that hath left house, or brethren, or sisters, or father, or mother, or wife, or children, or lands, for my sake, and the gospel's, 30But he shall receive an hundredfold now in this time, houses, and brethren, and sisters, and mothers, and children, and lands, with persecutions; and in the world to come eternal life. Mark 10:29–30**

I am going to offer you a possibility: if you are not around a good body of believers where there are some good fathers and mothers in the Lord, I pray God gives them to you quickly. They can fill you up with love you also need. You do not have to be violated in your spirit any more and you do not have to be cursed in it or guilty in it.

You can still love your parents, but you do not have to be victimized by the sin through them. God did not ask anyone, anywhere, to be a victim for any reason. Separate from the person and remove yourself if you have to. In a victimization situation, be it children, or husbands, or wives, I call for immediate separation. I would never send a wife back to an abusive husband. God has called us to peace and He said if it is at all possible, we are to live peaceably with one another.

> **If it be possible, as much as lieth in you, live peaceably with all men. Romans 12:18**

I won't tolerate victimization on any level. It is time out, it is separation time, time to declare where your treasure is and get it together in righteousness. There is no way God condones victimization under any name or under any title. He has called us to peace. In fact, Mark says when you go out, if you cannot leave your peace at the house you have entered into, shake the dust off your feet and go find a place where you can leave your peace.

> **10And he said unto them, In what place soever ye enter into an house, there abide till ye depart from that place. 11And whosoever shall not receive you, nor hear you, when ye depart thence, shake off the dust under your feet for a testimony against them. Verily I say unto you, It shall be more tolerable for Sodom and Gomorrha in the day of judgment, than for that city. Mark 6:10–11**

I know this Scripture pertains to evangelism, but the principles remain true. God has called us to peace, not to torment. This has nothing to do with loving your parents; it is following God. You can love someone who has evil, but you do not have to be a victim.

Separation from abusive situations is godly; it is not ungodly. There may be a time, after you have been sanctified and strengthened in the area of your weaknesses, when you can go back into the situation and be all right. You do not have to do this until you are healed and it may be that God won't ever want you to do it. I do not know. I do know when you go back prematurely to a place where you have been weakened by abuse or victimization on any level is not right. First, you need to get strengthened and healed in yourself. Give those who have wronged you to the Lord; you do not have to fix them.

When I minister to children who have been subjected to victimization, the worst thing I can do is send them back to the abusive parent. My position is for all victims to be removed *immediately until someone decides where their treasure is.*

**For where your treasure is, there will your heart be also. Luke 12:34**

This is true whether the victim is the husband, the wife or the child. We are not going to play games with victimization. The tragedy is just too high a price to pay. *If we had taken a stand at this level against victimization a long time ago, we would not have the tragedies it is causing today.* You cannot go back into a victimization situation in the name of love. It is **codependent.** It is further victimization. It is built-in guilt and you will not be able to have your peace. No one is spiritually strong enough to be a doormat for this type of thing and survive it for long. Remember my definition of codependency? Calling evil good in the name of love.

If God had made us able to handle evil, then we would enjoy it. We would enjoy murder, strife and jealousy. The reason evil behaviors and situations hurt so badly is because He did not create us to be victimized. God did not design this to be a part of our lives. This is why it is foreign to us and why it hurts so badly.

When dealing with abuse in a marriage, I tell the couple to either get it together or get out of it because everything else is fraud and sin. Be hot, be cold, but do not stay in it if you are only lukewarm. The Lord talked about His Church and His relationship with it as His wife:

**[15]I know thy works, that thou art neither cold nor hot: I would thou wert cold or hot. [16]So then because thou art lukewarm, and neither cold nor hot, I will spue thee out of my mouth. Revelation 3:15–16**

This concept brings everybody to a place of decision and it makes each party confess the answer to the question, "Where is your treasure?" Is the wife a man's treasure? If I tell him to get it together or get out of it, he is going to have to make up his mind. The Bible says, As a man thinketh in his heart, so is he.

**For as he thinketh in his heart, so *is* he: Proverbs 23:7**

It is the same for the wife; either "get it together," or "get out of it." I am not condoning divorce; I am also not condoning fraud. I am against fraud. Marriage is a sacramental union, or it is a fraud. God has called us to truth, not to fraudulent relationships.

Many marriages have been saved because I have taken this stand. I have had people come to me later and say, "Thank you for taking this stand because we wouldn't have survived it otherwise." Doesn't God bring us to this kind of decision? He said, Choose what you will have this day: blessings or cursings, life or death.

> **I call heaven and earth to record this day against you,** *that* **I have set before you life and death, blessing and cursing: therefore choose life, that both thou and thy seed may live: Deuteronomy 30:19**

I teach the **Ten Commandments of successful relationships**. Your relationship with God and others should be this way:

| | | | |
|---|---|---|---|
| 1. | Communicate | 6. | Communicate |
| 2. | Communicate | 7. | Communicate |
| 3. | Communicate | 8. | Communicate |
| 4. | Communicate | 9. | Communicate |
| 5. | Repent | 10. | Repent |

If we would do this with God and with each other, we could turn the world upside down, first beginning in our own lives, then in our families, our churches, our governments, our societies and the world.

I have been involved with many people, helping them in their lives and I came up with an incredible revelation. In my studies of the Word, in my studies of various things, I have never come up with a more astounding revelation than this in all of my life. It has set a standard for helping other people and it has set a standard in my own life.

I finally discovered **the root problem for misunderstandings**. Would you like to know what it is? This is awesome!

> ### *The root problem of a misunderstanding is that someone just did not understand.*

It seems very simple and if we could go directly to this level, we would eliminate all misunderstandings. If we try to find out who misunderstood, we end up in a war zone over the misunderstanding. All we need to do is go back and communicate. Then, if we need to, we repent and the misunderstanding is resolved. The Word is very clear: Do you have a problem with your brother? Go to your brother directly and communicate. If you need to repent about past actions, do so and then make peace with your brother. This is the Word. I like it, don't you?

> **[22]But I say unto you, That whosoever is angry with his brother without a cause shall be in danger of the judgment: and whosoever shall say to his brother, Raca, shall be in danger of the council: but whosoever shall say, Thou fool, shall be in danger of hell fire. [23]Therefore if thou**

> bring thy gift to the altar, and there rememberest that thy brother hath ought against thee; 24Leave there thy gift before the altar, and go thy way; first be reconciled to thy brother, and then come and offer thy gift. Matthew 5:22–24

## With Freedom Comes Great Responsibility

The Word says we see through a glass darkly.

> For now we see through a glass, darkly; but then face to face: now I know in part; but then shall I know even as also I am known. 1 Corinthians 13:12

So I would like to turn on a light in the darkness. I want you to have a better life. I want you to have a happier life, a saner life and a life filled with more health because the Word promises it to you.

But there are conditions. *With freedom comes great responsibility.* Freedom comes with a high price; it requires an effort. The Bible says,

> Submit yourselves therefore to God. Resist the devil, and he will flee from you. James 4:7

What does resisting require? An effort! I know God does the work in us, but He requires our participation. This is an effort. Why does God ask us to have discernment and put forth an effort in order to obtain freedom? Ezekiel and 2 Peter tell you why.

> For I have no pleasure in the death of him that dieth, saith the Lord GOD: wherefore turn *yourselves,* and live ye. Ezekiel 18:32

> The Lord is not slack concerning his promise, as some men count slackness; but is longsuffering to us-ward, not willing that any should perish, but that all should come to repentance. 2 Peter 3:9

In Ezekiel 18, God is defending the charge made by the people of Israel that He is not fair. Second Corinthians says that we are to cleanse ourselves from all filthiness of the flesh and the spirit.

> Having therefore these promises, dearly beloved, let us cleanse ourselves from all filthiness of the flesh and spirit, perfecting holiness in the fear of God. 2 Corinthians 7:1

*In each of these verses, an action on our part is required.*

**Condemnation is of the devil.** In the book of Revelation it says, The accuser of the brethren is cast down, who accused them before God day and night.

> And I heard a loud voice saying in heaven, Now is come salvation, and strength, and the kingdom of our God, and the power of his Christ: for the accuser of our brethren is cast down, which accused them before our God day and night. Revelation 12:10

Have you ever heard a voice in your head telling you how rotten you are and what a failure you always will be? Condemnation is of the devil.

Conviction is because of God's love for us. The Holy Spirit was sent to the earth some 2,000 years ago to dwell in each individual believer, to seal our spirits for God forever, to lead us into all truth, to be our comforter, our guide and to raise us up on that day (see John 14). Isn't this fantastic?

I hope that you are being nourished in my teaching. I hope you are being edified. I hope you are being built up. I hope I can represent a better life so 3 John 2 can be fulfilled: Dearly beloved, I wish above all things that you prosper and be in good health even as your soul prospers.

> **Beloved, I wish above all things that thou mayest prosper and be in health, even as thy soul prospereth. 3 John 1:2**

I am not into "name it and claim it." I'm not into being presumptuous. I do not believe God is a slot machine so you can put a nickel in and get something out. This is not what Scripture teaches.

God is faithful and He wants to bless you. You do not have to pump Him up. He is already pumped up. He came and died for you. He laid His life down, died for us and He wants to bless you. He wants to do more than bless you. He wants you to be like Him. From glory to glory we are being changed into His image.

> **But we all, with open face beholding as in a glass the glory of the Lord, are changed into the same image from glory to glory, *even* as by the Spirit of the Lord. 2 Corinthians 3:18**

God, *Elohiym*, said:

> **And God said, Let us make man in our image, after our likeness: and let them have dominion over the fish of the sea, and over the fowl of the air, and over the cattle, and over all the earth, and over every creeping thing that creepeth upon the earth. Genesis 1:26**

The work of God in the earth today is one of *sanctification*. Often you will not receive healing and deliverance from God without first submitting to God. Why do we call Him "Lord"?

Scripture gives us the answer in Romans 14:11: Every knee shall bow, every tongue shall confess that He (Jesus) is Lord.

> **For it is written, As I live, saith the Lord, every knee shall bow to me, and every tongue shall confess to God. Romans 14:11**

> **I have sworn by myself, the word is gone out of my mouth in righteousness, and shall not return, That unto me every knee shall bow, every tongue shall swear. Isaiah 45:23**

I am reminded of another Scripture about humbling yourself before God so He will raise you up in due season.

**Humble yourselves therefore under the mighty hand of God, that he may exalt you in due time: 1 Peter 5:6**

Also, Matthew 6:33 says, Seek ye first the kingdom of God and His righteousness and all these things shall be added unto you.

**33But seek ye first the kingdom of God, and his righteousness; and all these things shall be added unto you. Matthew 6:33**

What is the predicator? What action must come first? Seek God and His righteousness, then all things shall be added unto you (Matthew 6:33). Draw nigh to God and He'll draw nigh unto you. Humble yourself before the Lord and He will lift you up.

**8Draw nigh to God, and he will draw nigh to you. Cleanse *your* hands, *ye* sinners; and purify *your* hearts, *ye* double minded. 9Be afflicted, and mourn, and weep: let your laughter be turned to mourning, and *your* joy to heaviness. 10Humble yourselves in the sight of the Lord, and he shall lift you up. James 4:8–10**

1 Peter 5:6–9 says:

**6Humble yourselves therefore under the mighty hand of God, that he may exalt you in due time: 7Casting all your care upon him; for he careth for you. 8Be sober, be vigilant; because your adversary the devil, as a roaring lion, walketh about, seeking whom he may devour: 9Whom resist stedfast in the faith, knowing that the same afflictions are accomplished in your brethren that are in the world. 1 Peter 5:6–9**

*Wow!*

I want to remind you that Matthew, Mark, Luke, John and the book of Acts are a demonstration of God's love through the Lord and through the apostles in the early Church. Then, from Romans to Jude, God deals with our **sanctification**.

Without sanctification, you won't see Matthew, Mark, Luke, John and Acts made manifest in your life. There is little sanctification being taught today and this is why we do not see many healed or delivered. It wasn't because the Lord did away with miracles, healing and deliverance; it is that in the long-term, He could not perform them unless the Church submitted to Him in holiness. This teaching is given to us by the teachings of Paul.

## Jungian Psychology

Hebrews 4:12 teaches us the soul and the spirit are distinctively separate.

**For the word of God *is* quick, and powerful, and sharper than any twoedged sword, piercing *even to the dividing asunder of soul and spirit,***

**and of the joints and marrow, and *is* a discerner of the thoughts and intents of the heart. Hebrews 4:12**

This is what it says: "Is able to separate the spirit from the soul." One of the great tragedies of psychology in the teaching of Jungian psychology is it eliminates the spirit of man totally and inserts in its place the dualistic compartments of the soul.

In Jungian psychology and in modern-day psychology, there is no such thing as the spirit of man. There are the dualistic compartments of the soul called the "conscious" and the "collective unconscious." In the teachings of Jungian psychology, within the collective unconscious, you will find the archetypes and dark shadows. Jungian psychology identifies these dark shadows as the archetypes of our historic ancestry, bringing with them the darkness and the evil we need to come in contact with and identify with, so we can cohabit with the evil of our ancestral line generationally. This is classic Jungian psychotherapy.

I do not find these concepts anywhere in Scripture. What I do find in Scripture is the archetypes and dark shadows are in fact evil spirits, principalities, powers and the rulers of the darkness of this world.

**For we wrestle not against flesh and blood, but against principalities, against powers, against the rulers of the darkness of this world, against spiritual wickedness in high *places.* Ephesians 6:12**

I have a book about Carl Jung, written by a secular psychotherapist in Connecticut who did research on Carl Jung. Early on in Carl Jung's investigation into spiritualism (spiritism) and into Eastern mysticism, he became a channeler for invisible entities. It is in his writings. The principal entity he channeled was *a spirit entity called Philemon.* He also channeled two lesser spirit entities called Anima and Animus, who became the foundation of the male and female principles in Jungian psychology. In fact, these male/female principles of Anima and Animus can even be found in Christian ministry/counseling circles as a therapeutic model. These were invisible spirit entities Carl Jung channeled by using automatic handwriting (otherwise known as journaling) and they wrote much of our modern-day Jungian psychology through him. This means that much of modern Jungian psychology was written by invisible spirit beings. If you do not believe me, you can go to any public library and do your own research on the history of Carl Jung. Over the years I have done much research into his writings to substantiate what I have just said.

Carl Jung, early on in his investigation of spiritualism (spiritism) and mysticism, ran into invisible evil spirits and in his early writings he called them evil spirits. As he developed his precepts, he said that because of the failure of Christianity in dealing with the problems of the psyche or the soul of man and the body, or the diseases of man, *I will create an alternative to Christianity.* He considered Christianity to be a dead religion. In fact, Carl Jung was the son of a German Protestant minister and observed his minister-father preach a gospel that seemed to offer no solution for the diseases of the soul and body. He believed mankind had to be helped while they lived on planet earth.

> ***Modern-day psychology includes many Jungian principles and is the fruit of the failure of the Christian Church.***

Psychology has become a religion and psychologists have become the "pastors" of the Christian Church in matters of the soul. Many times, even Christian psychological counselors relegate everything to the dualistic concept of the soul to the exclusion of the *spirit of man.*

Jung believed modern man would not accept basic concepts of the Bible in view of their scientific way of thinking. He deliberately took the words "evil spirit," changed the concept and called them "archetypes" and "dark shadows" to accommodate himself to a more scientific approach and *he duped mankind, including the Christian Church, and lastly, even himself.*

I am not a psychologist. I am a student of God and His Word. I am a son of God by faith and I am a shepherd of the Most High God by His permission.

Hebrews 4:12 says the Word of God is able to separate the soul from the spirit.

> **For the word of God *is* quick, and powerful, and sharper than any twoedged sword, piercing even to the dividing asunder of soul and spirit, and of the joints and marrow, and *is* a discerner of the thoughts and intents of the heart. Hebrews 4:12**

*This Scripture makes the dualistic compartment of the soul taught by Jungian psychology a heresy.* Do you know what heresy is? It is a statement of truth that is not truth. It doesn't match up with the Word.

I am not into inner healing. I am not into inner healing taught by certain practitioners. I go far beyond it. *I am into the sanctification of the human spirit.* I **begin** with the sanctification of the human spirit. When we finally have it straight upstairs (spirit), then our bodies start to conform to the Word and the life of the living God. It comes from obedience (2 Corinthians 10:6) where Scripture tells us to have a readiness to revenge all disobedience.

> **And having in a readiness to revenge all disobedience, when your obedience is fulfilled. 2 Corinthians 10:6**

The focus of discernment is found in Hebrews 4:12 where we learn the Word of God is able to separate the soul from the spirit.

Now let's quote Hebrews 4:13, which is rarely ever quoted in conjunction with verse 12:

> **Neither is there any creature that is not manifest in his sight: but all things** *are* **naked and opened unto the eyes of him with whom we have to do. Hebrews 4:13**

What things are naked before Him? Who are the creatures who are manifested in His sight? I'll tell you who the creatures are in this verse: they are Satan and his kingdom of the second heaven who try to rule mankind. Satan is called the god of this world, the ruler of men's spirits and the ruler of men's minds. It is the principalities and powers, spiritual wickedness in high places, the rulers of the darkness of this world. These creatures are the rulers of men's spirits and the rulers of men's minds. These creatures are the archetypes and dark shadows of Jungian psychology who reside not in the collective unconscious compartment of the human soul but reside in the human spirit because they are spirit, comparing like with like. For example, 2 Timothy 1:7 says,

> **For God hath not given us the spirit of fear; but of power, and of love, and of a sound mind. 2 Timothy 1:7**

### *Fear is a spirit and can control our thoughts, both in spirit and in soul.*

But we have been called out of this darkness. We have been called out of occultism. We have been called out of it and into the new birth. We have been redeemed through the shed blood of our Lord, Jesus Christ. Did we come all the way out of the darkness so God could not reveal to us our enemies? You see, our enemies are not flesh and blood; our enemies are not the Russians or the Chinese. God loves the Russians and the Chinese. Our enemies are Satan and his fallen followers: the principalities, the powers, the spiritual wickedness in high places and the rulers of darkness of this world.

Second Timothy 1:7 says that God has not given us the spirit of fear. There is normal fear God has given, so we do not play in traffic or jump off a cliff, thinking we can fly. There is a normal *fight or flight* pattern God has developed in us.

There is also a kingdom out there wanting to be a part of your life. *The Church is incredibly ignorant about its enemy. "Out of sight, out of mind" seems to be a protective mentality in the Christian Church, but I'll tell you, "out of sight, out of mind" is not a spiritual principle.* Some spiritual warfare conferences are nothing more than shadow boxing. I am here to tell you we are going to defeat the devil and know him and his kingdom. Amen?

**The devil is *not* omnipresent.** We learned this from Job. The sons of God came to present themselves before the LORD and Satan came with them. The LORD said, "What have you been up to, big boy?" Satan said, "I've been walking up and down throughout the earth" (Job 1:7).

> **And the LORD said unto Satan, Whence comest thou? Then Satan answered the LORD, and said, From going to and fro in the earth, and from walking up and down in it. Job 1:7**

If he were omnipresent, he would not have to walk up and down on the earth. He's not omnipresent. He oversees a bureaucracy called the second heaven, which is invisible. You are living in the first heaven; the third heaven is where God is.

Paul said, I was caught up into the third heaven (2 Corinthians 12:2).

> **²I knew a man in Christ above fourteen years ago, (whether in the body, I cannot tell; or whether out of the body, I cannot tell: God knoweth;) such an one caught up to the third heaven. ³And I knew such a man, (whether in the body, or out of the body, I cannot tell: God knoweth;) ⁴How that he was caught up into paradise, and heard unspeakable words, which it is not lawful for a man to utter. 2 Corinthians 12:2–4**

If there is a first heaven and a third heaven, what comes in between? The second heaven. Satan is called the prince of the power of the air.

> **Wherein in time past ye walked according to the course of this world, according to the prince of the power of the air, the spirit that now worketh in the children of disobedience: Ephesians 2:2**

> **In whom the god of this world hath blinded the minds of them which believe not, lest the light of the glorious gospel of Christ, who is the image of God, should shine unto them. 2 Corinthians 4:4**

He's called the god of mankind. His domain is the second heaven.

You need to wake up! No more shadow boxing. Am I going to *resist* the devil today? No, I am not. I am going to *defeat* the devil in my life. That is my enemy. I am going to defeat fear in my life because that is my enemy. I am going to defeat bigotry in my life because that is my enemy. I am going to defeat self-hatred in my life because that is my enemy. I am going to defeat anger in my life because that is my enemy. These are powers answering to Satan and serving him.

If I am around someone who has violence, do you know what I am looking for? I do not tell them to stop being violent; they couldn't stop if they tried. When I am around people who are like that, I want to find out what happened. Where's the root? I am looking for the creature. I must divide. If I can get you right spiritually, then your mind will catch up.

I am a student of the psychology of man, not from a Jungian perspective but from a biblical perspective. We do ministry with many people once we get them changed spiritually and remove the critters and creatures. Then we have to come back and help them renew their minds.

## Teaching on Memory

We think on two levels. Did you know you are a spirit? Your spirit man thinks and your intellect thinks independently of your spirit man. This is why Hebrews 4:12 says that the Word of God comes to separate the soul from the spirit. Why? To get God's Word to enter into your human spirit so your mind is renewed by the washing of the water of the Word as you continually apply it. When your mind and your spirit were one in a way of thinking, it lined up with Satan's mind and you followed Satan.

As a work of the Holy Spirit who shall lead you into all truth, your spirit and your soul will now become one in God's way of thinking and following God. But in the process of becoming one in God's way of thinking, there is a great gap to be worked out. This stuff will tear you up. This is the stuff that doesn't want to let you change your way of thinking. Changing your thinking is really scary because your mind will pitch a fit.

Now, let me help you understand how this works.

When we have ministered to someone who has been subjected to some kind of tragedy or victimization and the result was wounding of their human spirit, they still remember the tragedy. We cannot take your memory away from you, because it is your soul. The Bible says your soul will be saved. How is your soul saved? Your brain cells are part of your soul. When you die, your brain cells die with your body, but the mirror image of the soul thoughts remain with your spirit which returns to God to await the resurrection. In fact, the Bible says, in that day (resurrection) you will be known as you were known.

> **For now we see through a glass, darkly; but then face to face: now I know in part; but then shall I know even as also I am known. 1 Corinthians 13:12**

> **I am the good shepherd, and know my *sheep,* and am known of mine. John 10:14**

> **But we are not of them who draw back unto perdition; but of them that believe to the saving of the soul. Hebrews 10:39**

> **Let him know, that he which converteth the sinner from the error of his way shall save a soul from death, and shall hide a multitude of sins. James 5:20**

This is how it works. We have short-term and long-term memory. Short-term memory and long-term memory are made up of units of memory called "memes." You have individual memes, you have mass memes and you have cultural memes (inherited or learned).

There is a Christian leader in the world right now named George Otis, Jr. I do not know if you know who he is. He is doing sociological and spiritual mapping of the planet with respect to spiritual bondage involving mass memes and cultural memes.

There are principalities who rule nations. We know this from Daniel. You know the prince of Persia and the prince of Grecia were invisible principalities ruling from the heavenlies on behalf of Satan over nations (Daniel 10). Another invisible principality who rules over nations is Gog, as found in Ezekiel 38–39. In my opinion, this invisible principality serves Satan today as the invisible ruler over Islam.

How is Satan the god of this world? He controls the minds of men with a gospel which is not the gospel of our Lord, but rules through the modalities of religiosity, ethnicity, sociology and the gods of this world. He controls minds, yet he and his kingdom are an invisible spirit form.

How many of you in your life have ever changed your theology?

How many of you have discovered in your life you had something called "stinkin' thinkin'"? Were you proud of it? How many of you have ever changed your mind? It is a woman's prerogative, but it is a little more difficult for the men. It is just a way of life for the women! Just kidding!

How many of you remember the erroneous thinking of your past? I am not asking you to meditate on it. How many of you would remember the error of your ways? You became born again and your heart opened up to God and you had a new life. The Word of God came to bring the mind and will of God to your life. So were you still able to remember your atheistic ways? We do not lose this memory. No, we do not, because it is part of your soul.

When someone has a broken heart and their spirit has been injured, we remove the pain in the heart through ministry. They still have the memory in their mind, but the pain in the heart no longer exists. How is it one day they have the memory and the pain and then, after the Lord comes to heal, they still have the memory but no pain? The creature inside, which was reinforcing the damage and the thought, was spiritually removed (Hebrews 12:13).

A meme is a unit of memory. Mass memes can include mass hysteria. Another mass meme is gossip. I want to help you think about this because some of you have been programmed in your long-term memory by your enemy and he wants you to follow his thinking all the way to the grave. Then, he can continue to keep these diseases that are the result of *stinkin' thinkin'* on you. Behind spiritually rooted diseases are always feelings, emotions and thoughts.

Your enemy is banking on the fact that he has you in your mind and in your heart. He has to have you because without you his kingdom cannot exist on this planet (Genesis 3).

*Do you know the enemy wants to use you as a medium of expression?* Does that scare you? Do you know many people are channelers for the devil and do not even know it? When you hate your brother, you are a channeler for the devil. When you slander your brother, you are an oracle for Satan. We're not always taught that, are we? This is why your mind needs to be renewed by the washing of the water of the Word.

**And be renewed in the spirit of your mind; Ephesians 4:23**

**That he might sanctify and cleanse it with the washing of water by the word, Ephesians 5:26**

In short-term memory, you "take a picture"—that is a meme. A unit of memory is an electrical, chemical occurrence that happens in the brain. In short-term memory, it doesn't become fixed. However, in long-term memory we have something happening and now being reinforced by meditation, being reinforced by repetition, being reinforced by a locking in of consciousness, so something happens in the electrochemical occurrence.

There is a factor of genetics that kicks in and involves RNA. Something called protein synthesis occurs and the memory becomes biologically a part of your brain cells, not just as a flash point or a picture in short-term memory. It has now become part of you biologically. That is how your soul is preserved. The mirror image is taken like a negative. The human spirit picks up on it and you become one with it spiritually and psychologically.

Proverbs says,

**For as he thinketh in his heart, so *is* he: Proverbs 23:7**

Well, I changed my heart recently and my poor head is catching up slowly. I follow God not just because my mind agrees; I follow God because my heart, mixed with faith, agrees based on the Word of God. The areas of your thinking that do not match God's knowledge need to become subjected to a superior way of thinking: God's thinking. Will you always remember your *stinkin' thinkin'* or your error or your ignorance? Yes, but as a work of the Holy Spirit, this old way of thinking, even though you remember it, is now inferior. This is how truth is established and error is dispelled.

Your enemy wants to control you through long-term memory. Do you know who else wants to control you through long-term memory? Do not be offended; God does! Would you rather be possessed by God or possessed of the devil? Would you rather have the mind of Satan or the mind of Christ?

We are to put on the mind of Christ.

**For who hath known the mind of the Lord, that he may instruct him? But we have the mind of Christ. 1 Corinthians 2:16**

What do you think that is? We go up and take His brain cells and stick them in our head? No, it means that we are to know the will of the Father and the Word of God: then we are able to conform to His nature and to His image, so when we think, it is like Him thinking; when we speak, it is like Him speaking; and when we act, it is like Him acting so it is the totality of the restoration of a man and a woman of God.

In the total restoration of a man and woman of God, this is how I see it in the Word of God: total expression of renewal and restoration from the works of darkness into the works of life. That is the way God sees me in my generation—my will should match the Father's will, and my word should match the Word of God, and my actions should be as if it were the Holy Spirit, so that the will and the Word and the action of God can be performed through me as a way of life. I am to be a total extension of the Word, the will and the action.

Isn't it amazing that we have been created in God's image? I want to break some past memes here, okay? Some of you have been conforming to the mind of Satan, the mind of death, the mind of antichrist, to things diametrically opposed to what God says. You have not been given the spirit of fear (2 Timothy 1:7). You are not to let a root of bitterness spring up and trouble you (Hebrews 12:15). We must guard what becomes a part of our long-term memory.

What is meant by holding every thought in captivity in 2 Corinthians 10? In your creation, the way you are, isn't it amazing we usually do things by thinking about them first? If you were to create something called a Styrofoam cup, an object to hold water, the first part of the concept would come from where? Your mind. Then you would find a friend and say, "I've just invented a cup." You would express what? The concept originating in your mind. Then, after you articulated it in writing or speech, the final stages should be what? Do it, create it, make it.

That is God's very essence: He thought it, He spoke what He thought and He did it. The three members of the eternal Godhead were in perfect agreement. *The Father willed it, the Word said it and the Holy Spirit did it.* If you are in fellowship with the Godhead and if you are in fellowship with God by His Word, you should be an extension of the will, the Word and the power as a way of life. When the world sees you, they ought to see an extension of the Godhead at every point they turn. Would that be something idealistic to think about or do you think it is scriptural?

We have a ways to go before we can unravel diseases. We need to be weighing and considering. I want you to be holding every thought in captivity. I want you to be doing some X-raying of your thoughts, emotions, parts and pieces of your existence. If you are afraid to go there, don't be. *You are already tormented into it anyway.* God wants to get inside you, so do not shut Him out. He wants you well, in your right mind, in health, sane and to be the fulfillment of 1 Thessalonians 5:23.

> **And the very God of peace sanctify you wholly; and *I pray God* your whole spirit and soul and body be preserved blameless unto the coming of our Lord Jesus Christ. 1 Thessalonians 5:23**

There is that word sanctify, there is that circumcision word, that burning fire of the Holy Spirit word and that conviction word. This is the thing that makes you whole. God wants to sanctify you wholly in spirit, soul and body. God just doesn't want you fixed in one dimension; He wants you fixed in every dimension of your creation. It begins deep on the inside—as a man thinketh in his heart, so is he.

> **For as he thinketh in his heart, so *is* he... Proverbs 23:7**

## Focus on Biblical Standard for Healing

I want to bring you into a place of focus. We have established, first, the biblical standard for healing. It is God's will to get involved in your life. The second thing we established is the Church has been a miserable failure in dealing with it. Third, in reading Ezekiel 34, we established that God the Father, by the Spirit of God (speaking through the prophet Ezekiel), revealed the fact that He was ticked off about it and He had a few things to say against the spiritual leaders. They were not healing the sick. They were not taking care of the diseased. They were not searching for the ones who were lost over the cliff.

We also found in both the Old Testament and the New Testament it is God's will that we prosper in spirit, soul and body. We have given you an insight into the reality of spiritual roots. We have established a foundation for our thinking about spirit and soul and how it affects our physiological existence. We are now moving into a place of looking into various diseases.

I want to say I represent the gap between allopathic medicine and no help at all. I deal with disease—with disease that has a spiritual root with various psychological and physiological manifestations. I deal with the etiology of hundreds of different, so-called incurable diseases in America and the world.

God and I have taken that word *incurable* and done this to it: *When you say incurable, you have made the devil greater than God.* I cannot bring myself to say this. I believe all things are possible. *I believe mankind has disease because we have become separated from God and His Word and fallen into disobedience to Him.*

*I consider all healing of spiritually rooted disease to be a factor of sanctification.* I believe all disease has a spiritual root that is a result of lack of sanctification in our lives as men and women of God. I believe all healing of disease and/or prevention is the process of being re-sanctified.

Remember what we read from 1 Thessalonians 5:23: "May the God of peace sanctify you wholly in spirit, in soul and in body." I also believe God cannot heal, He will not heal, unless we measure up to His standard of holiness. I do not think He has to. I do not think God is going to bless us and let us keep our sin. I am not into legalism. I am not into the works of righteousness. I am into a heart change—the circumcision of the human heart, the submission to the living God because we *want* to submit, not because we have to.

I believe there is a connection between sin and disease because Deuteronomy 28 says so. Disobedience to God and His Word and not staying in covenant with Him will open the door to the curse. In Deuteronomy 28, in the section on curses, we found all manner of disease. When men came to obedience to God and His Word, in covenant with Him as His children, we found blessings and I found not one disease listed. *I consider all disease to be a curse and not a blessing. I consider all absence of disease to be a blessing.* Choose this day what you shall have, blessings or curses, life or death:

> [19]**I call heaven and earth to record this day against you,** *that* **I have set before you life and death, blessing and cursing: therefore choose life, that both thou and thy seed may live:** [20]**That thou mayest love the LORD thy God,** *and* **that thou mayest obey his voice, and that thou mayest cleave unto him: for he** *is* **thy life, and the length of thy days: that thou mayest dwell in the land which the LORD sware unto thy fathers, to Abraham, to Isaac, and to Jacob, to give them. Deuteronomy 30:19–20**

With respect to forgiveness of sin and healing of disease, Psalm 103:3 says, The LORD who forgiveth us of all our iniquities and healeth us of all our diseases.

> **Who forgiveth all thine iniquities; who healeth all thy diseases; Psalm 103:3**

In one verse, we have forgiveness of sin and healing of disease together. In the New Testament, James 5:14–15, we're told concerning sick people in the Church:

> [14]**Is any sick among you? let him call for the elders of the church; and let them pray over him, anointing him with oil in the name of the Lord:** [15]**And the prayer of faith shall save the sick, and the Lord shall raise him up; and if he have committed sins, they shall be forgiven him. James 5:14–15**

There we have the connection between sin and healing. Jesus had just healed someone and He said:

> **Afterward Jesus findeth him in the temple, and said unto him, Behold, thou art made whole: sin no more, lest a worse thing come unto thee. John 5:14**

Right here in the harmony of just three Scriptures, I see a direct relationship between lack of sanctification, disease and sin.

I was recently reading in 2 Chronicles 29 and 30. It was really interesting, because in the days of King Hezekiah, he brought the Word of God back to God's people. The Levites had not been doing the sacrifices; there had been no shedding of blood for the remission of sins by the priests. The people had been serving the gods of pagan nations and Hezekiah the king came to reestablish the righteousness of God in God's people. It was interesting because they brought the Levites together. They brought the singers and the priests together and as they sacrificed for sin, worship went up to God. It was a spontaneous worship and thanksgiving in conjunction with establishing a fellowship and relationship with God and the sacrifice, which provided the shed blood for sin.

The LORD looked down and He heard:

> **And the LORD hearkened to Hezekiah, and healed the people. 2 Chronicles 30:20**

The LORD heard and He healed, but sanctification had to occur first. In order for you to be able to come to a place of receiving healing from God, you have to be in fellowship with Him. In fellowship, you are in contact with all three members of the Godhead. You are in fellowship with the Father, the Son and the Holy Spirit through the communion of the Holy Spirit:

> **The grace of the Lord Jesus Christ, and the love of God, and the communion of the Holy Ghost, *be* with you all. Amen. 2 Corinthians 13:14**

Much of the Church body today is trying to receive from God through prayers and petitions, but they are not in fellowship; they are not in obedience.

Jesus said loving Him involved obeying Him:

> **If ye love me, keep my commandments. John 14:15**

Fellowship with God involves being obedient to Him, not out of "Phariseeism" or legalism, but out of a heart that wants to know and be in fellowship with God by faith. Fellowship with the Father, fellowship with the Word, who is the Son and fellowship with the Holy Spirit is what God desires.

Out of the fellowship comes worship. We do not worship the Holy Spirit by Himself. We worship the Father and the Son, Who is Jesus. The work of the Holy Spirit is to confirm and execute the will of the Father and the Word of God. The Holy Spirit does not speak of Himself (John 16:13). He glorifies Jesus and the Father (John 16:14).

> **[13]Howbeit when he, the Spirit of truth, is come, he will guide you into all truth: for he shall not speak of himself; but whatsoever he shall hear, *that* shall he speak: and he will shew you things to come. [14]He shall glorify me: for he shall receive of mine, and shall shew *it* unto you. [15]All things that the Father hath are mine: therefore said I, that he shall take of mine, and shall shew *it* unto you. John 16:13–15**

All good things come down from the Father, in the name of Jesus, as a work of the Holy Spirit.

> **Every good gift and every perfect gift is from above, and cometh down from the Father of lights, with whom is no variableness, neither shadow of turning. James 1:17**

This is why we go to the Father, in the name of Jesus and the Holy Spirit performs it. We're only to contact one member of the Godhead in petition. Jesus said, In that day you shall ask Me nothing, but you shall ask the Father in My name and He shall give you what you ask.

> **[23]And in that day ye shall ask me nothing. Verily, verily, I say unto you, Whatsoever ye shall ask the Father in my name, he will give *it* you. [24]Hitherto have ye asked nothing in my name: ask, and ye shall receive, that your joy may be full. John 16:23–24**

Jesus said, Hitherto have ye asked nothing in my name: Ask and you shall receive that your joy may be full. And think not that I shall pray the Father for you. Then the disciples said, Teach us to pray and Jesus said, Boys, say it like this…

> **…Our Father which art in heaven… Matthew 6:9**

Petition is made to the Father in the name of the Lord Jesus Christ.

However, the Church doesn't seem to be getting many answers. This is a statement of the problem. I do not see a well Church trying to save a sick world. I see a sick Church trying to save itself. It should be a well Church trying to save a sick world. This is what I see in Scripture.

Reestablish your relationship with God and you will be in worship. When fellowship and worship are in place, then when you come before God in the name of the Lord, you are going to have His attention. It won't cost you anything.

*There will be people who hear this who will never be the same.* There are some of you who are dealing with things in your life. When you apply the principles that I have given you and you go before God and the Word, you will walk away from certain diseases just like you never had them. This does not happen to everyone because some of us are still working out our problems. We are still working them out, thinking about it, doing that circumcision, doing that repentance, getting before God, getting back in fellowship, getting to a place where we are going to be honest with God about our problem. We are getting to a place where we are ready to come before Him to deal with it.

The Bible tells me in John 8:36: "Who the Son makes free is free indeed." Support groups oftentimes will magnify what is going on in our lives without making a provision for freedom. Even though we are instructed to bear each other's burdens, support groups should ultimately have, as a part of their thinking, the possibility of freedom. Reflecting on this, support groups should include both dimensions: burden bearing and freedom.

## Knowing God's Word

When we get into certain difficulties, we find at some point in our family trees or in our own lives, our minds and our spirits have been opened up to the other kingdom. We have listened to those voices and we have followed modalities of thought and precepts that are diametrically opposed to what God has said in His Word. *The biggest problem I find in the Christian Church today is so often Christians do not know the Word of God.*

A workman that needeth not be ashamed, rightly dividing the word of truth.

**Study to show thyself approved unto God, a workman that needeth not to be ashamed, rightly dividing the word of truth. 2 Timothy 2:15**

This comes from sitting down with the Word and letting God speak to you. Study the Scripture for yourself. Do not be swayed by new doctrines or whims that come along—study!

When I first came back to God, I would sit down every morning at 6:00 until 7:30 before I went to my business. Week after week, month after month, for 1½ hours, I plowed into that Word. After months of study, the Bible exploded for me from cover to cover. This is where you begin. This is God's will. This is God's Word and, if you mix it with your faith and take it into your heart, you will never be the same. You will change your life, your family's lives, your city, your church and your world.

In *occultism*, the real thing is hidden and something false is offering itself as if it were the real thing.

Most of the mental diseases we have identified in mankind today are the result of separation from God's Word, which is the mind and will of God concerning all things. The revealed will of God and the living Word for mankind to follow can be found in the pages of Scripture. When we follow other ways of thinking, other gods and other spiritual leaders who are not set up by God, ordained by God, in covenant with God, anointed by God, or established by God, we have opened up our spirits to forces designed to steal our faith and bring us torment.

## *ALL FEAR COMES FROM NOT TRUSTING GOD AND HIS WORD.*

The Word says:

**Be careful for nothing; but in every thing by prayer and supplication with thanksgiving let your requests be made known unto God. Philippians 4:6**

**In every thing give thanks: for this is the will of God in Christ Jesus concerning you. 1 Thessalonians 5:18**

**Take therefore no thought for the morrow: for the morrow shall take thought for the things of itself. Sufficient unto the day *is* the evil thereof. Matthew 6:34**

*We are so busy dragging the past around with us and projecting it to the future that we forget to occupy today.*

If our minds, spirits and souls are filled with fear and confusion, projection and avoidance, we are no earthly good today. We are preoccupied with dragging this junk around and projecting it into the future. That is why we need Prozac, Valium and sleeping pills. That is why we have ulcers.

**Forget the past; forget the future.**

## *LET GOD BE GOD TODAY IN YOUR LIFE!*

The evil of today is sufficient unto itself.

**Take therefore no thought for the morrow: for the morrow shall take thought for the things of itself. Sufficient unto the day *is* the evil thereof. Matthew 6:34**

**Your life hangs in the balance.**

*Make sure you are in the right kingdom all the time.*

# Chapter Two
# **Spiritually Rooted Disease**

*Spiritually rooted disease is the result of separation on three levels:*

1. Separation from God, His Word and His love.

2. Separation from yourself.

3. Separation from others.

## 1. Separation from God, His Word and His Love

Mankind is diseased first of all because we are separated from God, His Word, His truth and His love—and this includes members of His Church. Do you know how many of the wonderful, believing saints I talk to who are not sure God loves them? They had earthly fathers who did not represent God the Father in their lives. God the Father is now guilty by association. He's a mean, bad dude.

Religion teaches that God the Father is sitting on the throne with lightning bolts, waiting to strike you dead if you are bad. This is not what I read in Scripture. Our God is a loving God. God is love (1 John 4:8).

> **And we have known and believed the love that God hath to us. God is love; and he that dwelleth in love dwelleth in God, and God in him. 1 John 4:16**

For God so loved the world that He gave...

> **For God so loved the world, that he gave his only begotten Son, that whosoever believeth in him should not perish, but have everlasting life. John 3:16**

Jesus said, If you've seen Me, you've seen the Father.

> **Then answered Jesus and said unto them, Verily, verily, I say unto you, The Son can do nothing of himself, but what he seeth the Father do: for what things soever he doeth, these also doeth the Son likewise. John 5:19**

> **Then said Jesus unto them, When ye have lifted up the Son of man, then shall ye know that I am *he*, and *that* I do nothing of myself; but as my Father hath taught me, I speak these things. John 8:28**

> **Jesus saith unto him, Have I been so long time with you, and yet hast thou not known me, Philip? he that hath seen me hath seen the Father; and how sayest thou *then*, Shew us the Father? John 14:9**

I like to have a little fun with religion. I love relationships, but to me religion is a killer. I try to bring people into a place of healing—a place of receiving. You see, healing doesn't ultimately come from Jesus. It comes from the Father. Jesus said, I only do the things I saw My Father doing. I only say the things I heard My Father saying.

> **I speak that which I have seen with my Father: and ye do that which ye have seen with your father.  John 8:38**

> **I can of mine own self do nothing: as I hear, I judge: and my judgment is just; because I seek not mine own will, but the will of the Father which hath sent me. John 5:30**

James 1:17 says that all good things come down from the Father of lights with Whom there is no variableness of turning.

> **Every good gift and every perfect gift is from above, and cometh down from the Father of lights, with whom is no variableness, neither shadow of turning. James 1:17**

Psalm 68:19 says, Blessed be the Lord, who daily loads us with benefits…the God of our salvation.

> **Blessed *be* the Lord, *who* daily loadeth us *with benefits, even* the God of our salvation. Selah. Psalm 68:19**

I get a real kick out of these "Jesus is Lord" signs on churches. I wonder what happened to the Father. He's not Lord? The Lord's prayer says, Our Father who art in heaven…

> **⁹After this manner therefore pray ye: Our Father which art in heaven, Hallowed be thy name. ¹⁰Thy kingdom come. Thy will be done in earth, as *it is* in heaven. ¹¹Give us this day our daily bread. ¹²And forgive us our debts, as we forgive our debtors. ¹³And lead us not into temptation, but deliver us from evil: For thine is the kingdom, and the power, and the glory, for ever. Amen. Matthew 6:9–13**

Jesus said in John 16:23, In that day you will ask Me nothing, but you will pray the Father in My name and He shall give you what you ask.

> **And in that day ye shall ask me nothing. Verily, verily, I say unto you, Whatsoever ye shall ask the Father in my name, he will give *it* you. John 16:23**

I like to see these, "Jesus is Lord" signs, but I'd like to see "Father is Lord" just above them. Jesus said, My Father and I are One…but He is greater than I.

> **I and *my* Father are one. John 10:30**

> **Ye have heard how I said unto you, I go away, and come *again* unto you. If ye loved me, ye would rejoice, because I said, I go unto the Father: for my Father is greater than I. John 14:28**

The order of the Godhead and the government of God is first, the Father; second, the Word Who came in the flesh as Jesus; and third, the Holy Spirit.

## 2. Separation from Yourself

Do you know how many people do not like themselves? Do you know how many people struggle with self-hatred, lack of self-esteem and guilt? It is a massive plague. How can you not love yourself if God loves you? He's greater than you are. He who is greatest and holiest of all, God the Father, says He loves you. Under what gospel do we have the audacity to say we do not love ourselves? If we do this, we make ourselves in opposition to God. We make ourselves a god unto ourselves. We deny His statement of love and open ourselves up to the enemy to agree with us. So instead of hearing God speaking to you, by His Word and by the Holy Spirit, telling you that you are loved and you are okay, you are going to hear this voice coming into your mind, telling you how rotten, stupid or worthless you are.

In this ministry, we deal with many autoimmune diseases: lupus, Crohn's, diabetes (type 1), rheumatoid arthritis and MS, to name a few. All autoimmune diseases have a spiritual root of self-hatred, self-bitterness and guilt. Diabetes can be defeated. Lupus and rheumatoid arthritis can be defeated. All autoimmune diseases can be defeated or can be prevented.

Do you know what really irritates me? When someone says, "This is incurable; they are just going to die anyway." Do you know what that does in my spirit? I am so grieved. This means to me that person believes Satan and death are greater than God and the Lord Jesus and His Word. I do not agree.

Do you think God needs a disease to get you to heaven? Do you think God needs to torment you so you can get over the great divide? Why have we become so acclimated to this kind of thinking and we have to die and move into Glory because of a disease? I think we have been had! I think we have been bewitched! I think we're following another gospel! Where did euthanasia come from, anyway?

**In Psalm 90, God, through Moses, prophesied that your lifetime should be 70 to 80 years. Anything less than that is a curse.**

> [10]**The days of our years *are* threescore years and ten; and if by reason of strength *they be* fourscore years, yet *is* their strength labour and sorrow; for it is soon cut off, and we fly away. [11]Who knoweth the power of thine anger? even according to thy fear, *so is* thy wrath. [12]So teach *us* to number our days, that we may apply *our* hearts unto wisdom. Psalm 90:10–12**

Where did this term "retirement" come from? Moses was 80 years of age before he even started his ministry.

## 3. Separation from Others

Separation opens the door to spiritually rooted diseases. Unforgiveness, or bitterness toward others, contributes to separation.

When you think of someone who has wronged you, do you feel it in the pit of your stomach? We need to start looking at those high-octane pings. You will always remember the individual and what they did to you, but you do not have to carry the thoughts of hate or bitterness. If you have truly forgiven them from your heart, these thoughts will be gone. You will still have the memory, but God will heal the pain so you can have victory over the situation. It doesn't need to ruin your life.

*We are not only into healing,*
*we are into disease prevention.*

Would you like to avoid certain diseases in your lifetime? *Newsweek* magazine (September 24, 1990) said, "The future of medicine does not lie in the treatment of illness but in preventing it."

**Family trees** are very important diagnostic tools. Behavior and health problems tend to repeat themselves. We see patterns repeated from mothers and fathers to their children. This is true in both biological and spiritual disease. Exodus 20 teaches about the sins of the father being passed on to the third and fourth generation. Psychologists also have observed certain personality characteristics and behaviors, such as rage, anger and molestation, that can roll over to the next generation(s).

> **Thou shalt not bow down thyself to them, nor serve them: for I the LORD thy God *am* a jealous God, visiting the iniquity of the fathers upon the children unto the third and fourth *generation* of them that hate me; Exodus 20:5**

> **Thou shalt not bow down thyself unto them, nor serve them: for I the LORD thy God *am* a jealous God, visiting the iniquity of the fathers upon the children unto the third and fourth *generation* of them that hate me, Deuteronomy 5:9**

Would you like to prevent disease in your children? Do you think it is possible? That would be *a more excellent way*™.

When I am involved with people who are about to be married, I look at the family trees from both sides to see what they are bringing into this family package. If you do not deal with what has happened in your family tree and if you do not deal with what is in your personal lives, your children will inherit your curses.

If we want to do something for our children, let's go before God and get our lives straightened out, so we can break the power of sin and so genetically inherited diseases no longer exist. In our ministry, globally, we have documented evidence of genetic code changes. When a disease was diagnosed through genetic investigation by an oncologist, after ministry and healing, the genetic pattern changed and this person could no longer have that specific disease again. Do you think that's possible?

Are we just going to go on this toboggan ride from generation to generation and do nothing about it? Look into your families and you will see some of the same diseases, personality traits and characteristics of relationships repeating: mothers and daughters not getting along, fathers and sons fighting with each other, etc. Broken relationships of some kind are passed along until someone decides "Enough" and breaks the cycle.

In an article in *USA Today*, a number of women were asked, "Where do you go when you are sick? Who do you talk to?" About half of all women said their primary care doctor is their main source of health care information. The other half reported as follows:

- 24 percent of all women learn about their problems and solutions from magazines and newspapers

- 7 percent from TV and radio

- 5 percent from a relative or a friend

- 5 percent from self-help books

- 4 percent from school courses

- 2 percent from a pharmacist

Not even a fraction of a percentage included a pastor, church, Bible or God. Yet God is the Creator. He is our Savior. He is our Healer and He is our Deliverer. If He created us, He knows what is wrong with us! Would we dare go there and ask Him to reveal this to His children? I have. I am just foolish enough (or smart enough) to believe He will answer me.

I am not against doctors, but I believe that in our ignorance and our separation from God, we have asked the medical community to do something they are not qualified to do—to pastor us and deal with spiritual issues. I do not find anywhere in Scripture, especially in Ephesians 4, where a doctor or a psychologist is considered to be a gift from the Lord Jesus in leadership to us.

**Wherefore he saith, When he ascended up on high, he led captivity captive, and gave gifts unto men. Ephesians 4:8**

> **And he gave some, apostles; and some, prophets; and some, evangelists; and some, pastors and teachers; Ephesians 4:11**

I have found the fivefold ministry mentioned includes apostles, prophets, evangelists, pastors and teachers as a gift to the body, but I did not find doctors or psychologists.

> **[27]Now ye are the body of Christ, and members in particular. [28]And God hath set some in the church, first apostles, secondarily prophets, thirdly teachers, after that miracles, then gifts of healings, helps, governments, diversities of tongues. 1 Corinthians 12:27–28**

### *These two professions are many times the result of the failure of the Christian Church and its leadership to execute its scriptural mandate in pastoral care.*

Psychologists have become the pastors of America, but God has not ordained them to be so. We have asked our medical community to be our healers of spiritually rooted diseases, but they are not qualified. This is why allopathic medicine is failing. The medical community does not know the etiology of over 80 percent of all diseases. If they do not know the cause, how can they cure the disease? They cannot. The best they can do is a little management of the disease and often with drugs which have terrible side effects.

While the Church has failed in this area, people are running to alternative and New Age modalities of disease management. These too are failing, because again they only offer "management" of the disease. People are beginning to come back to the Church for help and the Church should have the answers.

> **To the intent that now unto the principalities and powers in heavenly *places* might be known by the church the manifold wisdom of God, Ephesians 3:10**

People come for help from coast-to-coast and around the world and 45 percent of the people seeking help are unchurched and unsaved. They come in the back door asking, "Can you help?" The world is turning the corner and coming back to God, but the Church is turning the corner away from God. *I think it is time to let God be God in our midst with understanding and discernment.*

In our ministry brochure, there is a statement worth repeating:

> *The true etiology of many diseases reveals an often overlooked spiritual dimension. This dimension, more often than not, goes unaddressed by the afflicted, their health care providers and even their spiritual leaders.*

What would you think if I asked you to take responsibility for a spiritual root in exchange for healing? Would it be worth it? Would you dare believe it could happen? I want to tell you in God's Word it says that He who watches over His Word will perform it.

> Then said the LORD unto me, Thou hast well seen: for I will hasten my word to perform it. Jeremiah 1:12

> I have sworn, and I will perform *it*, that I will keep thy righteous judgments. Psalm 119:106

In the New Testament, Mark said the disciples went everywhere preaching the gospel and the Lord in Heaven worked with them, confirming the Word with signs and wonders following.

> And he said unto them, Go ye into all the world, and preach the gospel to every creature. Mark 16:15

> And they went forth, and preached every where, the Lord working with *them*, and confirming the word with signs following. Amen. Mark 16:20

*I do not chase signs and wonders, but I have discovered signs and wonders follow them that believe. If you do not believe, do not worry about it because it will never happen, but leave the rest of us alone who are believing.*

I learned something about God: He has created us with a free will and He is not going to force you to come to Him. He is not going to force you to become born again. He's not going to force you to go to heaven. He's going to deal with you, but you are going to have to do the responding.

Do you know people do not get born again if it is against their will? We are just like stubborn mules. You could not make us do something if you tried. I cannot make you do anything against your will. You would thrash me and you would not put up with it. God cannot make you do it either.

If I could sow seed in your lives and God could use it sometime in the eternal future to give you a better life, would it be worth it? Later in this teaching, I'll break down many diseases and tell you why people have those diseases. We will also tell you what it is going to take to move the hand of God and get healed.

A Jewish lady from New Jersey was healed before she was saved. Do you think God can heal people who are not born again? Do you have to become born again before He will heal you? I have noted God will heal people who are not born again. But when they are healed, they sure get born again quickly!

Another wonderful Jewish lady also came down from New Jersey. She had Chronic Fatigue Syndrome, Electromagnetic Field Sensitivity and

Environmental Illness. She could not even live in her home. She was allergic to heat, electricity, could not read a book and could not have a light bulb on. She then learned of someone who had been healed. She called me and said, "I want to come down to Georgia and I want you to heal me."

I said, "Oh, I do not heal anyone; God does."

Well, that brought up another subject. She asked, "Do you have to talk about Jesus if I come down there?"

I said, "No, we do not have to talk about Jesus."

She said, "Well, you are a Christian."

I said, "You are Jewish, so I'll talk about the God of Abraham, Isaac and Jacob. Will that be okay?"

She said, "Well, sure!"

I said, "He is the same God you know. I will talk about the God of Abraham, Isaac and Jacob and I'll pray for you in the name of the God of Abraham, Isaac and Jacob. Could I pray for you in the name of the Lord? Could you handle that?"

She said, "That sounds pretty good, but do I have to accept this Jesus? You said, you do not heal anyone. If I am healed and it is this Jesus who did it, do I have to accept Him when He heals me?"

I said, "No, but it would be a good thing to consider because He is going to be the One who does it."

In the following four months, we never discussed her disease. She was so mad at me. She came into my office and asked, "What are we going to talk about today?"

I would say, "The God of Abraham, Isaac and Jacob. Let's go to the Torah, let's go to Isaiah, let's go to Jeremiah."

During the four months, I revealed to her the identity of the national God of Israel, the promised Messiah who came in the flesh to die for her. She would take what I said back to her husband and her rabbi and they would try to prove me wrong. They couldn't do it. I showed them the Godhead in the Old Testament Torah, in Isaiah, in Psalms—the plural unity of God, the Echad of Deuteronomy 6:4, the One, the plural unity.

**Hear, O Israel: The Lord our God *is* one Lord: Deuteronomy 6:4**

They couldn't prove me wrong.

Finally, one day she came back after four months and said, "I'm only 90 percent convinced that Jesus is the promised Messiah, but I am 100 percent convinced that He is God Who came in the flesh. I am ready to receive Him as my Savior and my Lord." I then led her in the sinner's prayer. We had a happy time. She is a wonderful lady and within 60 days, she was well. After six months of being at our retreat center receiving ministry, she went home. She is well today, marvelously healed by her Creator, her Savior, her God and the Father Who sent Him and Who loved her from the foundation of the world with an everlasting love.

There was another Jewish lady in New Jersey, 60 years of age, who had advanced osteoporosis. She contacted our ministry through our National Ministry Line. There is osteoporosis from estrogen deficiency because of menopause and there is osteoporosis which is non-menopausal and comes from a spiritual root. Do you know what the Bible says the spiritual root is for non-menopausal osteoporosis? I'll tell you—envy and jealousy are the cause of rotting of the bones:

> **A sound heart *is* the life of the flesh: but envy the rottenness of the bones. Proverbs 14:30**

Do you think there is a connection and a spiritual root?

When we cracked Environmental Illness in 1990, seven words in the Bible, having been there for 3,000 years, were the insight God gave me to unravel this bizarre disease. Today our ministry is internationally recognized in the healing of MCS/EI because I took God at His Word. Our success in the healing of this disease coast-to-coast and worldwide is second to none. I do not mean to be presumptuous. No, I am just letting you know how our wonderful God has done this.

I was flying across America to see someone who had MCS/EI. I did not know anything about the disease at that time. This person told me pesticides had destroyed their immune system and then allergies developed. I did not know; I thought it could possibly be true. I was sitting in an airplane with my Bible, talking to God.

I said, "God, talk to me. Here I am, flying across America to see somebody who doesn't know me. I do not know them and they are expecting You to heal them from a disease that I know nothing about." I had told this individual, "I'll give you ten days of my life to see what God will do. I'll drop what I am doing and I'll fly across America. I'll come see what God will do." As I was browsing in my Bible, in Proverbs, I saw the answer from God for the healing of MCS/EI.

> **A merry heart doeth good *like* a medicine: but a broken spirit drieth the bones. Proverbs 17:22**

Do you know laughter can strengthen the immune system? It has been documented. Laughter causes the body to manufacture T cells and killer cells.

"A merry heart doeth good like a medicine, but a broken spirit drieth the bones." I stared at this verse in Proverbs 17:22 and all of a sudden the lights came on. I thought, "Wait a minute; a broken spirit drieth up bones!" Bones, bones, what is in bones? Couldn't be osteoporosis, this person is too young and not diagnosed. Bones, drying up of bones. The immune system. It started to click!

(In college, I was a premed student, majoring in biology with a minor in psychology, so I had a little background in medicine.) Wait a minute—the immune system. This person told me their immune system had been compromised by pesticides, but this verse in the Bible did not say it was pesticides destroyed the immune system. It was a broken spirit that dried the bones or destroyed the immune system.

So when I got to the person's home, this individual asked, "Has God shown you anything about my disease?" I said, "I'm not sure, but I need to ask you a question. I wonder who broke your heart. I wonder who damaged you on the inside so severely you now have a compromised immune system. I have a feeling the pesticides and the allergies are just a by-product."

Today we have found this to be true. It is not chemicals or odors causing MCS/EI. *The immune system is compromised because of fear and anxiety coming out of a broken heart.* When you have a compromised immune system, you automatically have allergies.

The lady with osteoporosis in New Jersey did not know God. Though she was Jewish, she was separated from God. When we were able to be involved in her life, we knew that she had envy and jealousy coupled with some bitterness coming out of some tragic circumstances of life.

My staff dealt with her over the phone. I have never met her in my life; my staff has never met her. This illustrates how for a long time, a large number of people have gotten well in America through our telephone ministry or by applying the principles in our teaching material.

Do you know there is no distance in the Spirit? In the story about the centurion, Jesus said, "I'll come and heal your servant."

He said, "No, no, I'm a man of authority, I tell my servants to go here, do this, do that. I perceive you are a man of authority. Simply speak the word and my servant shall be healed."

When the centurion got back to his hometown, he inquired and the man was well. What hour was it? It was the same hour Jesus had spoken.

**⁵And when Jesus was entered into Capernaum, there came unto him a centurion, beseeching him, ⁶And saying, Lord, my servant lieth at home sick of the palsy, grievously tormented. ⁷And Jesus saith unto him, I will**

come and heal him. ⁸The centurion answered and said, Lord, I am not worthy that thou shouldest come under my roof: but speak the word only, and my servant shall be healed. ⁹For I am a man under authority, having soldiers under me: and I say to this *man,* Go, and he goeth; and to another, Come, and he cometh; and to my servant, Do this, and he doeth *it.* ¹⁰When Jesus heard *it,* he marvelled, and said to them that followed, Verily I say unto you, I have not found so great faith, no, not in Israel. ¹¹And I say unto you, That many shall come from the east and west, and shall sit down with Abraham, and Isaac, and Jacob, in the kingdom of heaven. ¹²But the children of the kingdom shall be cast out into outer darkness: there shall be weeping and gnashing of teeth. ¹³And Jesus said unto the centurion, Go thy way; and as thou hast believed, so be it done unto thee. And his servant was healed in the selfsame hour. Matthew 8:5–13

What did this show me when I was growing up in the Lord? There is no distance in the Spirit. I can minister over the telephone as well as I can in person most of the time, but not always. Isn't that amazing?

What makes this testimony so incredibly significant is she was on prednisone. You do not have any chance of defeating osteoporosis while you are on prednisone because it prevents bone density increase as a side effect. She was still taking the drug when she went back to her doctor to have her annual tests. I have in my files the documentation by her doctor about this healing. This is a documented healing by the medical community.

She was age 60 with progressive osteoporosis. She had contracted this disease in her thirties and by her early forties, she was in the advanced stages of osteoporosis. They did the bone scans and the tests. When she went for her results, her doctor told her this: "I do not know what has happened to you. I have been in this business for years. I have been your doctor for years and all osteoporosis has been halted. Not only has it been halted, but in all bone scan areas of your bones, structure-wise, you have an average bone density increase of 15 percent to 18 percent. *You have the bones of a 30-year-old woman.*" In Psalms it says, He will renew our youth like the eagle's.

*...so that* thy youth is renewed like the eagle's. Psalm 103:5

It happened to her!

That is what God did when she lined up with these principles. You cannot have strong bones and not deal with the spiritual root. Remember, I read this to you from Jeremiah. If we follow after the opposite of God and His precepts, then we shall bring to ourselves the opposite of the blessings. The opposite of the blessing is a curse.

## Blessings and Curses

In Deuteronomy 28 (read the whole chapter), there is a whole section on blessings and curses. God said: **If** you do this, **then** I'll do this, **but** if you do not, then all these curses shall come upon you.

> **And said, If thou wilt diligently hearken to the voice of the Lord thy God, and wilt do that which is right in his sight, and wilt give ear to his commandments, and keep all his statutes, I will put none of these diseases upon thee, which I have brought upon the Egyptians: for I *am* the Lord that healeth thee. Exodus 15:26**

It is important to note that curses do not come from God. They come from Satan.

> **Let no man say when he is tempted, I am tempted of God: for God cannot be tempted with evil, neither tempteth he any man: James 1:13**

On the cursing side is all manner of disease (Deuteronomy 28:15–68). On the blessing side it says this:

> **28:1And it shall come to pass, if thou shalt hearken diligently unto the voice of the Lord thy God, to observe *and* to do all his commandments which I command thee this day, that the Lord thy God will set thee on high above all nations of the earth: 2And all these blessings shall come on thee, and overtake thee, if thou shalt hearken unto the voice of the Lord thy God. Deuteronomy 28:1–2**

*There are conditions to healing.* You do not just get healed by barging in and making demands. The condition is obedience to God. Obedience is better than sacrifice.

> **22And Samuel said, Hath the Lord *as great* delight in burnt offerings and sacrifices, as in obeying the voice of the Lord? Behold, to obey *is* better than sacrifice, *and* to hearken than the fat of rams. 23For rebellion *is as* the sin of witchcraft, and stubbornness *is as* iniquity and idolatry. Because thou hast rejected the word of the Lord, he hath also rejected thee from *being* king. 1 Samuel 15:22–23**

I am not into legalism. I am into something much deeper than legalism. I am into something called "heart change."

I want to tell you something. I do not serve God because I have to; I serve God because I want to. I do not love God because I have to; I love God just because I love Him. I am not obedient to God because I am afraid of hell; I serve God because I want to be an obedient son. I have been a rebel too many years. I am a sinner saved by the grace of God. I am worthy of death, but God chose otherwise. I am a grateful prodigal and I am a grateful son. I know what I have been saved from. I am not going back. You can go back if you want, but I am not going back with you. I just came from there. I know what it is like. I am not going back into cursings; I am going on into blessings.

Choose this day what you shall have: blessings or curses, life or death.

> [19]I call heaven and earth to record this day against you, *that* I have set before you life and death, blessing and cursing: therefore choose life, that both thou and thy seed may live: [20]That thou mayest love the LORD thy God, *and* that thou mayest obey his voice, and that thou mayest cleave unto him: for he *is* thy life, and the length of thy days: that thou mayest dwell in the land which the LORD sware unto thy fathers, to Abraham, to Isaac and to Jacob, to give them. Deuteronomy 30:19–20

It is your choice. In Deuteronomy 28, you will find the three key words in Scripture: they are "**IF**," "**THEN**" and "**BUT**." One day I am going to teach a sermon called "If, Then and But."

### *Freedom requires responsibility.*

There is a required action on our part in order to receive God's blessings. You cannot have your sin and also have your blessings (doctrine of Balaam).

I want to teach you something, if you have ears to hear. In Scripture, when the children of God were coming across the Jordan, Joshua separated God's people around two mountains, **Mount Gerizim** and **Mount Ebal.** Mount Gerizim was the Mount of Blessings; Mount Ebal was the Mount of Curses. In Deuteronomy 11:26–29 it says,

> [26]Behold, I set before you this day a blessing and a curse; [27]A blessing, if ye obey the commandments of the Lord your God, which I command you this day: [28]And a curse, if ye will not obey the commandments of the Lord your God, but turn aside out of the way which I command you this day, to go after other gods, which ye have not known. [29]And it shall come to pass, when the Lord thy God hath brought thee in unto the land whither thou goest to possess it, that thou shalt put the blessing upon mount Gerizim, and the curse upon mount Ebal. Deuteronomy 11:26–29

As God's people came into promise, they were immediately brought into a place of *discernment.* What was the discernment? *Choice!* You are going to choose what you are going to believe. You are going to choose which path you shall follow.

God was bringing a very powerful truth to His people—in your obedience to Me and My commandments, which is best for you, the blessings are immediate and close by. However, if you are disobedient, the curse shall surely come. God built into this a type and shadow: this fact is in His grace and mercy He would build into our lives time for reflection, time for conviction and time to work it out. So I am building into your consciousness today, precepts, concepts, the theology of God to bring you to a place of focus to recover yourself from the snare of the devil, not only for the healing of disease but for the prevention of it.

In Deuteronomy 28, there are a bunch of blessings and then there are a bunch of curses. *Under curses are all manner of disease:* then it says, and other diseases not written shall come upon you.

> **Also every sickness, and every plague, which *is* not written in the book of this law, them will the LORD bring upon thee, until thou be destroyed. Deuteronomy 28:61**

For every disease allopathic medicine thinks they have cured, five more brand-new ones pop up. Do you realize this?

This is a mess. The *Merck Manual*[1] I have is getting thicker every year, because there are more and more new plagues surfacing. ***The study of disease is bigger than my Bible.*** The book on *Pathophysiology: The Biologic Basis for Disease in Children and Adults*[2] is thicker than my Bible. The PDR (*Physician's Desk Reference)*[3] on drugs and their side effects is bigger than my Bible. I think we need to pay attention.

*On the blessing side of Deuteronomy 28, not **one** disease is mentioned.* Do you consider disease to be a blessing or a curse? I consider all disease to be a curse. Why? Because the Bible says so. *It says, when there is blessing, there is no disease (and when there is a curse, all manner of disease is listed).*

You say, "I thought we were freed from the power of sin and death at the cross. I thought Christ said, 'It is finished.'"

If it was finished and the penalty of the curse was paid, and you call yourself a believer yet you have a disease, you must not be born again. I do not find one Christian today who does not have some type of disease in their life in America, to some degree. If it's finished, then why do we have disease?

I teach something, which may not be your position, but I teach something called *appropriation* of what was done at the cross. It is the only thing making any sense. It is called appropriation and was granted when Christ died. He died for all the sins of the world. Did He? Did He pay for all sins once and for all? Is everyone saved? (No.) But it was finished. If it was

---

[1] *Merck Manual*, 16th edition. Rahway, NJ: Merck & Co., 1992.

[2] McCance, Kathryn L. and Sue E. Huether. *Pathophysiology: The Biologic Basis for Disease in Adults And Children*, 5th Edition. St. Louis, MO: Mosby, 2005.

[3] *Physician's Desk Reference*, 55th edition. Medical Economics Company, 2001.

finished, then why isn't everyone saved? *Because you have to appropriate it by faith.*

It is the same way with healing. When it says by His stripes we were healed and He bore the penalty of the curse, it does not mean you keep your sin and have your freedom.

> But he *was* wounded for our transgressions, *he was* bruised for our iniquities: the chastisement of our peace *was* upon him; and with his stripes we are healed.  Isaiah 53:5

If we were totally free at conversion, then why would we need to be sanctified? So why would we listen to Paul tell us about circumcision of the heart? *Then would Paul say to cleanse ourselves from all filthiness of the flesh and spirit?*

> Having therefore these promises, dearly beloved, let us cleanse ourselves from all filthiness of the flesh and spirit, perfecting holiness in the fear of God.  2 Corinthians 7:1

I just raise the question. I do not know what your walk with God is, but I have learned I am working out my own salvation daily with fear and trembling.

> Wherefore, my beloved, as ye have always obeyed, not as in my presence only, but now much more in my absence, work out your own salvation with fear and trembling. Philippians 2:12

> Blessed *be* the Lord, *who* daily loadeth us *with benefits, even* the God of our salvation. Selah.  Psalm 68:19

I am appropriating His grace and mercy in His Word and by the circumcision of my heart and this is an ongoing process. God is continually cutting away the part of me and my nature He did not create from the beginning.

Here in Deuteronomy 28, it talks about barrenness, divorce, losing your cows and your goats and in verse 58 it says "If thou wilt not observe to do all the words of this law written in this book..." How do we know when we are under the law? Do you think God's nature has ever changed? Does He say, "I change not"?

> For I *am* the LORD, I change not... Malachi 3:6

Did Christ come and change certain aspects of the law? Yes, He did. He rewrote certain aspects of the law concerning dietary rules, concerning Sabbath, concerning an eye for eye and tooth for tooth. But principles of righteousness have never changed!

> [58]If thou wilt not observe to do all the words of this law that are written in this book, that thou mayest fear this glorious and fearful name, THE LORD THY GOD; [59]Then the LORD will make thy plagues

wonderful, and the plagues of thy seed, *even* great plagues, and of long continuance, and sore sicknesses, and of long continuance. ⁶⁰Moreover he will bring upon thee all the diseases of Egypt, which thou wast afraid of; and they shall cleave unto thee. ⁶¹Also every sickness, and every plague, which *is* not written in the book of this law, them will the LORD bring upon thee, until thou be destroyed. ⁶²And ye shall be left few in number, whereas ye were as the stars of heaven for multitude; because thou wouldest not obey the voice of the LORD thy God. ⁶³And it shall come to pass, *that* as the LORD rejoiced over you to do you good, and to multiply you; so the LORD will rejoice over you to destroy you, and to bring you to nought; and ye shall be plucked from off the land whither thou goest to possess it. Deuteronomy 28:58–63

⁶⁶And thy life shall hang in doubt before thee; and thou shalt fear day and night, and shalt have none assurance of thy life: ⁶⁷In the morning thou shalt say, Would God it were even! and at even thou shalt say, Would God it were morning! for the fear of thine heart wherewith thou shalt fear, and for the sight of thine eyes which thou shalt see. Deuteronomy 28:66–67

Being a doer of the Word is an Old Testament and a New Testament principle!

## Spiritually Rooted Disease is a Result of Separation on Three Levels

What do you think the solution is? Removing the separation! These three root "**causes of disease**" are:

1. Separation from God and His Word, His person and His love.

2. Separation from yourself—not accepting yourself, not loving yourself, and having guilt and condemnation.

3. Separation from others—breaches in relationships, hatred, bitterness, envy, jealousy, competition, performance, drivenness, lack of nurturing, lack of love, and on and on the list goes.

I have found there is a breakdown on these three levels in all diseases with a spiritual root.

## The Power of the Tongue

The Bible teaches that if you gossip or slander about your neighbor, it is equal to murder. Do you know murder with the tongue is equally as damaging as killing someone with a gun?

Do you remember the saying, "Sticks and stones may break my bones, but words will never harm me"? Whoever wrote this was delusional. They were in denial.

The Bible says words can pierce to the very penetrating of the human spirit.

> **The words of a talebearer *are* as wounds, and they go down into the innermost parts of the belly. Proverbs 18:8**

They are arrows of destruction. They are words of death or words of life. The Bible says life and death are in the power of the tongue.

> **Death and life *are* in the power of the tongue: and they that love it shall eat the fruit thereof. Proverbs 18:21**

I am either blessing you or cursing you with what I say. I am either building you up or tearing you down. Has everyone always built you up? Has everyone always built you up? I thought we were supposed to be gifts one to another. I practice being a gift to you because I practice being a gift to my wife and children. After I practice there, I come out and practice on you.

## Generational Blessings and Curses

### Generational Sins and Genetically Inherited Disease

In Exodus 20, the Bible says the sins of the fathers shall be passed on to the third and fourth generation of them that hate the LORD.

> **Thou shalt not bow down thyself to them, nor serve them: for I the LORD thy God *am* a jealous God, visiting the iniquity of the fathers upon the children unto the third and fourth *generation* of them that hate me; Exodus 20:5**

This Scripture becomes the spiritual basis for all spiritual, biological and genetically inherited diseases. In Nehemiah 9:2, we read about the children of the captivity—those who came out of Babylon in the days of Nehemiah and Ezra. Ezra the priest brought the law and the Word of God before the people and they stood there. They were mommies and daddies and children in Nehemiah 8:1–8, and Ezra the scribe gave cause and reason and understanding of the Word of God.

> **8:1And all the people gathered themselves together as one man into the street that *was* before the water gate; and they spake unto Ezra the scribe to bring the book of the law of Moses, which the LORD had commanded to Israel. 2And Ezra the priest brought the law before the congregation both of men and women, and all that could hear with understanding, upon the first day of the seventh month. 3And he read therein before the street that *was* before the water gate from the morning until midday, before the men and the women, and those that could understand; and the ears of all the people *were attentive* unto the book of the law. Nehemiah 8:1–3**

> [7]...and the people *stood* in their place. [8]So they read in the book in the law of God distinctly, and gave the sense, and caused *them* to understand the reading. Nehemiah 8:7–8

> [2]And the seed of Israel separated themselves from all strangers, and stood and confessed their sins, and the iniquities of their fathers. [3]And they stood up in their place, and read in the book of the law of the LORD their God *one* fourth part of the day; and *another* fourth part they confessed, and worshipped the LORD their God. Nehemiah 9:2–3

They realized why mommy and daddy, grandma and grandpa had been in captivity. They had been disobedient to the Word of God. In Nehemiah 9:2, the children of the captivity stood and confessed their sins and the sins of their fathers.

> And the seed of Israel separated themselves from all strangers, and stood and confessed their sins, and the iniquities of their fathers. Nehemiah 9:2

Why did they confess the sins of their fathers? They confessed them because they were the product of their parents' disobedience.

## Family Tree of Abraham

Now, I want to give you a family tree history. You will be shocked, because I am about to go to the founding father of our faith. The founding father of the Jewish faith is Abraham. You can read this for yourself in Genesis. Father Abraham was called out of Ur of the Chaldees. God appeared to him, and he came with Sarai his half sister and wife, and Lot the son of Haran, into Terah (an area of Turkey). They hung out there for a while, then went south, into the land of promise, but there was a famine in the land, so they couldn't stay. Then they went down into Egypt, the land of Pharaoh (Genesis 12).

Abram's name was later changed to Abraham and Sarai's name changed to Sarah in Genesis 19. Abram said to Sarai his wife, "You are the most beautiful woman in the whole world. I want you to tell the Pharaoh you are my sister and I am going to tell him you are my sister. If I say that you're my wife, he will kill me for you because you're so beautiful." Abram enticed his wife to lie and he also lied to the Pharaoh. The root problem behind people who lie is *fear of man, fear of rejection and fear of failure; primarily it is the fear of man.*

When you have children who lie, it is because they are afraid of judgment. The root behind all liars is *fear of man, fear of rejection and fear of judgment.* Father Abraham had a spiritual problem. First of all, *he had fear and he was a liar.* This is a good place to start. God came and dealt with this issue and Abram had to repent. But Abram did not get the message.

He left the land of Egypt and moved north into the land of the Philistines, where Abimelech was king (Genesis 20). He came into the land of the Philistines and told Sarah again that she was still very beautiful and he was afraid he was going to lose her. He said, "Abimelech is a heathen king, so let's tell him you're my sister." He told the same lie to Abimelech that he had told to the Pharaoh. He got in trouble all over again. He had to repent all over again. Now we have Abraham caught in a double lie. He did not learn the lesson the first time or the second time. We find that Abraham continued to have *fear of man and* he had a *lying spirit*.

That was just the beginning. Later, Abraham had a son named Isaac, who married Rebekah. Rebekah and Isaac, we are told in the book of Genesis, took a little vacation and went down into the land of the Philistines, where Abimelech was still king forty years later (Genesis 26).

Forty years after Abraham had stood there before Abimelech, king of the Philistines, Isaac and Rebekah stood before King Abimelech. Isaac said to Rebekah, "You're beautiful, you're a real fox and I am afraid if I say you're my wife, Abimelech will kill me and want you. Tell him you're my sister." *When you read it in Genesis, Isaac said word for word what his father Abraham had said forty years before* (Genesis 26). Now we have a second generation of fear and lying. It didn't stop there. We are just seeing a good story continuing.

Isaac had two sons, Esau and Jacob. Rebekah came along; she and her husband Isaac had already lied in their encounter with King Abimelech. She got into a discussion with Jacob over the birthright and together they deceived Isaac and lied to him (Genesis 27). Now we have another generation of liars, Abraham, Isaac and Jacob. It doesn't stop there.

Jacob had twelve sons. Ten of the sons were jealous over Joseph, killed an animal, kidnapped Joseph, dipped his coat of many colors in the blood, took it back to daddy and said, "Daddy, an animal just killed Joseph" (Genesis 37). They lied to Jacob. If it had not been for the intercession of Judah to sell Joseph into slavery, Joseph would have been killed.

Now we have four generations of liars. Not only that, Jacob's wife Rachel lied to her father Laban over the issue of idols (Genesis 31:35). Now we have men and women and children lying.

This is where our faith begins—with a bunch of fear-filled, lying saints. Abraham, believe it or not, was called a "friend of God" (Isaiah 41:8; James 2:23). There is hope for you and me, isn't there? Amen!

These biblical histories are the foundation of understanding inherited spiritual dynamics. They become a foundation of understanding and tell us why, in Exodus 20:5, God said the iniquities of the father shall be passed on to the third and fourth generation.

> **Thou shalt not bow down thyself to them, nor serve them: for I the LORD thy God *am* a jealous God, visiting the iniquity of the fathers upon the children unto the third and fourth *generation* of them that hate me; Exodus 20:5**

The fathers are the holders of blessings and curses in the family. What about the females? They have daddies, too, you know.

In Numbers 30, it says that if a man standing by hears his wife bind her soul with a vow and he holds his peace and allows the words of his wife to stand, she's bound her soul to a curse. If a man standing by hears his wife bind her soul to a vow and he disallows the words of his wife, he has released her from the curse.

If a man standing by hears his daughter bind her soul with a vow with her words and holds his peace and does not disallow the words of his daughter, she's bound her soul to the penalty of the curse. If he is standing by and hears his daughter bind her soul with a vow and he disallows it and says, "Daughter that's not cool," and she agrees, he has saved his daughter from the penalty of the curse. *There is no such provision for boys.*

> **[3]If a woman also vow a vow unto the LORD, and bind *herself* by a bond, *being* in her father's house in her youth; [4]And her father hear her vow, and her bond wherewith she hath bound her soul, and her father shall hold his peace at her: then all her vows shall stand, and every bond wherewith she hath bound her soul shall stand. [5]But if her father disallow her in the day that he heareth; not any of her vows, or of her bonds wherewith she hath bound her soul, shall stand: and the LORD shall forgive her, because her father disallowed her. [6]And if she had at all an husband, when she vowed, or uttered ought out of her lips, wherewith she bound her soul; [7]And her husband heard *it,* and held his peace at her in the day that he heard *it:* then her vows shall stand, and her bonds wherewith she bound her soul shall stand. [8]But if her husband disallowed her on the day that he heard *it;* then he shall make her vow which she vowed, and that which she uttered with her lips, wherewith she bound her soul, of none effect: and the LORD shall forgive her. Numbers 30:3–8**

### *The beginning of all healing in this planet is the salvation of all men.*

If you want to get this thing turned around, men, get right with God and tell every man you see to do the same. Get right with God because the curse is upon us because of our failures.

Adam had a similar problem as Abraham. When it came time to choose between God and his woman, he chose his woman and not God. He did not disallow her words concerning the eating of the fruit and the action. I firmly believe Adam could have changed the destiny of mankind and taught us obedience, not disobedience.

The Bible says the head of the woman is the man (spiritual covering), the head of the man is Christ and the head of Christ is God the Father.

**But I would have you know, that the head of every man is Christ; and the head of the woman *is* the man; and the head of Christ *is* God. 1 Corinthians 11:3**

I myself have had to get right with God and I am still working on it. We have generations of bondage and entrapment behind us. The man is supposed to represent God the Father to his entire family and the man is supposed to be to the woman as Christ is to the Church in all matters. It's amazing that we can talk to Jesus but not to our husbands. It's amazing in church to say "Our Father," but we go to our earthly fathers and we're told to sit down, shut up and be quiet. I think we have lost our way.

Each of you should build your own family tree. Were your family members in past generations Christians? Were they righteous or unrighteous? What were their personalities like? Were they filled with fear, hate, envy, strife, bitterness, etc.? What did they do for a living? Were they into alcohol, drugs and pornography? Did their lives contain any of the elements we are learning, which are the roots for disease? Go back as many generations as you can. This will give you an idea of what is in your family.

Every time you step outside of the covenant, you open yourself to the law and the penalty of the law. The good thing about the new birth and the provision of grace and mercy under Christ is that you are not dead by sundown. You have this time to maintain your forgiveness and your relationship with God in the area of sanctification.

All of the people in your family tree bring into the picture good and evil, blessings and curses. The reason I know this is because many Christians have diseases that are genetically inherited. Where did you get that genetically inherited disease? You received it from whom? Your parents. If it's not dealt with before the Lord, you will pass it on to your seed. *Would you like to prevent disease in your children?* Wouldn't that be *a more excellent way™?*

### *One thing I represent is disease prevention, not just the healing of disease.*

Do you think it is possible the inherited genetic disease can be prevented if the parents line up with God before conception? I do! Do you think  the unborn generation can be sanctified by believing parents who come before

God honestly and humbly and know exactly what they are up against and why? Do we just shut our eyes, have children and hope to God they turn out all right?

I'll tell you what the Word says: Foolishness is bound up in the heart of a child.

> **Foolishness *is* bound in the heart of a child; *but* the rod of correction shall drive it far from him. Proverbs 22:15**

What does this mean? It means a child is born with evil. I know mommies and daddies do not like to think about this, but by age three you know it is there. Foolishness and rebellion do not just go away. In fact, it gets worse at age 15.

King David said his mother conceived him in sin.

> **Behold, I was shapen in iniquity; and in sin did my mother conceive me. Psalm 51:5**

Did you ever meditate on that? King David was a man after God's own heart. He had a man murdered, stole his wife, lusted and tempted Israel, but he was called a man after God's own heart. You figure this one out. David's family was a tragedy; one son raped a daughter and one son rose up in sedition, in anarchy against him. One son died at childbirth because of the sins of the father David.

The *male lineage* traces ancestry through your father, his father and his father's father. What do they have in common with you that could be considered sin? How many of you had parents who did not know God? You are a miracle if your parents did not teach you about God. Do you know anything about your family tree that is not right? Did you ever hear rumors?

The *female lineage* traces ancestry back through her father and what he brought into it and then all the males before him. Your mother had a father and this line channels right down through the male. Wherever you find a male, you find the curse channeling down through the female.

This is why you can inherit things from your mother even though they were in the family tree of her father. Why is this? At any point, if there had been a man of God in that home, he would have taken every step to sanctify his wife and children. God holds the men responsible for all matters of the family, home and everything.

Do you have your family tree written on paper? We want you to be able to look at the inherited parts of your family tree. Start thinking about the desolation in the generations in your family. Mark down the characteristics: bootlegger, pirate, warlock, wife beater, molester, adulterer, fornicator, or murderer—it is all there. Slanderer, division maker; do you think this is what God created? Do you think God created this mess we have to unravel? NO!

There may be some things you are dealing with in your life that you inherited. You say, "That's not fair." Well, it's not fair, but that's the price we pay for separation from God and opening ourselves to the devil and allowing him to be our father and our leader and our truth.

> **Ye are of your father the devil, and the lusts of *your* father ye will do. He was a murderer from the beginning, and abode not in the truth, because there is no truth in him. When he speaketh a lie, he speaketh of his own: for he is a liar, and the father of it. John 8:44**

This is the price we pay.

Proverbs 26:2 says that as a bird by wandering and the swallow by flying, so the curse causeless does not come.

> **As the bird by wandering, as the swallow by flying, so the curse causeless shall not come. Proverbs 26:2**

In spiritually rooted diseases there is always a spiritual defect.

### *The spiritual defect is an area lacking sanctification.*

## Generational Sins and Children

Fear can be inherited. Allergies can be inherited. Many of the things we deal with can either develop in our lifetime or we can inherit them from our family tree. Now, when I see this happening in a child, I can go back to the father and mother, grandfather and grandmother—both sides—and I'll find some abuse. I'll find victimization and rejection; I'll find someone not being nurtured somewhere. That can be inherited not only from a genetic standpoint, but it can also be inherited from a spiritual standpoint. The Bible says in Ezekiel 18:19 that the children do not have to die for the sins of the father. Exodus 20:5 says that the curse which is the result of the iniquity shall be passed on to the third and fourth generation.

We have a ministry to children and we do minister to children. We come before the Lord and ask God to heal the child. But we have discovered something else very powerful. If we see the child having a disease or problem that is the direct result of the parents, then we can get the parent to come before God and have the sin resolved. We have seen children instantly healed of diseases and prayers have never even occurred on their behalf. When the curse is broken at this level, it is an amazing thing to see God's provision for children who are not yet at the age of understanding. It is amazing. The Bible says the children are sanctified by the believing parents.

> For the unbelieving husband is sanctified by the wife, and the unbelieving wife is sanctified by the husband: else were your children unclean; but now are they holy. 1 Corinthians 7:14

Yes, they can be healed. (See the story of the Syrophenician woman and her intercession for her daughter with Jesus in Mark 7.)

## Healing Spiritually Rooted Diseases

All healing of spiritually rooted diseases begins with:

1. Your coming back in alignment with God, His Word, His person, His nature, His precepts and what He planned on this planet for you from the beginning. The solution is restoration.

2. Accepting YOURSELF in your relationship with God; getting rid of your self-hatred, getting rid of your self-bitterness, getting rid of your guilt and coming back in line with who you are in the Father through Jesus Christ.

3. Making peace with your brother, your sister and all others, if at all possible.

### *So, the beginning of all healing is restoration.*

The Bible says this about relationships in Matthew 22:37–40: You shall love the Lord thy God with all of thy heart, with all of thy soul and all of thy mind, and you shall love your neighbour as yourself.

> [37]Jesus said unto him, Thou shalt love the Lord thy God with all thy heart, and with all thy soul, and with all thy mind. [38]This is the first and great commandment. [39]And the second *is* like unto it, Thou shalt love thy neighbour as thyself. [40]On these two commandments hang all the law and the prophets. Matthew 22:37–40

You cannot love your neighbor if you do not love yourself. It is not possible. If you say you do, you are kidding yourself. It's not possible. You bring the strength of God into your life and then you bring the strength of God into others' lives, in this order.

Any breakdown in this sequence over a long term produces many, many diseases. Why? Because God commanded that you shall love your neighbor as yourself.

When I started to get involved with disease, I found disease to be a result of separation from God, first and foremost. It was right there in Deuteronomy 28. I said to God, "Okay, you're telling me something. We have curses and blessings, so what does that mean to me? Blessings and curses...so we either blew it or we didn't blow it." God led me to Proverbs 26:2 in my thoughts, where He said, the curse without a cause does not come.

**As the bird by wandering, as the swallow by flying, so the curse causeless shall not come. Proverbs 26:2**

I went, "Hmm, what are you telling me, God?" In my understanding and in my mind, I felt God was saying this: *"If you see any disease, Mr. Henry Wright, you see a curse and if you see a curse, there is a reason for it. Did you get the point, son?"*

Cause and effect, *"if, then, and but."* "Are you telling me, God, if I see a disease, it's like a bird that has landed and a swallow that has landed, but it had a right to?" He said, "That's what I said over in 2 Timothy 2:24–26."

**24And the servant of the Lord must not strive; but be gentle unto all *men,* apt to teach, patient, 25In meekness instructing those that oppose themselves; if God peradventure will give them repentance to the acknowledging of the truth; 26And *that* they may recover themselves out of the snare of the devil, who are taken captive by him at his [the devil's] will. 2 Timothy 2:24–26**

In order to get the disease removed, I must remove the cause. This is being sanctified. God said, That is what I have called my people to—a people who are sanctified without spot or blemish.

**26That he might sanctify and cleanse it with the washing of water by the word, 27That he might present it to himself a glorious church, not having spot, or wrinkle, or any such thing; but that it should be holy and without blemish. Ephesians 5:26–27**

**7Let us be glad and rejoice, and give honour to him: for the marriage of the Lamb is come, and his wife hath made herself ready. 8And to her was granted that she should be arrayed in fine linen, clean and white: for the fine linen is the righteousness of saints. 9And he saith unto me, Write, Blessed *are* they which are called unto the marriage supper of the Lamb. And he saith unto me, These are the true sayings of God. 10And I fell at his feet to worship him. And he said unto me, See *thou do it* not: I am thy fellowservant, and of thy brethren that have the testimony of Jesus: worship God: for the testimony of Jesus is the spirit of prophecy. 11And I saw heaven opened, and behold a white horse; and he that sat upon him *was* called Faithful and True, and in righteousness he doth judge and make war. 12His eyes *were* as a flame of fire, and on his head *were* many crowns; and he had a name written, that no man knew, but he himself. 13And he *was* clothed with a vesture dipped in blood: and his name is called The Word of God. 14And the armies *which were* in heaven followed him upon white horses, clothed in fine linen, white and clean. 15And out of his mouth goeth a sharp sword, that with it he should smite the nations: and he shall rule them with a rod of iron: and he treadeth the winepress of the fierceness and wrath of Almighty God. 16And he hath on *his* vesture and on his thigh a name written, KING OF KINGS, AND LORD OF LORDS. 17And I saw an angel standing in the sun; and he cried with a**

loud voice, saying to all the fowls that fly in the midst of heaven, Come and gather yourselves together unto the supper of the great God; [18]That ye may eat the flesh of kings, and the flesh of captains, and the flesh of mighty men, and the flesh of horses, and of them that sit on them, and the flesh of all *men, both* free and bond, both small and great. [19]And I saw the beast, and the kings of the earth, and their armies, gathered together to make war against him that sat on the horse, and against his army. **Revelation 19:7–19**

I have called them to holiness.

**For God hath not called us unto uncleanness, but unto holiness. 1 Thessalonians 4:7**

I have called them to walk before Me because I am their God.

**And as for thee, if thou wilt walk before me, as David thy father walked, and do according to all that I have commanded thee, and shalt observe my statutes and my judgments; 2 Chronicles 7:17**

And I have called them to be cleansed.

**Having therefore these promises, dearly beloved, let us cleanse ourselves from all filthiness of the flesh and spirit, perfecting holiness in the fear of God. 2 Corinthians 7:1**

*The curse without a cause does not come* (Proverbs 26:2).

When I find any evidence of disease today, what am I looking for? *The cause.* I go to the Word to find it and I go to the medical community to find out what they know. I am teaching in America: "Ministers, you need more than *Vines, Ungers, Strong's* and a Bible. Instead of getting 14 translations, why don't you buy a *Merck Manual*, a pathophysiology manual and an anatomy and physiology book and do a little laymen's study on disease?"

Fibromyalgia for example: is anyone interested in this?

Let me read you something: *Fibromyalgia* is what the medical community calls pain in fibrous tissues, muscles, tendons, ligaments and other connective tissue. Do you know why it is there? I'll tell you why. You ladies have not been nurtured. You are paying a high price for your insecurities and your fears. Let me read this thing here, "The condition occurs mainly in females…primary fibromyalgia syndrome (PFS) is particularly and likely to occur in healthy young women who tend to be stressed, tense, depressed, anxious, and striving…" and driven (*Merck Manual*, 16th edition, pp. 1369–1370).

How long did it take me to get into position against this disease? As long as it took for me to read what I just read! Immediately, I came to realize the cause. Okay, *fibromyalgia: the result of fear, anxiety and stress;* unresolved conflict and stresses and you know this is true. When the anxieties and the insecurities issues are dealt with, many times the fibromyalgia goes away. Similarly, when I deal with bitterness, many times the arthritis goes away. When I deal with self-hatred and guilt, many times lupus and other autoimmune diseases go away. When I deal with a broken heart and those wounds, many times allergies will go away.

*I want to conclude this teaching with a mandate.* The mandate comes out of Ezekiel chapter 34 with a statement from the Father concerning the shepherds of Israel:

> ¹**And the word of the LORD came unto me, saying, ²Son of man, prophesy against the shepherds of Israel, prophesy, and say unto them, Thus saith the Lord GOD unto the shepherds... Ezekiel 34:1–2**

Who are these shepherds? Pastors. What am I? I am a shepherd boy. I take care of sheep; I put salve on their wounds. I go over the cliff all over America and I pull them up to save their lives.

All over America, I find them abandoned by the Church, abandoned by their leaders, abandoned by their families. I used to be able to fly across America to help keep one person from dying more than one time. In fact, we said the other day we were going to change the name of our ministry to "Over the Cliff Ministries." I am "over the cliff" with someone who is dying and separated. That's why I started the For My Life™ program.

Do you remember what the Lord said about the 99 sheep safe in the fold versus the one who went over the cliff?

> ¹¹**For the Son of man is come to save that which was lost. ¹²How think ye? if a man have an hundred sheep, and one of them be gone astray, doth he not leave the ninety and nine, and goeth into the mountains, and seeketh that which is gone astray? ¹³And if so be that he find it, verily I say unto you, he rejoiceth more of that *sheep,* than of the ninety and nine which went not astray. ¹⁴Even so it is not the will of your Father which is in heaven, that one of these little ones should perish. Matthew 18:11–14**

He placed a great premium on the isolated, dying ones and my mission is to gather them into the fold. My mission is to keep them from going over the cliff to begin with and this should be your mission to mankind.

### *This is a more excellent way™:*
### *healing and prevention of disease.*

Ezekiel 34 says (italics added),

> ²**Son of man, prophesy against the shepherds of Israel, prophesy, and say unto them, Thus saith the Lord GOD unto the shepherds; *Woe be to the shepherds* of Israel that do feed themselves! Should not the shepherds feed the flocks? ³You eat the fat, you clothe yourself with wool but you kill them who are fed. *You do not feed the flock.* ⁴The diseased have you not**

*strengthened, neither have you healed that which was sick, neither have you bound up that which was broken, neither have you brought again that which was driven away, neither have you sought that which was lost;* but with force and with cruelty have you ruled them.

[5]And they were scattered, because there is no shepherd: and they became meat to all the beasts of the field, when they were scattered. [6]My sheep wandered through all the mountains, and upon every high hill: yea, my flock was scattered upon all the face of the earth, and none did search or seek after them. [7]Therefore, ye shepherds, hear the word of the LORD; [8]As I live, saith the Lord GOD, surely because my flock became a prey, and my flock became meat to every beast of the field, because there was no shepherd, neither did my shepherds search for my flock, but the shepherds fed themselves, and fed not my flock;

[9]Therefore, O ye shepherds, hear the word of the LORD; [10]Thus saith the Lord GOD; Behold, I am against the shepherds; and I will require My flock at their hand, and cause them to cease from feeding the flock; neither shall the shepherds feed themselves any more; for I will deliver my flock from their mouth, that they may not be meat for them.

[11]For thus saith the Lord GOD; Behold, I, even I, will both search my sheep and I will seek them out. [12]As a shepherd seeking out his flock in the day that he is among his sheep that are scattered; so will I seek out My sheep, and I will deliver them out of all the places where they have been scattered in the cloudy and dark day. [15]I will feed My flock, I will cause them to lie down saith the Lord GOD. *[16]I will seek that which was lost, and bring again that which was driven away, and I will bind up that which was broken and I will strengthen that which was sick: but I will destroy the fat and the strong; I will feed them with judgment.* Ezekiel 34:2–12, 15–16

Isaiah reflects the compassion of the LORD for the brokenhearted:

The Spirit of the Lord GOD *is* upon me; because the LORD hath anointed me to preach good tidings unto the meek; he hath sent me to bind up the brokenhearted, to proclaim liberty to the captives, and the opening of the prison to *them that are* bound; Isaiah 61:1

The healing of MCS/EI is the healing of a broken heart.

A merry heart doeth good *like* a medicine: but a broken spirit drieth the bones. Proverbs 17:22

We spend more time healing broken hearts in America than you can imagine.

Of the people looking for help, 85 to 90 percent have been female. God has used me to heal many females from their abandonment by fathers and husbands and to get them back in line with their heavenly Father and the Lord who sought them and bought them. More and more men are coming forward with the same problem.

You can thank God for my intensity because I am a warrior. I am out to destroy the works of the devil and to reclaim God's precious flock from the hands of Satan and reestablish you into praising His glory here and now, not when you get to heaven. Then, when you get to heaven, you can give Him thanks for it. Amen!

Isaiah continues to talk about God's healing and restoration that has been provided.

> ¹**The Spirit of the Lord GOD** *is* **upon me; because the LORD hath anointed me to preach good tidings unto the meek; he hath sent me to bind up the brokenhearted, to proclaim liberty to the captives, and the opening of the prison to** *them that are* **bound; ²To proclaim the acceptable year of the LORD, and the day of vengeance of our God; to comfort all that mourn; ³To appoint unto them that mourn in Zion, to give unto them beauty for ashes, the oil of joy for mourning, the garment of praise for the spirit of heaviness; that they might be called trees of righteousness, the planting of the LORD, that he might be glorified. Isaiah 61:1–3**

Isaiah 61:4 is generational in nature and provides for the healing of generations. This is the breaking of inherited genetic curses. This is breaking inherited familiar spirits from your family trees, the rollovers, with specifics, meaning spiritually, psychologically and biologically inherited diseases.

> **And they shall build the old wastes, they shall raise up the former desolations, and they shall repair the waste cities, the desolations of many generations. Isaiah 61:4**

I am going to tell you there is a revival coming to this planet. There is a revival coming to this nation, but it will not be the type of revival you may think it is.

The revival coming is one of *sanctification and purification*. I'll tell you with all the authority in my heart. I know, the only way it will be ushered in is the same way it was ushered in the first time: by the Lord when He came. This is the healing of diseases, the casting out of evil spirits and the establishment of His grace and His mercy—you can read about it from Romans to Jude.

A lot of people struggle with this: why don't we see healing of diseases and the great teaching of healing of diseases and casting out of evil spirits after the book of Acts? The reason for it is this: Matthew, Mark, Luke and John record how the Lord showed us God's love in spite of sin. John demonstrated God's power through Christ over evil in spite of sin—all to demonstrate God's love for us.

The Word in Acts demonstrated the early Church's power over the same thing.

After the demonstration was done, sanctification was taught as we read in Romans to Jude. Without sanctification, you cannot have Matthew, Mark, Luke, John and the book of Acts happening at all. It is not going to happen.

When you have Romans to Jude in your life, the blessings will come; the showers of blessing will come. Then the knowledge of God will flow *because God is not going to bless disobedient children over the long-term.*

*I have had to learn this the hard way. Would it be a fair exchange— obedience for disease? Would it be a fair exchange—sanctification for disease? Would it be a fair exchange—obedience for insanity? Would it be a fair exchange—trust in God for fear and anxiety? Would it be a fair exchange to believe and receive God's love versus an unloving, unclean spirit of self- hatred? Would it be a fair exchange to forgive your brother in exchange for the healing of cancer? Would it be a fair exchange to deal with fear and anger in exchange for a heart attack?*

**This is *a more excellent way*™!**

You know what the Word says, don't you, about fear and heart attacks?

> **Men's hearts failing them for fear, and for looking after those things which are coming on the earth: for the powers of heaven shall be shaken. Luke 21:26**

This is what it says.

I can go to a pathophysiology text and find one of the basic causes for most heart attacks is *fear and anxiety.* How about *aneurysms, strokes, hemorrhoids, varicose veins?* Do you know what the cause is for these? *Anger and rage.*

Do you want to prevent *aneurysms* and *strokes* in your life? Get anger and rage out of your life as fast as you can. Rage, anger and hostility, with the deep root of bitterness needs to be dealt with, because you are going to explode at some point. *As you are exploding spiritually, your body will respond in your lifetime.*

Some people teach there were certain spiritual attacks in Scripture God did not remove, such as the attack on Job and Paul's thorn in the flesh. Proverbs teaches us there is a reason (Proverbs 26:2). Let's take a look.

Job had spiritual problems. Job's first spiritual problem—he told us about his fear:

> **For the thing which I greatly feared is come upon me, and that which I was afraid of is come unto me. Job 3:25**

The second thing Job feared was evidenced when he became preoccupied with the spiritual safety of his children.

> **⁴And his sons went and feasted *in their* houses, every one his day; and sent and called for their three sisters to eat and to drink with them. ⁵And it was so, when the days of *their* feasting were gone about, that Job sent and sanctified them, and rose up early in the morning, and offered burnt**

**offerings** *according* **to the number of them all: for Job said, It may be that my sons have sinned, and cursed God in their hearts. Thus did Job continually. Job 1:4–5**

This was an open door for fear. Then, in Job 40 and 41, when we look at the characteristics of Behemoth and Leviathan, we find Job had pride and spiritual arrogance (Behemoth).

**He** *is* **the chief of the ways of God: he that made him can make his sword to approach** *unto him.* **Job 40:19**

**He beholdeth all high** *things:* **he** *is* **a king over all the children of pride. Job 41:34**

In his great discourse with God about his own righteousness, as he saw it, God cut him back down to size (Job 40:1–14). When Job prayed for his friends, God removed the power of Satan and restored to him twice what he possessed previously (Job 42:7–17).

In the case of Paul's thorn in the flesh, we are not exactly sure it was a disease. The word "flesh" is a Greek word, but the word "flesh" as found in Romans 7 also has to do with our spiritual nature. It could also mean the human body. Greek is a very limited language as compared to Hebrew. In fact, in Greek, you will find one word having more than one meaning.

In the Old Testament, there are almost 9,000 different Hebrew words used. The Greek Scriptures used a little over 5,500 words in the writing of the New Testament. The reason for this is the Jews, in the Hebrew, have a word for just about every meaning. This is not the case with the Greeks. Even in the English language we sometimes have a word with more than one meaning.

The teachings of Paul on the *flesh* have to do with the carnal nature; this is the part unrenewed within us called "the flesh." However, the word *flesh* can also mean your human body. Paul's thorn in the flesh may not necessarily have been a biological disease.

In Romans 7:15, Paul is talking about a spiritual battle he is having or has had. The good that I want to do, I do not do it and the evil that I do not like doing, that's what I do. So in the day that I want to do good, I do not do it; and the evil that I wish I would not do, I do it. The day that I do the evil, it is no longer I that am doing the evil, but sin that dwelleth in me (is doing it).

**¹⁵For that which I do I allow not: for what I would, that do I not; but what I hate, that do I. ¹⁶If then I do that which I would not, I consent unto the law that** *it is* **good. ¹⁷Now then it is no more I that do it, but sin that dwelleth in me. ¹⁸For I know that in me (that is, in my flesh,) dwelleth no good thing: for to will is present with me; but** *how* **to perform that which is good I find not. ¹⁹For the good that I would I do not: but the evil which I would not, that I do. ²⁰Now if I do that I would not, it is no more I that do**

it, but sin that dwelleth in me. ²¹I find then a law, that, when I would do good, evil is present with me. ²²For I delight in the law of God after the inward man: ²³But I see another law in my members, warring against the law of my mind, and bringing me into captivity to the law of sin which is in my members. Romans 7:15–23

This is an apostle, with 20 plus years as an apostle, saying that he had the indwelling presence of sin. In fact, he went on in the chapter and said that there was a war, a kingdom at work within him that wars against the law of God, bringing him into captivity to the law of sin (as a believer).

It would seem to be, if we looked at Paul's discourse in Romans 7, his thorn in the flesh may not have been a biological disease; it may have been an area of his carnal nature he just never got under control.

He did say it was a "Messenger of Satan" and it was not removed. The Word tells us why it wasn't removed: because there was a chance Paul might be over exalted in pride because Paul was a Pharisee. He was a "Pharisee of Pharisees," and the chance of Paul having spiritual pride would have been very good. I do not have a specific answer. We do know that it was a messenger from Satan.

> And lest I should be exalted above measure through the abundance of the revelations, there was given to me a thorn in the flesh, the messenger of Satan to buffet me, lest I should be exalted above measure. 2 Corinthians 12:7

We do know that Paul prayed for God to remove it and God's answer was that it wouldn't be removed. But I only offer this as a possibility; I do, however, consider Paul's discourse in Romans 7 showing us how he had spiritual battles and the indwelling presence of sin.

Peter's problem was a little different. Jesus said to Peter, Satan desires to sift you like wheat and when you have recovered yourself, strengthen the brethren.

> ³¹And the Lord said, Simon, Simon, behold, Satan hath desired *to have* you, that he may sift *you* as wheat: ³²But I have prayed for thee, that thy faith fail not: and when thou art converted, strengthen thy brethren. Luke 22:31–32

Jesus did nothing to prevent the sifting of Peter by Satan. Why? Because Peter had spiritual problems.

## The Chastening of the Lord

I have a particular opinion about the chastening of the Lord. I read in the Bible that when we follow our enemies, God gives us over to the blessings of our enemies, which are curses (Deuteronomy 28:15). When we have had enough, or when the Old Testament saints had finally had enough of the blessings of their enemies (which, in fact, were oppression and bondage), they would cry out to God. They would repent; He would end their captivity and He would bless them. He would release them when they repented and turned back to Him.

*Keep this in mind: the Lord is not putting evil on us, but giving us over to the devices of our own heart until we have had enough.* When we recognize the spiritual defects of our life through conviction by the Holy Spirit and through the washing of the Word, the spiritual defect is then purified. Some call it the "Baptism of Fire"—the purging work, the sanctifying work of the Holy Spirit.

God did not give the spiritual defect. How could He put sin into our lives? This would be contrary to His holy nature.

> **Let no man say when he is tempted, I am tempted of God: for God cannot be tempted with evil, neither tempteth he any man: James 1:13**

He wants to purge us from it.

> **He that committeth sin is of the devil; for the devil sinneth from the beginning. For this purpose the Son of God was manifested, that he might destroy the works of the devil. 1 John 3:8**

Acts says:

> **38How God anointed Jesus of Nazareth with the Holy Ghost and with power: who went about doing good, and healing all that were oppressed of the devil; for God was with him. Acts 10:38**

So it is very clear God wants to destroy the works of the devil and to heal all who are oppressed by the devil.

## Chapter Three
# Bitterness

Bitterness is a principality of the enemy. Ephesians 6:12 says that our battle is not against flesh and blood but against principalities, powers, spiritual wickedness in high places and the rulers of the darkness of this world.

> **For we wrestle not against flesh and blood, but against principalities, against powers, against the rulers of the darkness of this world, against spiritual wickedness in high *places*. Ephesians 6:12**

If we are in conflict with one another, I am not your enemy. You are not my enemy. Do you know the problem we have? *We are not able to separate the person from their sin. Their sin is our enemy—**NOT THEM!***

When someone violates us, we make him or her evil along with the evil they did, don't we? *You have to be able to separate people from their sin.* God didn't create you from the foundation of the world as a sinner. He created you from the foundation of the world as saints before Him and as His sons and daughters forever. Because of sin, we have become separated from Him. Even after conversion, we still have many things to work out. I want to help you begin to do this today.

**Bitterness is a principality; under it and answering to it are seven spirits that reinforce bitterness.**

## 1. Unforgiveness

When the root of bitterness in Hebrews gets a foothold, the first thing that happens is a record of wrongs.

> **Looking diligently lest any man fail of the grace of God; lest any root of bitterness springing up trouble *you,* and thereby many be defiled; Hebrews 12:15**

How many of you are still having flashbacks about things having been done against you? If I mention Aunt Sally's name, you would probably be able to give me 15 reasons why you do not like her. This is unforgiveness. After unforgiveness gets a foothold and creates a record of wrongs, there's another dimension of the spiritual dynamics. What I am talking about is called resentment.

## 2. Resentment

Resentment is the record of wrongs being fueled by feelings of holding onto it and starting to meditate or chew on it. It is amazing to me that when we have feelings of resentment, we think about Aunt Sally up here (in our mind), but we feel her down here (in our heart). Why is it that you think about Aunt Sally up here but you feel her down here? It is because your mind is where your soul is and your spirit is where your heart is. You are a spirit being; you have a soul and you live in your body.

Resentment is a spiritual problem, not a psychological problem. Bitterness, unforgiveness and resentment are spiritual problems, not psychological problems. You can take these keys and use them in any spiritual conflict you have in your life. This gets us right here in our heart. This is what separates us from others and it is the foundation of fear which may come later: fear of man, fear of rejection, fear of failure, and fear of abandonment. We go hide!

## 3. Retaliation

After resentment gets a foothold, then we have retaliation. I saw a bumper sticker the other day saying, "I DO NOT FORGIVE, I JUST GET EVEN." Maybe you saw it too. After resentment has started to simmer, we find ways to get back at the person who caused it. Retaliation wants to make the person pay. It's time to get even!

## 4. Anger

After retaliation gets a foothold, then anger starts to set in. Unforgiveness, resentment and retaliation have been building and now a real strong feeling of anger comes along.

Has anyone ever experienced anger toward someone in your lifetime? Did all this other stuff come with it too?

## 5. Hatred

After anger sets in, there comes hatred. Hatred says this: "Because I'm remembering what you did to me, because I have really been meditating on it and I really resent it, I'm going to get even. I'm going to get the pressure cooker going because I'm going to add fuel to this thing and now at this stage you do not have any reason to exist anymore, especially in my presence." Hatred says, "There's not even room on this planet for you and me at the same place at the same time." Hatred says, "You and I cannot stay in the same room together."

Hatred starts to develop into the elimination modality.

## 6. Violence

After hatred comes violence. Violence says this: "Before I eliminate you, you are going to feel my pain. You are going to hear my voice. You are going to know my hatred. You are going to experience it."

## 7. Murder

Once violence erupts, the final fruit of bitterness is murder.

This can be actual physical murder, or murder with the tongue, which is character assassination or verbal abuse. Whenever I find any of these in a person's life, all the stuff from here (the mind) to here (the heart) is there. I know if we do not deal with it, it's going to go to the heart and take up residence. So what am I giving you right now? Discernment.

When hatred, violence and murder are in someone's life, they feel they are justified and everybody else is going to pay the price. Have you been a victim of this? Did you feel defiled? Have you perhaps made a victim of someone else on this basis?

I have found that if any one of these seven areas answering to bitterness exists, all of the preceding ones will be there from the one area. I noticed; if left unchecked, all the rest will surely come. For example, if you see hatred in a person, unforgiveness, resentment, retaliation and anger always precede. Also, each of the seven is progressively worse than the one just preceding it. For example, violence is a much more serious problem than resentment.

## Forgiveness: What God Expects of Us—70 x 7

What does God expect of us when we're forgiving someone else?

Peter and Jesus had an interesting conversation. Jesus was teaching and Peter asked the Lord, How often should I forgive my brother? Up to seven times? Jesus said, No, I do not say until seven times; I say to you seventy times seven.

> **Jesus saith unto him, I say not unto thee, Until seven times: but, Until seventy times seven. Matthew 18:22**

One day in my prayer time, I asked the Lord, "What did you mean by that?" This came into my heart and into my understanding: our days are 24 hours long—8 hours for work, 8 hours for family and 8 hours for sleep. 8-8-8. If you take 8 hours of the day, whether it's for business, family or yourself, this is the whole dimension of human existence, others, yourself and so on. If you take 8 hours, how many minutes are there to an hour? Sixty. Sixty times 8 is 480. What is 70 x 7? 490.

I feel the Lord saying it this way: "Every minute of your day when your brother blows it regarding the same issue—minute by minute, hour by hour, day by day—release him." But you say, "Lord, what if he does the same thing again?" Do you know how many people come to me and say, "I went to them, they repented and then they did it all over again"?

"How often, Lord, should my brother sin against me and repent to me and I should still be expected to forgive him?" Minute by minute, hour by hour, day by day, release him. In releasing him, you have released yourself. Besides, when you go to other Scriptures, you quickly see that the Lord is his judge, not you.

> **Judge not, that ye be not judged. Matthew 7:1**

> **But why dost thou judge thy brother? or why dost thou set at nought thy brother? for we shall all stand before the judgment seat of Christ. Romans 14:10**

You forgive others because He has forgiven you. He has told you to forgive and you are His obedient child. When you have forgiven your brother his trespass, then God releases you because you have released your brother from his trespass.

You are now released from the spirit of bitterness and the antagonistic high-octane ping on the inside goes away. When you think about your Aunt Sally and her trespasses tomorrow or the next day, when the work of the Holy Spirit has been completed in your life, you do not feel her down here in your gut anymore. You do not have that high-octane ping. You will always remember the evil that was done to you but you do not have to carry it as a sin in your own life.

You do not have to carry someone else's sin inside of you. This is their sin. God will be their judge. Your job is to release them, get back before God, get your heart right with God, then keep on moving. *Your freedom does not depend on their resolution—it depends on your resolution.*

When you forgive others, you are not letting them off the hook but giving them to God, still wiggling *on* the hook. *You* are now off the hook.

When you forgive someone, you continue to hate their sin, but you are commanded to love them. **To forgive, you do not have to condone their sin.**

Is that liberating? It was for me! God said to me, "Henry, my son, when I forgave you, I did not condone your sin. I bore it. I took it." I said, "Thank You, Lord."

You see, you are not the judge. If you make yourself the judge, then you tell God to go sit down and shut up. I do not think this is what we want to do. God might want to save someone down the road and you do not want to be in the way.

There are only two future judgments found in Scripture: the judgment seat of Christ and the white throne judgment of the Father.

> **But why dost thou judge thy brother? or why dost thou set at nought thy brother? for we shall all stand before the judgment seat of Christ. Romans 14:10**

> **And I saw a great white throne, and him that sat on it, from whose face the earth and the heaven fled away; and there was found no place for them. Revelation 20:11**

Scripture says one day we shall judge angels.

> **Know ye not that we shall judge angels? how much more things that pertain to this life? 1 Corinthians 6:3**

The only other judgment I have found in Scripture is to judge yourself so you do not have to be judged by God.

> **For if we would judge ourselves, we should not be judged. 1 Corinthians 11:31**

This leaves out judging others. We are going to judge ourselves and we are going to judge angels. The Lord is going to judge the saints. The Father is going to judge the unrighteous and that's it! There is no provision for you to judge anyone. Paul said it—no man has judged me, but God the Father has judged me.

> **For I know nothing by myself; yet am I not hereby justified: but he that judgeth me is the Lord. 1 Corinthians 4:4**

When we get right down to it, why are we judging someone to begin with? Because we want retaliation! Earlier we taught you the seven factors of bitterness. The third was retaliation, the "I'm going to get even" mentality.

Whether a person responds to you in forgiveness or not, it's their problem and their sin. Walk away, keep your heart right, pray and ask God to bring reconciliation. Do what you can to bring it about and if you cannot have your peace, keep on moving.

## Chapter Four
# Insights into Healing and Prevention of Disease

## Pathways of Thought

### Your Construction

In order to help give you the tools you need, we need to talk about your construction. It will help you to understand how an invisible kingdom can tempt you, speak to you and try to control you by forming its personality as part of your personality. If it can become part of your personality, it will seem normal and you will not resist it. That kingdom makes what is abnormal to seem like normal.

You are a triune being. You are a spirit. You have a soul. Your body is your mobile home. But your body is not the real you. As a believer, your body is the temple of the Holy Ghost. Your body is how you get around in a physical world, but you are a spirit. You cannot see your spirit with your physical eyes, but it's in you. If your spirit leaves your body, you are dead.

Those who have had "out of body" experiences or astral-projection say they left their body. They didn't. There was an evil spirit within them that had access to their human spirit. The evil spirit was able to project pictures into the soul so the person *thought* they had left, when in fact, they went nowhere. The evil spirit projects through theta brainwave activity, giving pictures and images to reinforce the experience. In the spirit world, there is no dimension of time as we know it.

When Jesus died, His spirit left His body. It was when Jesus "gave up the ghost" that His spirit left His body. When His spirit left, His body hung on the cross with no life in it. They took His body off the cross, wrapped it in grave clothes, put a napkin over His face and took Him to the tomb. His body lay three days and three nights in the tomb. But "He" wasn't in His body. His spirit had left.

> [18]**For Christ also hath once suffered for sins, the just for the unjust, that he might bring us to God, being put to death in the flesh, but quickened by the Spirit:** [19]**By which also he went and preached unto the spirits in prison; 1 Peter 3:18–19**

This Scripture tells us Jesus went into hell and preached to the spirits who were disobedient in the days of Noah—to everyone who had died in the flood. When His spirit entered back into His body, God raised Him from the dead. He was seen by up to 500 people at one time. For 40 days He walked up and down the streets of Israel and, by many infallible proofs, proved that He was the risen Christ.

I mentioned an evil spirit can have access to the human spirit. How? They access our thoughts through our brainwaves. There are four types of brainwaves: alpha, beta, theta and delta. We won't talk about delta, because we are not discussing the dream state. These brainwaves operate in the realm of your physiological brain. But each of these brainwaves is necessary for our comprehension in thought. These three brainwaves facilitate images, thought and how we process it as a living being. This gives us our deductive reasoning, our personality and the compositeness of our existence.

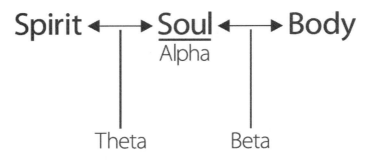

Your soul is the bridge between the spirit world and the physical world. You comprehend what I am saying through two of your five physical senses: sight and hearing. As you are listening to me, your beta brainwaves are being activated. They allow your brain to pick up images of sight and sound through an electrochemical process. You're actually taking snapshots, pictures. It is short-term memory. Your brain records the experience from the physical world. This process programs your soul.

Your soul involves: your *intellect*, your mind; your *emotions*, the recording of your good and bad experiences in life; and your *will*, to make decisions.

In ministry, we can deal with the spirit world and its influence on your mind and your emotions. The invisible kingdom may have taught you something that opposes God's will for your life.

> **For God has not given us the spirit of fear; but of power, and of love, and of a sound mind. 2 Timothy 1:7**

For example, if that kingdom has taught you fear because of experiences you've had in your life, fear will rule your thoughts, your emotions and the decisions you make. That is not God's will for you. Through ministry I can remove the driving influence of the spirit of fear. The spirit is removed but your long-term memory still remembers everything fear taught you. A renewing of the mind must occur.

> **...be ye transformed by the renewing of your mind... Romans 12:2**

How does your mind become renewed? Your mind is renewed or cleansed by the washing of the water of the Word. This means you begin to meditate on the Word of God day and night, studying thoughts and comparing them to how God thinks.

The Word of God teaches you how to think. This thinking now confronts the bad thinking. If you have fear/anxiety/stress disorders, this is the process of getting free. This begins to make us correct spiritual people in how we think, speak and act. It is the journey of sanctification. We call it Walk Out. You can learn how God wants you to think and apply it to your life. I ask God our Father to join you in your journey so you can be reformed into His image.

## The Process of Protein Synthesis

As you think about things over and over again, protein synthesis occurs. It involves RNA and DNA, but specifically RNA. The thought that is recalled over and over again actually becomes permanently part of your biology. God wants to train you so that His law is not just in your spirit, but so that His law is part of your personality as a human being.

The enemy wants to train you too and he uses the same pathway. He wants to give you the law of sin as part of your personality, as opposed to the law of God. There is a battle because both laws are in your members according to Scripture.

Even as Christians, we have the law of sin in our members. For example, do you ever experience strife in your families? Is the distance between your brain and your tongue ever zero? Are the words that come out of your mouth words of life or words of death?

The law of sin is reinforced by a being (sin by its fallen nature) or because your mind has not been renewed. Everything you perceive externally is recorded in your long-term memory, which becomes part of your biology.

Many Christians serve sin. That does not mean they are possessed. It means they are under the influence of the law of sin and they follow it as if it were truth.

## Theta Brainwaves

Theta brainwave is the pathway of impressions, thoughts and pictures allowing your brain, to be connected to your spirit man. Theta brainwaves are about four and a half beats per second. It is the drumbeat used by the Shaman. The Shaman knows if he can get the adherents to yield their minds to him, the drumbeat will activate the pathway between the soul and the spirit allowing evil spirits access to the human soul through thought.

If you didn't have theta brainwaves, you would never have a conscience that would speak to you. You would never hear the voice of the Holy Spirit bearing witness to truth, you would never be convicted of anything and you could never be tempted by the devil and his kingdom. Satan used the serpent because he needed a physiological body and its vocal cords to speak.

Mental telepathy is spiritual activity. It is actually two evil spirits giving information to two humans as if it were between them. It is a very easy exercise by spirits of divination and occultism to work through the human spirit. An evil spirit can speak to your spirit. You perceive its thoughts at the soul level through theta brainwave activity. Your spirit knows everything your soul does and your soul knows everything your spirit does because of theta.

If you were to die today, your body would go back to the dust. Where would your soul go? Your soul goes back to the dust because your soul is made up of brain cells.

So how is your soul saved? Your soul is saved by the consciousness of your identity known in your spirit man. In the first resurrection, the Holy Spirit forms a brand new body around your spirit man. That includes a brand new glorified soul. Because of this, there is an instant consciousness as if you always had a body. This way you can continue to operate in both the spirit world dimension and the physical dimension as Jesus did in His glorified body.

Many of you have been taught *stinkin' thinkin'*. You have experienced the mind-set of others, been influenced by others' thinking or been victims of others.

Many people don't realize that temptation can come in the form of emotion and feeling. Temptation is not just some thought that comes to you like, *Go murder someone, Go commit adultery* or *Go rob a bank*. We think that's temptation. We don't understand that Satan will come to us through his kingdom with aspects of human failure to try to get us to become a personality of human failure.

Here is how *stinkin' thinkin'* works. Adam and Eve were in the garden. They were immune to Satan's kingdom. Eve ate of the fruit and nothing happened. She gave the fruit to her husband and said, "If you eat of this fruit, it will make us wise." Adam ate of the fruit. Something did happen. They were taught the knowledge of sin, the law of sin.

Humans only know what they have been taught. You are not a creature of instinct. From a baby, you only know what you have learned. But how are you taught? You were taught from external sources and from internal sources.

This involves a tremendous amount of discernment to help you hold every thought captive.

There once was a barrier between Adam and Eve and Satan's kingdom. His kingdom could not have access to them unless they gave permission. Adam gave that kingdom permission when he disobeyed God's command. When Adam ate of the fruit, their eyes were opened—their spiritual eyes. Spiritual understanding came to them and they knew good and evil. They saw they were naked. They were ashamed of their nakedness. When the LORD came to walk with them in the cool of the evening they hid. They had shame. They had guilt. They had fear.

The LORD came and couldn't find them. He said, "Adam, where are you?" "I heard your voice and I was afraid because I was naked," Adam said. The LORD said, *"Who* told you that you were naked?"

Notice that the LORD didn't say, "Adam, you have developed a psychosis." "Adam, you are chemically imbalanced." "Adam, where did you get that negative emotion?" The LORD never indicated that the source of Adam and Eve's thoughts were their own psyches. The LORD said, *"Who* told you that you were naked?"

You have been trained the same way. *Who* told you?

You have been trained in your families for almost 6,000 years to think just the opposite of God. You have been taught to relate to each other in an improper way, to *be* victims, to *make* victims, to be afraid, to be rejected, to be bitter, to have inappropriate feelings, and then when you go to a shrink, he blames *you* anyway.

God did not ask, "Who told you to be afraid?" or "Who told you to be depressed?" God asked Adam, *"Who* told you that you were naked?" He could have asked, *"Who* told you to be afraid?" *"Who* told you to be depressed?" You are not the problem. You have been trained in the law of sin. Adam and Eve's thoughts were not their own. Are your thoughts your own?

God wants to remove the things that are not of Him. This will begin to renew your mind. You will begin to have the mind of Christ and to have ways of thinking that are superior to the law of sin.

God wants to teach you. The Holy Spirit wants to bear witness of truth. As you read the Scriptures, alpha waves give you the ability to have cognitive, deductive reasoning. The alpha waves record all the things that you've perceived externally and internally, integrated to produce deductive reasoning. This becomes the compositeness of the identification of your personality and your soul.

### Wholeness

Are you able to do a spiritual inventory of your personality without fear? I want to give you some tools to overcome stinking thinking. I want you to begin to see yourself as a triune being.

**And the very God of peace sanctify you wholly; and I pray God your whole spirit and soul and body be preserved blameless unto the coming of our Lord Jesus Christ. 1 Thessalonians 5:23**

May the God of peace sanctify you wholly is important. We know sanctification means holiness and the word sanctify means to make holy. But it says the very God of peace sanctify you to make you wholly that you can be made whole. We are talking about wholeness—spirit, soul and body.

We know that 80 percent of all disease has its origin in the spirit level. At this level the wrong way of thinking triggers the body to respond into disease.

*In fact, all your enemy has to do to produce over 100 major syndromes and diseases is control the activity of your hypothalamus through the mind-body connection.*

Let's say I'm your enemy and I want to give you high blood pressure. It is easy if the enemy can get your thoughts captured and make his spirituality part of your spirituality. So, let's say a spirit of fear begins to speak to you. A spirit of fear knows it cannot put a disease on you unless you are disobedient to God's Word. It cannot touch you like Satan could not touch Adam and Eve until you say amen to the thought process of Satan. Adam and Eve disobeyed God's Word and opened the spiritual door for Satan to work in their lives.

So, how can a spirit of fear put high blood pressure on you? It is going to need your permission. How can it get your permission? The first thing it is going to do is begin to give you thoughts. It will speak to you, spirit-to-spirit, out of the spirit world because it is a spirit. This is temptation. Yet, temptation is not sin. Most of us don't realize feelings and thoughts can be temptation.

That's why 2 Corinthians 10:5 says you are not only to hold every thought captive, but every imagination. These are your feelings, apprehensions, emotions, trepidations and uneasiness. You are being tempted to believe that it is real. It wants to train you in the law of sin so it can put a disease on your body. You are taught when you have these feelings that it is a negative emotion, a psychological defect. You are not taught there is a kingdom assigned to you that wants to get you to disobey God's Word.

High blood pressure comes out of disobedience to God's Word. Medical science says hypertension is a stress disorder. When you go to a doctor with hypertension or high blood pressure, he doesn't discuss the fact that you have a stress disorder. He puts you on medication. Is he concerned about the pathway of your thoughts that produced that disease? Do you think the medication has sanctified you? Let me explain this to activate your discernment.

> **[12]For when for the time ye ought to be teachers, ye have need that one teach you again which be the first principles of the oracles of God; and are become such as have need of milk, and not of strong meat. [13]For every one that uses milk is unskillful in the word of righteousness: for he is a babe. [14]But strong meat belongs to them that are of full age, even those who by reason of use have their senses exercised to discern both good and evil. Hebrews 5:12–14**

This Scripture says that he who is on milk is unskillful in the Word of righteousness. But he who is of full age, he who is able to handle strong meat, is he or she who has their senses exercised, to discern thoughts, of whether these thoughts are good or evil.

Are your feelings and thoughts good or evil? You say, well, it's just human nature. Human nature is not evil. Something has joined human nature and made it less than what God had intended.

If we can remove what is not of God, we have human nature that has been sanctified to produce wholeness as it says in 1 Thessalonians 5:23. God wants to sanctify you wholly; wholeness in spirit, soul and body. God wants to sanctify your spirits. It begins in the conversion of the human spirit. Then your mind is renewed by the washing of the water of the Word. So before, you were one with the law of sin, spirit and soul. Now, you are one with the law of God, spirit and soul and your body is about to conform to health, not disease.

I want you to understand your feelings are not always you. At times, you have become one with something as if it were you. A spirit of fear can teach you to be so afraid through the spirit, soul (mind) and body connection that your body can shake. Your body can even go into anaphylaxis or catatonic states, get rashes, hives, hyperventilate, heart palpitations, start to sweat and you are convinced this is real. It is only real because you bought the law of sin as a way of thinking.

I mentioned high blood pressure. How can the enemy put this disease on you? He is going to give you feelings of worry, pictures of things that can go wrong in the future, get you to worry about the economy, worry about the mother-in-law who wants to come live with you, worry about finances and the six o'clock news is certainly going to stir you up.

As a result, the enemy has trained you in your long-term memory to make worry part of your personality.

But the Scripture says in Matthew 6:34:

> **Take therefore no thought for the morrow: for the morrow shall take thought for the things of itself. Sufficient unto the day is the evil thereof. Matthew 6:34**

All of the worry was to get you to violate this one Scripture. You are worrying, taking thought for tomorrow and the enemy is training you to be afraid. He is not only going to give you thoughts and feelings; he is going to let it feel like it's really you. After a period of time, that thought, through protein synthesis, will become permanently part of your biology. Now, not only are you being tempted, you have the law of sin working as part of your existence.

We not only want you to get healed, we want to equip you with tools to stay well and help others get well. This cannot be a selfish journey. We must redefine health and healing in the world because it isn't working.

So, what happens in high blood pressure is this: As you become one with worry, the mind-body connection, through the limbic system, puts things in motion. The hypothalamus integrates a pathway to produce all kinds of neurological misfirings. The central nervous system, endocrine system and homeostasis are affected until finally you're like a scarecrow flapping in the wind of a hurricane. All of this is because you think that is just who you are and physiological manifestations are occurring to prove it.

An imbalance of the sympathetic nervous system occurs. This causes the cell membrane of the cardiovascular system to narrow. The opening is not large enough to accommodate the volume of blood. That increases blood pressure. So you take a drug that is a beta blocker. That opens up the blood vessels. It appears you are out of danger.

But, do you still worry? Do you still have fear? Have you been sanctified? Are you a doer of the Word? You are actually being maintained by the same kingdom who gave you the disease.

In Galatians 5, Paul called *pharmakeia* witchcraft, a work of the flesh, because it offers itself as a healing. It is not. It is disease management. Disease management means you're not healed. You might be out of danger, but you are not healed. God does not want you to be managed; He wants you to be free of disease.

**You can prevent and defeat high blood pressure if you understand how this kingdom speaks to you.** Are you able to be honest with yourself, about yourself? Self-accusation and guilt are going to hammer you. Then you are going to go into denial because you don't want to face your battleground. Out of sight, out of mind is not a spiritual principle.

The ostrich sticks his head in the sand because he figures that if he can't see you, you can't see him. That's denial. What he doesn't realize is that when he does that, his big fluffy tail is straight up in the air and he is a bigger target to his enemy. Denial exposes you to the enemy.

God wants you to be awake and alert. He's called you to hold every thought captive. He's called you to redefine and look at every fabric of your personality. Is it really of God? Did you inherit it? Do you really understand? These are the questions that I'm asking you. Are we really discerning the source of our thoughts?

## The Misunderstanding of Possession

There is a big debate over whether or not a Christian can have an evil spirit. The misunderstanding is of possession versus servitude to sin. The evil spirit could be inside, outside or on Pluto with a megaphone; the point is, you've been listening. Being born again doesn't make you immune to evil spirits.

The only way your soul knows anything is through theta or beta brainwave activity. Satan's invisible spirit world knows this. The only way it can access or influence your thinking is through temptation. It either has to materialize in the physical world, where you can see it and perceive it through your five physical senses through beta, or it speaks to your spirit. You hear it and apprehend it through thoughts, impressions and feelings through theta brainwave activity. Your soul is the bridge. There is no entrance to it except through these two brainwaves.

So, to say an evil spirit is not speaking to you means you don't understand temptation. Temptation is not you tempting yourself. Jesus told Peter that Satan desired to sift him like wheat.

> [31]**And the Lord said, Simon, Simon, behold, Satan hath desired to have you, that he may sift you as wheat:** [32]**But I have prayed for thee, that thy faith fail not: and when thou art converted, strengthen thy brethren. Luke 22:31–32**

Jesus knew the thoughts that came into Peter's mind were not his own. The evil genius of the thought that caused Peter to speak and rebuke the Lord was not original to Peter's psychology or his psyche. Jesus knew Satan communicated that thought spirit-to-spirit to Peter. He knew Peter picked it up through theta, at the soul level, and then his mouth opened and spoke it. That's why Jesus addressed the *source* of the thought.

## Moving on to Maturity

Are you able to address the source of your thoughts? You have to ask, "Is this really me? Is this really how I think? Is this God's nature in me? Or is it some other nature that has taught me?"

We are to discern both good and evil according to Hebrews 5:14:

> ...to them that are of full age, even those who by reason of use have their senses exercised to discern both good and evil. Hebrews 5:14

Paul said the law of sin resided in his members—his spirit, soul and body.

> For I delight in the law of God after the inward man. But I see another law in my members, warring against the law of my mind, and bringing me into captivity to the law of sin which is in my members. Romans 7:22–23

He said he had two laws: the law of God and the law of sin. He said that with his mind he served the law of God, but with the flesh the law of sin. I want to help you get out of denial and for you to not be afraid. I know it's hard to ask you to look at the things that make you feel unhappy on the inside. I know it's not fun to have to face the things that make you feel unlovely and afraid, that torment you, accuse you. I know it's not fun, but I want you to understand—it is not you.

You have a choice to make. You hold the law of God in one hand and the law of sin in the other. When someone comes against you, you have a choice to make. You are either going to repay evil with evil, or repay evil with good.

In Proverbs 15:1, the Bible says a soft answer turns away wrath. The law of God says forgive them—don't pay attention when wrong is done to you. It's hard, isn't it? Why? It's difficult because you have been trained by the law of sin screaming in your head, tempting you to repay evil with evil.

It's not easy to be led by the Spirit of God when you have so much other stuff ingrained in you demanding your attention. When you feel like being bitter, hateful toward yourself, bitter at others, or when you have rejection, fear, unloveliness, envy and jealousy, that is temptation. If it has become part of your personality, then you are serving sin. You need to recognize it, repent to God for serving it and be delivered. Then you can have your mind renewed. Otherwise, you are stuck with it and the torment that comes with it.

God is not going to sovereignly overtake you. You are going to have to work with God in your journey. Can you do this? Can you practice discernment? Can you hold up forgiveness in one hand and unforgiveness in the other? Can you choose to forgive them, not because you feel like it, but because it is God's will? Forgiveness is superior to unforgiveness. Love is superior to hate. Being a peacemaker is superior to being a troublemaker. Having mercy is superior to showing no mercy. Having patience is superior to showing impatience. But it's your choice.

Do you really want to change? If so, God will help you be transformed through the renewing of your mind. He will work through your pathways of thought.

## Insights to Disease

The Bible tells us where disease comes from. A lot of people say it comes from God.

Why would God destroy what He created? After God finished creation, He didn't say it was good; He said it was very good.

Disease actually means dis-ease. Dis-ease means "not at ease," or "not at peace." Yet, this was not God's intention for our lifestyle.

Jesus said in John 14:27:

**Peace I leave with you, my peace I give unto you... John 14:27**

James 1:17:

**Every good gift and every perfect gift is from above, and comes down from the Father of lights... James 1:17**

The Psalmist says our Father daily loads us with benefits in Psalm 68:19:

**Blessed be the Lord, who daily loads us with benefits, even the God of our salvation. Selah. Psalm 68:19**

The first benefit of the Father, *Adonay Yhovih* (ad-o-noy' yeh-ho-vee'), is Jesus, *Yhovah Elohiym* (yeh-ho-vaw' el-o-heem'), who is the God of our salvation.

Early death is not God's plan. Do you think God would take a Christian brother at the age of 48 and leave behind a wife and four children? No. But some Christians will justify it by saying, "You are going to get a perfect healing in heaven...so it's not so bad to die." That is bad theology. If you die today as a believer, you end up in heaven, disembodied.

Where does your body go when you die? To the dust. Where does your spirit go? Back to God who gave it.

In 2 Corinthians 5:8, Paul said he would rather...

**... be absent from the body, and to be present with the Lord. 2 Corinthians 5:8**

The spirit of man returns to God. If a disease has taken you out of this world, how can you get a perfect healing in heaven when your body doesn't go there with you? You don't get your glorified body until the resurrection.

God's perfect will is not to heal you. His perfect will is that you don't get sick. Pathways of disease and health are taught in Scripture. Divine health is a principle of Scripture. We have been so trained to expect disease that health is almost a surprise. The Word of God does not teach this.

We should be interested in what God has said, not what man has said. Since God honors only His Word, then what He has said is the only thing we should be concerned about. Anything you think or believe that does not match what God has said or how He thinks is a form of insanity; it is not sane thinking.

Fear is a form of insanity because it falls short of the soundness of God's mind. God says He has not given you the spirit of fear, but of power, love and a sound mind.

> **For God hath not given us the spirit of fear; but of power, and of love, and of a sound mind. 2 Timothy 1:7**

Error is being taught in the body of Christ today. Some teach that healing passed away 2000 years ago. For them…it did. If you say you don't believe God heals, then for you, He won't.

We believe the Scriptures indicate God does heal today. Some teach there is no connection between the human spirit and the physical body.

Yet, Proverbs 17:22 says,

> **A merry heart does good like a medicine: but a broken spirit dries the bones. Proverbs 17:22**

This Scripture shows the connection between the health of the human spirit and the health of the marrow of your bones. As you recall, those seven words, "A broken spirit dries the bones," are how God revealed to me the roots to Environmental Illness. These seven words unraveled the most bizarre disease known to mankind. Be in Health™ is considered an international expert in the healing and prevention of Environmental Illness.

The same verse in Proverbs also reveals the pathway into the compromising of the immune system that produces allergies.

What causes allergies? They do not come out of nowhere. There is a pathway. Allergies are a by-product of your spirituality. In allergies, the first things you lose are dairy products and sugars. Then you lose the wheat.

God granted all foods to be eaten—with thanksgiving. When it comes to food, the Bible says:

> ³...men forbidding... and commanding to abstain from meats, which God hath created to be received with thanksgiving of them which believe and know the truth. ⁴For every creature of God is good, and nothing to be refused, if it be received with thanksgiving: 1 Timothy 4:3–4

Isn't it amazing? When the spies went into the Land of Promise that God provided for them, they found it was flowing with milk and honey. Yet these are the first two products to be lost in allergies: milk and honey.

The Bible says God's people have gone into captivity.

> ¹³Therefore my people are gone into captivity, because they have no knowledge: and their honorable men are famished, and their multitude dried up with thirst. ¹⁴Therefore hell hath enlarged herself, and opened her mouth without measure: and their glory, and their multitude, and their pomp, and he that rejoices, shall descend into it. Isaiah 5:13–14

Why have the people gone into captivity? Because they have no knowledge...and hell hath enlarged herself. Did you think God's people were immune to hell? The Scripture says hell hath opened her mouth. Does that mean they lost their salvation? I don't know...it doesn't say. It does show us the captivity of what hell represents is part of their life.

Do you think God intended for you as a believer to be tormented and destroyed by what hell represents? Do you think that's really what the gospel is all about? I don't think so.

However, there is a consequence to disobedience. Some say that because we are New Testament saints, hell has no power over us in our disobedience. This is not true. There are consequences to disobedience of God's ways whether you are believers or not. That's why the sinner has the same diseases you have and you have the same diseases as the sinner. You are practicing the same sins! Someone said, "Why is that sinner in better health than I am?" Because he is more righteous than you. He is practicing greater deeds of righteousness from his conscience than you are with truth.

The book of Hosea shows the importance of knowledge. Isaiah tells of people who went into captivity because they had no knowledge.

> My people are destroyed for lack of knowledge: because you have rejected knowledge, I will also reject thee, that you shall be no priest to me: seeing you have forgotten the law of your God, I will also forget your children. Hosea 4:6

God said, *My* people are destroyed...because *you* have rejected knowledge. He also said, you shall be no priest to me. We are supposed to be the priesthood of believers. You ask, "Can I be rejected by God?" It's not that you are rejected by God. It is that *you* have rejected God. When you listen to rejection, it forces Him to withdraw until you are tired of following another god. Remember your true Father and what He has said and return to Him.

Notice this verse also says, I will forget your children. This is the foundation for generational inherited disease—the loss of blessing passed from generation to generation.

There is a connection between sin and disease. If God says you should forgive your brother, is that a commandment or a suggestion? A commandment.

What if you don't want to? Is there a consequence? Yes. Because when you practice unforgiveness, you're not a doer of the Word. You're a doer of some other word.

> **Also every sickness, and every plague, which is not written in the book of this law, them will the LORD bring upon thee, until thou be destroyed. Deuteronomy 28:61**

Deuteronomy 28:15–68 describes all manner of disease known to mankind and it says there are others not written.

The examples of diseases and dis-eases listed in Deuteronomy 28 are known to mankind today and include everything from infertility to miscarriages, psoriasis to itching, losing your home and farms to foreclosure, losing your wife to another man, panic attacks, phobias, famines and all manner of disease from histamine release and cancers right down to hemorrhoids.

Isaiah chapter one also talks about the connection between sin and disease. Verses 2 and 3 tell us we have sinning saints…

> **[2] Hear, O heavens, and give ear, O earth: for the LORD hath spoken, I have nourished and brought up children, and they have rebelled against me. [3] The ox knoweth his owner, and the ass his master's crib: but Israel doth not know, my people doth not consider. Isaiah 1:2–3**

Verses 4–6 tell us that these sinning saints are sick because of sin…

> **[4] Ah sinful nation, a people laden with iniquity, a seed of evildoers, children that are corrupters: they have forsaken the LORD, they have provoked the Holy One of Israel unto anger, they are gone away backward. [5] Why should ye be stricken any more? ye will revolt more and more: the whole head is sick, and the whole heart faint. [6] From the sole of the foot even unto the head there is no soundness in it; but wounds, and bruises, and putrifying sores: they have not been closed, neither bound up, neither mollified with ointment. Isaiah 1:4–6**

Here, all manner of diseases are covered: everything psychological, physical, even drugs—the ointments—and nothing has fixed God's people.

> **[16] Wash you, make you clean; put away the evil of your doings from before mine eyes; cease to do evil; [17] Learn to do well; seek judgment, relieve the oppressed, judge the fatherless, plead for the widow. [18] Come now, and let us reason together, saith the LORD: though your sins be as scarlet, they shall be as white as snow; though they be red like crimson, they shall be as wool. Isaiah 1:16–18**

You are going to have to do something! You are going to have to cleanse yourself.

## All Disease is a Curse

Is disease a curse? Yes. If you have disease that is also in your children, then you have passed down an inherited disease from your generation. This is a curse from generation to generation. You have not only gone into captivity because you have no knowledge, but you are now dying before your time because of ignorance.

The Word of God in Deuteronomy 28 has clearly said that all disease is a curse. When we choose to not believe inherited disease is a curse, we do not believe the Bible.

We have found that 80 percent of all incurable disease has a spiritual root. That spiritual root has corresponding psychological and biological manifestations. So we are not just talking about physical healing.

Not dealing with the spiritual root is why the Church has less than a five percent healing rate. Some pastors will agree with these statistics, but they don't want to talk about it. Perhaps they don't have the knowledge.

So who gets discouraged? The people who walk out as sick as they came in and the minister of God who is trying to obey the Word.

What if God healed you of a disease that had a spiritual issue behind it without requiring you to acknowledge that sin? He would be establishing evil in the earth through you in the name of love by overlooking your sin. If He did heal you of a disease that had a known spiritual root behind it, you wouldn't stay well. The spiritual issue would cause your body to break down again. The disease would come right back on you and then He would get blamed for you losing the healing.

What happened with King Saul? He didn't go insane because he had an organic defect. The Spirit of God departed from him and the spirit of insanity came. His insanity was caused by an evil spirit, according to 1 Samuel 16:23. When the anointed man of God came with his music, the evil spirit left King Saul and he was back in his right mind. When the music stopped, the evil spirit came back. King Saul did not have a sound mind; he eventually committed suicide on the battlefield.

A sound mind comes from gaining knowledge from the Bible. It's important to read the Bible in context.

> **Is any sick among you? let him call for the elders of the church; and let them pray over him, anointing him with oil in the name of the Lord: James 5:14**

That is the Scripture, but people often don't quote the rest of it. We need to be sure to read everything before and after a specific verse so we have the knowledge and understanding God has provided for us. The next verse says:

> **And the prayer of faith shall save the sick, and the Lord shall raise him up; and if he has committed sins, they shall be forgiven him. James 5:15**

Jesus healed a man in John 5:14 and then told him, "go your way and sin no more, lest a worse thing come upon you."

> **…Who forgives all your iniquities; who heals all your diseases;…**
> **Psalm 103:3**

What precedes healing of disease? Forgiveness of iniquities. Forgiveness…and then healing.

## Blessings and Curses

Are there conditions for blessings and curses? Yes.

> [1] **And it shall come to pass, if thou shalt hearken diligently unto the voice of the LORD thy God, to observe and to do all his commandments which I command thee this day, that the LORD thy God will set thee on high above all nations of the earth:** [2] **And all these blessings shall come on thee, and overtake thee, if thou shalt hearken unto the voice of the LORD thy God. Deuteronomy 28:1–2**

The blessings are funneled through one word: IF. *If* in Hebrew is *"im"* (i-m). It's conditional. Are the blessings conditional? YES. How many? ALL of them. Some will say this is Old Testament, but it is found in the New Testament also:

> **But be ye doers of the word, and not hearers only, deceiving your own selves. James 1:22**

If you are a doer of the Word, you cannot stop the blessings from overtaking you. As you become a doer of the Word, you are not thinking about the blessings—you are just blessed! The blessings are listed in Deuteronomy 28:1–14. For those who are doers of the Word, there is not one curse or disease listed.

### Testimony of Healing

A lady attended the For My Life™ program. She forgave herself for self-hatred and became a doer of the Word by loving herself. The Word says we are to love ourselves as we love our neighbor, right? She began to love herself and repented to God for this dead work of self-hatred and that very day, the cancer fell off her face onto the floor. She doesn't have face cancer anymore. No one prayed for her!

When she became a doer of the Word, the blessings came upon her and overtook her. God stripped death from her, stripped disease from her, the thing fell to the floor and she gives God glory.

This testimony is documented and is one of hundreds of testimonies of healing on file at Be in Health™.

There are conditions for curses also.

> As the bird by wandering, as the swallow by flying, so the curse causeless shall not come. Proverbs 26:2

If you are NOT a doer of the Word, what shall come to pass? The curses found in Deuteronomy 28:15–68.

> But it shall come to pass, if thou wilt not hearken unto the voice of the LORD thy God, to observe to do all his commandments and his statutes which I command thee this day; that all these curses shall come upon thee, and overtake thee. Deuteronomy 28:15

Who gave the right to the curses? We and our ancestors did…and now the curses have a right to come to us. This is important because people want to know *why* they are sick.

The definition of *blessing* is found in *Strong's Concordance* #1288. In the Hebrew, *blessing* means benefit from God. A blessing is the opposite of a curse! Some say you are free from the curse. If you are free from the curse, why do you still have hemorrhoids?

The definition of *curse* is found in *Strong's Concordance* #7045. The first definition is vilification. What does vilification mean? Vilification means abatement or lessening of the benefit; all the curse means is the abatement or lessening of the benefit. In this word study, the word villain can be found, vilifying the benefit. The Word identifies the villain. The villain is the devil.

> The thief cometh not, but for to steal, and to kill, and to destroy: I am come that they might have life, and that they might have it more abundantly. John 10:10

So who gave the right to the villain to vilify you? You and your ancestors did. Why do we want to be forgiven of the iniquities of our ancestors? Because it precedes healing.

You and I are caught between two kingdoms. One kingdom produces blessings and the other kingdom produces curses. If you repent and become a doer of the Word, then all the blessings will come and overtake you; you will have His broken body working for you and you can be healed of all your diseases.

If you do not repent for participating with sin, then you are NOT a doer of the Word and all these curses shall come and overtake you.

The connection between sin and disease can be found in Psalm 103.

**Who forgiveth all thine iniquities; who healeth all thy diseases; Psalm 103:3**

The Church is trying to be healed without obedience. They don't realize that forgiveness, healing and deliverance are appropriated by faith, which requires obedience!

## Healing is for Today

Scripture clearly says healing is for today. We get the gift of healing for someone else's benefit.

**But the manifestation of the Spirit is given to every man to profit withal. 1 Corinthians 12:7**

Healing is still the children's bread. It belongs to you first as a believer so you can teach what you've received to others!

**But Jesus said unto her, Let the children first be filled: for it is not meet to take the children's bread, and to cast it unto the dogs. Mark 7:27**

Some say healing passed away with the disciples 2000 years ago. This is not true because the one who taught on healing was NOT one of the 12 disciples. It was Paul! This becomes a block to healing for those who say healing passed away.

Whom are we told to go to for healing? We are told to call for the elders of the Church. We are told to confess our faults (our dead works) one to another in order to be healed.

**¹⁴Is any sick among you? let him call for the elders of the church; and let them pray over him, anointing him with oil in the name of the Lord: ¹⁵ And the prayer of faith shall save the sick, and the Lord shall raise him up; and if he have committed sins, they shall be forgiven him. ¹⁶ Confess your faults one to another, and pray one for another, that ye may be healed. The effectual fervent prayer of a righteous man availeth much. James 5:14–16**

So we see here that it may be a sin issue.

What can interfere with health and healing or even contribute to disease?

Not being a doer of the Word by participating with sin. In *A More Excellent Way*™, there are 33 blocks to healing listed along with possible spiritual roots.

In Isaiah 58:4, people were sick and diseased because they were filled with strife, debate and conflict with each other. These are blocks to healing.

> Behold, ye fast for strife and debate, and to smite with the fist of
> wickedness: ye shall not fast as ye do this day, to make your voice to be
> heard on high. Isaiah 58:4

In the story of the boy born blind, Jesus was asked, Who sinned? Father or mother?

> [1]And as Jesus passed by, he saw a man which was blind from his
> birth. [2]And his disciples asked him, saying, Master, who did sin, this man,
> or his parents, that he was born blind? [3]Jesus answered, Neither hath this
> man sinned, nor his parents: but that the works of God should be made
> manifest in him. John 9:1–3

They asked a correct theological question because they knew sin and sickness were connected. In the Old Testament days, they knew the connection. Jesus knew that not all sickness is because of sin and told them the boy was born blind for the glory of God. This is not saying that disease is for glory of God, but the *healing of the disease* was for the glory of God.

## Not All Disease Has a Spiritual Root

Disease may or may not have a spiritual root. In many cases, we know when it's a spiritually rooted disease and when it is not. In our findings, less than five percent are healed of incurable disease in churches today.

We don't teach that *all* disease has a sin issue. Only 80 percent of disease that's called incurable is rooted in the spiritual and that is according to medical science. We call these dead works, with corresponding psychological and biological manifestations. Oft infirmities are things common to man, such as a cold (unless they are chronic—then there is another issue).

A quote by Dr. McLaughlin of the Women's Medical College in Philadelphia from *The Unshakeable Kingdom and the Unchanging Person* by E. Stanley Jones:

> Dr. McLaughlin of the Women's Medical College in Philadelphia says
> that from sixty-five (65) percent to eighty-five (85) percent of all diseases are
> rooted in the mental and spiritual, ninety-nine (99) percent of headaches,
> seventy-five (75) percent of stomach disorders, seventy-five (75) percent of
> asthma, and seventy-five (75) percent of skin diseases.

And this was written just about 35 years ago. It has been my experience that about 80 percent of all incurable diseases have spiritual root issues with corresponding psychological and biological manifestations.

In this same book, there was a surgeon that said to this author,

> You could have headed off, with the kind of religion you are
> proclaiming, eighty-five (85) percent of the cases that come to me for
> surgery. They begin with functional disturbance through wrong mental and

spiritual attitudes and actions, then the functional pass into the structural, and then we surgeons get them.

At Be in Health™ we understand pathways of disease. We understand how the enemy causes disease. We understand the molecular parts of our bodies, our minds and our souls, hormonal imbalance, neurotransmitter imbalance, nerve activity, mutation of cells in mitosis for cancer, viruses.

We want you to know how to get free and stay free so you can help others understand the gospel. That brings realistic fruit to your life, not just spiritual theories. We offer that which is already found in the Bible and the study of science. We share practical application of the Word of God.

We are prepared to let God work through us in creative miracles. There are nine gifts of the Holy Spirit. One is the gift of healing. One is the gift of miracles. They are both misunderstood. If you have a disease in your organs, we would waste our time ministering healing to you. It is going to take a creative miracle.

Do you know what a creative miracle is? God intervenes by creating something in your body that is not there. It can be body parts being reformed. There are parts of your body that will not heal. Organs do not heal. Brain cells do not heal. Nerve cells generally do not heal. You can speak new nerve endings into place in the name of Jesus. Anything that will happen will be a work of the Holy Spirit. There are parts of your body that will heal. This requires operating in the gift of healing.

Some people have disease resulting from their ancestors' sin issue. We all carry the biological or spiritual results of our ancestors' participation with the enemy.

> **...for I the LORD thy God am a jealous God, visiting the iniquity of the fathers upon the children unto the third and fourth generation of them that hate me; Exodus 20:5**

We have a pathway of psychological and biological diseases that our ancestors have had for generations. This pathway must be faced and dealt with. If they did not deal with it, they passed it on to you. Be in Health™ has evidence of genetic code change through ministry. Not only was a person healed of the disease they inherited, but the gene that was responsible for it was made normal. So the person is no longer a carrier. Their children will no longer inherit the genetic defect.

God wants us to prosper and be in health.

> **Beloved, I wish above all things that you may prosper and be in health, even as your soul prospers. 3 John 1:2**

When you are obedient to God, you have psychological and biological health. The fruit of obedience is health. The fruit of disobedience is disease. Which gospel do you want to follow? If God says to forgive your brother, do you think there will be a benefit to forgiving your brother? Yes. A large number of diseases won't come your way. Do you think there is a consequence to not forgiving your brother? Yes. There are diseases headed your way due to the pathways affected by your unforgiveness. This is taught in Scripture.

Did God give you the disease? No. Satan did through his kingdom. You are going to reap the benefits of one kingdom or the other. If you follow the thinking of Satan and his kingdom, he will bless you with the fruit of disobedience, which is disease. The law of God has fruit and the law of Satan has fruit. The law of God produces health. The law of Satan produces disease. When you make Satan your lord in a certain area of your life, you force God to withdraw from that area of your life. It is your choice.

There is more to the gospel than being born again. The gospel is filled with Scriptures that indicate God's will is to be done on earth. The Lord's prayer says, "Thy will be done in earth as it is in heaven." The gifts of the Holy Spirit are not for you in heaven; they are here for you now. Healing is still the children's bread.

Disease follows relationship breakdown. Relationship breakdown involves separation on three levels. 1) Separation from the Godhead. Many of you don't have your peace with God the Father. 2) Separation from yourself. Many people don't like themselves. Remember the woman with the face cancer? When she dealt with self-hatred, the curse was broken and healing came. 3) Separation from others. This could be due to bitterness, envy and jealousy, or it could be anger or fear of another.

Healing begins with reconciliation. If 80 percent of all disease involves separation, then 80 percent of all healing begins with reconciliation to God, the Father, the Son and the Holy Spirit, to yourself and to others.

> **And he answering said, you shall love the Lord your God with all your heart, and with all your soul, and with all your strength, and with all your mind; and your neighbor as yourself. Luke 10:27**

> **On these two commandments hang all the law and the prophets. Matthew 22:40**

The foundation for the entire Word of God, in the Old and New Testaments, has to do with relationships. These are the three areas Satan uses to destroy the peace of mankind. No peace produces dis-ease that leads to disease.

## Where Does Peace Come From?

Where does peace come from?

> **And the very God of peace sanctify you wholly; and I pray God your whole spirit and soul and body be preserved blameless unto the coming of our Lord Jesus Christ. 1 Thessalonians 5:23**

True Peace comes from God.

Not from Yoga, Transcendental Meditation or Prozac.

> **Peace I leave with you, my peace I give unto you: not as the world giveth, give I unto you. Let not your heart be troubled, neither let it be afraid. John 14:27**

> **Thou wilt keep him in perfect peace, whose mind is stayed on thee: because he trusts in thee. Isaiah 26:3**

"Thee" is the Lord—the Word of God. A lot of Christians use the name of Jesus, but they do not know what He said. You cannot meditate on His name. You must meditate on what He said because what He said is for you. It's for your peace. Jesus is not going to come and live your life for you. We cannot say, "Well if God loves me, He'll just have to fix me." God is looking for relationship, working together.

What does it mean to be wholly? W-h-o-l-l-y sanctified? Sanctification means holiness, h-o-l-y. First Thessalonians 5:23 is saying, "May the God of peace make you holy, h-o-l-y, so that you can be made whole, w-h-o-l-e." No holiness…no wholeness. A lack of holiness leads to lack of wholeness. "So that you can be made whole" includes spirit, soul and body.

We do not promote inner healing or physical healing. We offer wholeness: the sanctification of the human spirit [spirit]; the renewal of the human mind [soul]; and the healing of the mobile home [body] that carries us where we need to go. This is a wholeness approach.

Jesus was our example. When the evil one came to Jesus, in His hour of temptation, he found nothing to connect with in Jesus to cause Him to sin. In our lives, there is stuff the enemy is already connected with. It is in all three dimensions—spirit, soul and body. The work of the Holy Spirit is to remove those things that give the enemy a legal right to our lives. So your whole spirit, soul and body can be preserved blameless unto the coming of our Lord Jesus Christ.

Has the Lord Jesus Christ come back for us yet? No. Then this work to be made whole is here—now—in your generation on three dimensions. We are going to help you face the stuff you have been avoiding in denial or ignorance. Your diseases are the fruit of avoiding that stuff. So, we are going to talk about the cleansing of spirit, soul and body.

To help you understand this, let's look at high blood pressure. If you have high blood pressure, you are participating with the spirit of fear. The medical community says that high blood pressure or hypertension is a stress disorder. What do you think stress is? A type of fear. There are over 4000 kinds of fear listed in the April 2, 2001, issue of *Time Magazine.* High blood pressure is a result of fear. That fear is in violation of one Scripture:

> **Take therefore no thought for the morrow: for the morrow shall take thought for the things of itself. Sufficient unto the day is the evil thereof. Matthew 6:34**

People with high blood pressure are always projecting into the future what could go wrong. Am I going to have enough money? Am I going to have a house? What about this, what about that? High blood pressure causes them to be scattered and smothered. They wonder why they have high blood pressure. Then they go to the doctor and he gives them medication...so they don't have a stroke and die. He tells them they have to stay on it the rest of their life. Then they really do have fear!

Let's settle this once and for all.

> **¹And it shall come to pass... ²And all these blessings shall come on thee, and overtake thee... Deuteronomy 28:1–2**

"And it shall come to pass...." That means something is going to happen. "If" you shall hearken unto the voice of the Lord...all these blessings shall come on you.

The Bible tells us to be doers of the Word. So, if you will be a doer of what God said, all these blessings shall overtake you. There is not one disease listed in Deuteronomy 28:1–14. So to not have a disease is a blessing.

Starting in verse 15, it says, "But it shall come to pass, if you will not hearken unto the voice of the Lord thy God, then all these curses shall come upon you." Everything from biological and psychological disease...to losing your house...to foreclosure...to divorces...to hemorrhoids...is listed as a result of not being a doer of the word. So the spiritual conclusion is that disease is a curse.

God does not give us disease. Disobedience brings about the curse, which is disease. Some say they believe God gave them their diseases. However, they are going to the doctor to become well. Why? Isn't that hypocritical?

If God gave you something, why would you try to get rid of it? Disease is a curse. At the cross, Christ paid the penalty for the curse. Some say, "I am a new covenant saint and Jesus paid the penalty on the cross for me, so I am free from the curse."

Did Jesus pay the penalty for all sin at the cross? Yes. Is everybody saved? No. Why not? They have not appropriated it. By His stripes we were healed. Is everyone healed of disease? No. Why not? They have not appropriated it. But was it finished? Yes, it was finished, but we have the responsibility to appropriate it.

Here's something else Paul taught in Hebrews. If you willfully continue in your sins after the knowledge of the truth, you crucify Christ all over again. You put Him to an open shame and put Him back on the cross. What He did for you in His obedience, you negate in your disobedience. Until you repent, what He did for you at the cross is unavailable to you until you come to your knees. When you respond to what He did for you at the cross, the Scripture may be fulfilled.

**If we confess our sins, he is faithful and just to forgive us our sins, and to cleanse us from all unrighteousness. 1 John 1:9**

But some of the Church is trying to appropriate what Christ did while they are in rebellion to His Word and it is not working. God is looking for obedience. This is not legalism. Legalism tries to make you righteous. But Jesus said, "If you love me, you will keep my commandments." We want your love for Jesus and the Father to be increased. We want to give you knowledge so that you can love Him more…in obedience.

*It is God's will that we be healed.* Disease does not come without a cause.

**As the bird by wandering, as the swallow by flying, so the curse causeless shall not come. Proverbs 26:2**

The curse—disease—is not going to land unless something has caused it.

Do you remember Job? What he feared greatly came upon him. Fear is an open door, a doorpoint. Participation with sin, generationally and personally, allows Satan the right to bless you with disease as a result of disobedience.

Maybe your generations have been practicing sin for generations. So in this understanding, disease is the fruit of continual yielding to sin. Healing is the fruit of repentance. Wholeness is the fruit of sanctification.

If you have a disease, we want to bring you to a place of recognizing why you are bound, to recognize what caused it, to recognize the open door and to help you deal with the spiritual roots so that your healing can begin.

Medication does not sanctify us. Medication can help in times of need. When it becomes our "source," then we are bound by another sin—sorcery. If you are on medication for a disease, do not come off your medication without your doctor's supervision.

The drug you take will not help you deal with the fear issue behind high blood pressure. You are being maintained by a drug instead of being sanctified by God's peace. God would want you to be delivered from fear of tomorrow. Then you wouldn't have high blood pressure and you wouldn't need the drug. That would be to His glory! That is the fruit of the gospel!

## Insights to Prevention of Disease

I want you to understand: **God's perfect will is not to heal you; His perfect will is that you don't get sick.**

### Is It Possible to Prevent Disease?

Earlier, we discussed a *Newsweek* article dated 9/24/90 and titled "Greater Expectations," which said, "The future of medicine lies not in treating illness but in preventing it." It's not healing and disease management but disease prevention. Continuing:

"Throughout the 20th century, medicine has advanced primarily by improving curative care....But curative care has its limits....

"Accompanying the use of more refined technology to prevent and treat illness, psychoimmunology, the science that deals with the mind's role in helping the immune system to fight disease, will become a vitally important clinical field—perhaps the most important field in the 21st century....

"Healthy thinking may eventually become an integral aspect of treatment for everything from allergies to liver transplants."

Another article in *Newsweek*, dated 9/24/90 and called "The Power to Heal," said, "The fate of the spirit is relegated to religious specialists who have little to say about their followers' physical well-being. For most societies around the world today, priest and physician are still one. The state of the body is inseparable from the condition of the spirit. Sickness is disruption, imbalance, the manifestation of malevolent forces in the flesh.

"Western medicine tends to dismiss the ideas that lie at the heart of traditional healing—ideas concerning the spiritual realm, mind-body interactions, the interplay among humanity, the environment and the cosmos—for they don't fit readily into its scientific model. Yet there is a growing recognition that the mysteries of health and healing cannot be separated from the totality of the human experience."

### How Do We Prevent Sickness from Coming Our Way?

When we can get the dead works out of our life, then the diseases that were headed our way won't come.

Deuteronomy 7:15 says the Lord will take away all sickness from you. But, this is conditional upon Deuteronomy 7:12: "If ye…."

> [12]**Wherefore it shall come to pass, if ye hearken to these judgments, and keep, and do them, that the LORD thy God shall keep unto thee the covenant and the mercy which he sware unto thy fathers:** [13]**And he will love thee, and bless thee, and multiply thee: he will also bless the fruit of thy womb, and the fruit of thy land, thy corn, and thy wine, and thine oil, the increase of thy kine, and the flocks of thy sheep, in the land which he sware unto thy fathers to give thee.** [14]**Thou shalt be blessed above all people: there shall not be male or female barren among you, or among your cattle.** [15]**And the LORD will take away from thee all sickness, and will put none of the evil diseases of Egypt, which thou knowest, upon thee; but will lay them upon all them that hate thee. Deuteronomy 7:12–15**

Diseases are evil, NOT God. Verse 15 calls diseases evil: "…will put none of the evil diseases…." God did not give you a disease. God is not evil, He is good. He is the author of good and all good things come down from the Father.

> **Every good gift and every perfect gift is from above, and cometh down from the Father of lights, with whom is no variableness, neither shadow of turning. James 1:17**

Some say God created evil because of Isaiah 45:7.

> **I form the light, and create darkness: I make peace, and create evil: I the LORD do all these things. Isaiah 45:7**

In *Strong's Concordance*, the Hebrew word for *create*, under #1254, is *bara*. It is the same word that is used when God created. But the second meaning for the Hebrew word *create* is "to break down, tear down, cut down like wood."

Now, let's read the Scripture again with the *Strong's* definition in it.

> **I form the light, and** *I tear down and destroy darkness.* **I make peace and I** *tear down and cut down like wood everything that's evil.* **I am the author of the destruction of evil.**

God did not create evil.

You have to choose to love the Lord your God…that you may obey His voice and that you may cleave unto Him. He is your life and the length of your days. But we all have to choose!

> **I call heaven and earth to record this day against you, that I have set before you life and death, blessing and cursing: therefore choose life, that both thou and thy seed may live: Deuteronomy 30:19**

Ezekiel 18:31–32 says,

> [31]**Cast away from you all your transgressions, whereby ye have transgressed; and make you a new heart and a new spirit: for why will ye die, O house of Israel?** [32]**For I have no pleasure in the death of him that**

**dieth, saith the Lord GOD: wherefore turn** *yourselves*, **and live ye.
Ezekiel 18:31–32**

The principles that will move the hand of God to heal are the same ones that will prevent many of the diseases.

## What about Disease Prevention?

[11]**You shall therefore keep the commandments, and the statutes, and the judgments, which I command you this day, to do them.** [12]**Wherefore it shall come to pass, if you hearken to these judgments, and keep, and do them, that the LORD your God shall keep unto you the covenant and the mercy which he swore unto thy fathers: Deuteronomy 7:11–12**

Verse 11 means you are to be a doer of the Word, not just a hearer only. Verse 12 means something is going to happen, *if* you hearken to these judgments and keep and do them.

So by being a doer of the Word and not just a hearer only, the Lord will keep His covenant with you. You will be blessed above all people.

**And the LORD will take away from you all sickness, and will put none of the evil diseases of Egypt, which you know, upon you; but will lay them upon all them that hate you. Deuteronomy 7:15**

**How much sickness will He take away?** All! Do you think it is God's will to heal all of your diseases? Yes. It says so in Psalm 103:3, 3 John 2 and 1 Thessalonians 5:23. "The Lord will *take away from you…*"—which means you have it in you—"*all* sickness and will put none of the evil diseases of Egypt which you know…."

Are diseases good or evil? They are evil. Where do they come from? Egypt. What is Egypt? It is a type and shadow of the world and Satan's rule of the world. More specifically, not under God's rule. God says, "I will take it away. I will put none of the evil diseases of Egypt which you know upon you, but will lay them upon all them that hate you." Deuteronomy 7 is a provision for divine health.

God says, "I change not." God's character, His nature and how He thinks have never changed. A measure of time has been provided for us to get right with Him.

[26]**Behold, I set before you this day a blessing and a curse;** [27]**A blessing, if ye obey the commandments of the LORD your God, which I command you this day:** [28]**And a curse, if ye will not obey the commandments of the LORD your God, but turn aside out of the way which I command you this day, to go after other gods, which ye have not known. Deuteronomy 11:26–28**

Your disease manifests according to the choices you make. You actually can choose your health and He will work with you. You can make yourself a new heart and a new spirit as we saw in Ezekiel 18.

Proverbs 25:28 says,

**A man who has no rule over his own spirit is like a city with its walls broken down.  Proverbs 25:28**

You are to rule over your own spirit. You choose life or death. You have a choice. Deuteronomy 30:19 says,

**I set before you this day life or death, blessings or curses. Deuteronomy 30:19**

It's *your* choice.

You receive a blessing if you obey the commandments. That means a blessing if you are a doer, not just a hearer, of the Word. You receive a curse if you will not obey or will not be a doer of the Word.

There are two meanings of the Hebrew word "if" in Deuteronomy 11:27–28. In verse 27, the word "if" is *"asher"* in the Hebrew. It is *Strong's Concordance* #834. It means the blessing *comes quickly*. In verse 28, the word "if" is *"im"* in the Hebrew. It is *Strong's Concordance* #518. It means the curse *will not come quickly*, but it will *surely* come.

You cannot blame God and you cannot blame the devil. God hasn't called you to be leavened. He has called you for purity. He has called you to establish His kingdom.

Here is the verse transliterated:

Behold I set before you this day a blessing and a curse.  If you obey the commandments of your God, the blessings shall come and they shall come quickly. That's *asher*.

In verse 28, if you will not obey the commandments of your God, the curse does not come quickly but it shall surely come. That's *im*.

You hold the keys to both kingdoms. You decide which kingdom moves in your life. You decide whether or not to remove the other kingdom that shouldn't be there. You do it and God will work with you.

In conclusion, 80 percent of incurable disease comes from disobedience to God. Healing is not yours in disobedience, although we have seen God heal people who didn't qualify because He said:

**... I will have mercy on whom I will have mercy, and I will have compassion on whom I will have compassion. Romans 9:15**

When He does that, it makes some of the rest of us angry.

Our theology includes healing of disease and prevention of disease. Healing is a provision made possible for you by the cross. Divine health is a scriptural principle.

> *The principles that bring you healing*
> *are the same principles that keep you in divine health.*

## Pathways to Spiritual Wholeness

Many people have received healing just by reading this book. The truth alone set them gloriously free. This section will help you apply these truths to your life so you too can walk in the same freedom.

> **Then Peter opened his mouth, and said, of a truth I perceive that**
> **God is no respecter of persons: Acts 10:34**

### How Do We Get There? What is the Path?

Which path are you going to choose to walk down? The one bathed in light or the one obscured by darkness? The one that offers wholeness or the one that offers only disease, distress and division? Every step moving forward will be a choice. You are not, however, left without direction. The road map for the journey ahead is God's Word.

In order for us to walk in freedom, victory and health, we must first be able to discern what is good from what is evil. Our definitions of good and evil, however—what is sin and what is not—may have to be expanded. Who thought before that fear was a sin? Who knew before that some of our methods of getting healed were not from God? Now, thankfully, we have the tools of knowledge and discernment.

> **But strong meat belongeth to them that are of full age, even those**
> **who by reason of use have their senses exercised to discern both good and**
> **evil. Hebrews 5:14**

Once we have discerned those unwanted areas within ourselves, we need to acknowledge them before God and take the appropriate steps to remove them from our lives. This may require some serious house cleaning. It requires a conscious change of lifestyle—including our thoughts, relationships and our reasons for living.

This process is called sanctification.

> *Walking in sanctification means actively choosing*
> *to be a partaker of God's kingdom in Christ*
> *and removing the presence of evil from our lives.*

You can now begin to walk out of those old paths and patterns of darkness and disease and walk into all the blessings of health God's Word has promised us.

> **Beloved, I wish above all things that thou mayest prosper and be in health, even as thy soul prospereth. 3 John 2**

Anything less than the fulfillment of God's plan for our lives is compromise. Remember, if disease or calamity has come upon your life, then there is a reason for its presence.

> **As the bird by wandering, as the swallow by flying, so the curse causeless does not come. Proverbs 26:2**

## What is Disease?

Disease is the result of separation on three levels:

- Separation from God and His Word, His person and His love

- Separation from yourself by not accepting yourself, suffering from guilt and shame

- Separation from others by breaches in relationships

Disease is obviously a curse. Deuteronomy 28 states very clearly that if we choose not to obey the statutes of God, the diseases of Egypt will be upon us as a curse. Therefore, the curse of disease must have some type of spiritual cause behind it. We call it a "root." The bad fruit is the disease; the root (sin issue) is the cause. Why pray against the fruit when you can chop it off at the root once and for all? It is our responsibility to identify the spiritual root of the disease and resolve it before God.

## What is Blocking Our Paths?

Remember: our enemy is a master deceiver. The Word tells us not to be ignorant of his wiles and devices.

> **Lest Satan should get an advantage of us: for we are not ignorant of his devices. 2 Corinthians 2:11**

> **Put on the whole armour of God, that ye may be able to stand against the wiles of the devil. Ephesians 6:11**

Satan is able to harvest bad fruit in us because he has long ago planted some bad roots in us, such as ungodly belief systems, negative programming, *stinkin' thinkin' and* a lack of proper discernment. All of these wiles have managed to separate us from healthy relationships with God, ourselves and others.

Learning how to recognize these roots is the first step toward gaining our freedom (see Teaching Unit 5 on the 8 Rs). The process of sanctification will bring us closer to God, ourselves and others. With Satan's master plan (devices) exposed, his weapons (wiles) laid out and the battlefield (our minds) clearly drawn, we are well on our way to victory.

## What Are the Steps on the Path?

- Recognition

- Repentance

- Walk Out!

The key roots behind disease are: bitterness, accusation, occultism, envy and jealousy, rejection, unloving spirits, addictions and fear.

## Bitterness

> **Looking diligently lest any man fail of the grace of God; lest any root of bitterness springing up trouble *you*, and thereby many be defiled; Hebrews 12:15**

Bitterness corrodes like acid, eating away at our soul. It poisons first the mind and then the body. It is often marked by cynicism and animosity toward others. Bitterness is a strong man kept in place by several underlings. Each underling is given entry into our lives by the one preceding it. The severity of the evilness of each underling is progressive in nature.

**Unforgiveness** would say, "I am not willing to forgive the offense against me. I will remember what has been done to me." This unforgiveness actually invites bitterness to become a part of our lives, entertaining the next six spirits.

**Resentment** is a feeling of ill will. It says, "I do not like him. I will never forgive him for what he did to me." Resentment keeps unforgiveness in place.

**Retaliation** will now come and speak his piece, "It is time to get even. He should pay for what he did…I am going to get even with him."

**Anger and Wrath** wait on retaliation to become strong and then they will break out. Anger can be both seen and felt.

**Hatred** will come forth with the idea of elimination and it sounds like this: "He does not deserve to live. He does not deserve to be on this planet."

**Violence** is anger and hatred in action. It might take the form of striking, throwing things, screaming, and physical, sexual and emotional abuse.

**Murder** may be actual murder or premeditated, which is murder in the heart, or murder with the tongue, such as gossip.

### Why is Bitterness Sin?

By holding onto bitterness, you are telling God He is not needed in this situation. You have placed yourself in His shoes by judging someone else for what they have done, either to you or to someone close to you. Your heart says, "God, I will execute judgment here." But, Scripture clearly tells us vengeance belongs to the Lord (Romans 12:19).

God's Word states that unless we forgive those who trespass against us, God will not forgive us our sins (Matthew 6:15; Mark 11:26). This is why bitterness (which is rooted in unforgiveness) must be eliminated first.

## Accusing Spirits

**Now is come salvation, and strength, and the kingdom of our God, and the power of his Christ: for the accuser of our brethren is cast down, which accused them before our God day and night. Revelation 12:10**

We have all experienced the destructive work of accusation. It accuses us to ourselves, to others and to God. Accusing spirits are subtle in their charges. Remember, even 90 percent truth mixed with just a 10 percent lie still equals error. This mixture is deadly because it can subject believers to condemnation instead of conviction.

It is important to distinguish between conviction and condemnation. Conviction is specific and endorses our value in God. Condemnation, on the other hand, tends to be vague and brings with it feelings of worthlessness. Conviction brings us to a point of wanting to get closer to God and in line with His Word, while condemnation drives us away from God and brings feelings of wanting to give up.

Some of the fruits of accusation are: holding a record of wrongs, murder with the tongue (gossip and slander), mind control, scrambling thoughts, chaotic thinking, jumbled thought patterns, misunderstandings, projected fear, accusing another in your own sin, burden bearing and becoming codependent in another's sin by attempting to be their Holy Spirit.

### What Makes Accusation a Sin?

By accusing someone, you are telling God He is not needed in a particular situation. You have placed yourself in His shoes by deciding what would be right or wrong for someone else. Your heart says: "God, I will decide good and evil here." Then you take great joy in sharing your "valuable" opinion with all.

**Knowledge puffeth up, but charity edifieth. 1 Corinthians 8:1b**

## Occultism

**And no marvel; for Satan himself is transformed into an angel of light. 2 Corinthians 11:14**

Satan's counterfeits offer up different ways of thinking than are revealed in the Scriptures. They offer up another Jesus and another kingdom.

They may outwardly appear good, but beware of our enemy's disguises as an angel of light.

## What Makes Occultism a Sin?

In occultism, the real truth is obscured—something or someone has been set up to be your god. You are worshipping a *part* of creation (either God's or man's) while you may be under the impression you are worshipping God. Be it blatant or subtle, it is still idolatry. Your heart says, "This is where I place my trust, God. I do not need You anymore."

## What Makes Alternative Medicine a Sin?

Alternative medicine also provides an answer outside of God. It is not saying these modalities have no power, but where is the power coming from? When all hopes are put on such practices for healing, there is no place for God. One then chooses to put all trust in a practitioner, his potions and abilities, instead of in God. This again is a subtle form of idolatry.

> Beloved, believe not every spirit, but try the spirits whether they are of God: because many false prophets are gone out into the world. 1 John 4:1

> [7]Which is not another; but there be some that trouble you, and would pervert the gospel of Christ. [8]But though we, or an angel from heaven, preach any other gospel unto you than we have preached unto you, let him be accursed. [9]As we said before, so say I now again, If any man preach any other gospel unto you than that ye have received, let him be accursed. Galatians 1:7–9

## Envy and Jealousy

> A sound heart is the life of the flesh: but envy the rottenness of the bones. Proverbs 14:30

> For wrath killeth the foolish man, and envy slayeth the silly one. Job 5:2

> And he said unto them, Take heed, and beware of covetousness: for a man's life consisteth not in the abundance of the things which he possesseth. Luke 12:15

Envy, jealousy and covetousness take your eyes off of God and fix them upon a person, a place or a thing. The person or material object will then become the source of your supply of value and fulfillment. This is idolatry! God will not share us with false gods or idols.

Whatever you worship is your god. Thus God, in His jealousy, will release you to your own devices without His protection. If money is your god, then money will have to protect you.

Envy produces strife. Not listening to envy produces peace. Remember, Satan's mission is to divide the body of Christ, destroy relationships, wreck marriages, break up families and cause animosity between neighbors.

## What Makes Envy and Jealousy Sin?

By harboring envy and jealousy, you compare yourself to others. This brings discontentment as you accuse God of being a respecter of persons. Your heart says: "God, I know my needs better than You do. Why are You not supplying them?"

Envy and jealousy really are subtle forms of unbelief and doubt. You do not really trust God to provide for you.

> Let your conversation be without covetousness; and be content with such things as ye have: for he hath said, I will never leave thee, nor forsake thee. Hebrews 13:5

> Pleasant words are as an honeycomb, sweet to the soul, and health to the bones. Proverbs 16:24

## Rejection

> The spirit of a man will sustain his infirmity; but a wounded spirit who can bear? Proverbs 18:14

The Word of God tells us we are loved, adopted and accepted, but rejection has an assignment to steal those truths away from us. We all know the deep sting of rejection, because we are all born with an innate longing for love and acceptance. The effects of agreeing with rejection can be physically and psychologically devastating.

## What Makes Rejection a Sin?

Accepting rejection (real or imagined) disagrees with who God says we are. It places man's acceptance as more important than God's. Your heart says: "God, You lied when You said that I was worthy. I would rather believe what other people think of me."

Rejection will lead us on a desperate search, striving for the love that will complete us. This love cannot be found in people, places or things, but only in God!

> [4]According as he hath chosen us in him before the foundation of the world, that we should be holy and without blame before him in love: [5]Having predestinated us unto the adoption of children by Jesus Christ to himself, according to the good pleasure of his will, Ephesians 1:4–5

## Unloving Spirits

> [37]Jesus said unto him, Thou shalt love the Lord thy God with all thy heart, and with all thy soul, and with all thy mind. [38] This is the first and great commandment. [39] And the second is like unto it, Thou shalt love thy neighbor as thyself. Matthew 22:37–39

The unloving spirit rejects everything God has said about you in His Word (you are fearfully and wonderfully made, etc.) and replaces God's Word with Satan's blatant lies. These deceptions will prevent you from loving God, loving yourself and loving others. It blocks you from receiving this love as well as from giving it.

Many of us have not grown up in a godly, loving environment. This hinders us from an early age in receiving the very love we crave so much.

### What Makes Unloving Spirits a Sin?

You only believe yourself. This can occur two ways. In one way, you may believe you are not worthy of God's love or acceptance. In the other way, you may believe yourself to be better than everyone else. You are God's gift to mankind. This is self-idolatry. Your heart says: "Step aside, God. I am in charge here."

> No man hath seen God at any time. If we love one another, God dwelleth in us, and his love is perfected in us. 1 John 4:12

## Addiction

> Now the works of the flesh are manifest, which are these; Adultery, fornication, uncleanness, lasciviousness, Galatians 5:19

Remember, one can be addicted to almost anything: drugs, alcohol, sex, food, shopping, or anything to distract us from the feelings of being unloved.

Each person is created to know and to receive God's perfect love. When people have not received true, unconditional love as a foundation, they are always in search of getting a need fulfilled. The need to know God's love can open us up to look for love in all the wrong places. This need leaves us vulnerable to the deception of Satan, who seduces us into believing the world offers us a better substitute.

### What Makes Addiction a Sin?

You are saying through your actions that God is not able to meet your needs. Your heart says: "God, I need a fix that You cannot supply. I will get it myself." Our comfort must be in God, not in people, places or things.

> **Peace I leave with you, my peace I give unto you: not as the world giveth, give I unto you. Let not your heart be troubled, neither let it be afraid. John 14:27**

## Fear

> **For God hath not given us the spirit of fear; but of power, and of love, and of a sound mind. 2 Timothy 1:7**

Fear means being afraid, scared, worried, anxious and concerned that a bad thing is going to happen. It is projecting into the future. Fear, then, is the opposite of faith. Fear and faith are equal. They both project into the future and both demand to be fulfilled. The bottom line is: which authority are you going to listen to?

## What Makes Fear a Sin?

God's Word tells us over 365 times to "fear not."

By entertaining the spirit of fear, your actions are saying you cannot trust God and you have to take control of your own life. Your heart says: "God, I just do not trust You. You cannot meet my needs as my protector."

> **And he said unto his disciples, Therefore I say unto you, Take no thought for your life, what ye shall eat; neither for the body, what ye shall put on. Luke 12:22**

## Traumas and Doorpoints

God has set parameters of protection around mankind against the devil. Yet there are ways he can get a foothold. We call these doorpoints of entry.

Traumas and doorpoints are the incidences in your life giving entry to these bad roots. These points of entry could be in your own life or in your family tree.

Different phases or events of life bring their own traumas. Doorpoints around birth and early childhood could be issues of abandonment in the event of unwanted pregnancy. This allows a spirit of rejection to enter into the unborn child. When parents divorce, children question their own worth and this may give entry to unloving spirits. Due to sickness, we may engage in alternative therapies, giving entry to occultic spirits.

## Repentance

Now that we have identified these roots of sin, we have to break association and agreement with them. This requires repentance and renouncement. (See Teaching Unit 5 on the 8 Rs to Freedom.)

Gaining freedom from these roots of sin is not a ritual. Even though we have included a sample prayer, repentance must first come from the heart. David talked about the humility God respects in his psalms. Rote words are meaningless to God. It is a relationship He's looking for.

> **The Lord is nigh unto them that are of a broken heart; and saveth such as be of a contrite spirit. Psalm 34:18**

A broken spirit cries out, "God, I need you. I cannot do this by myself."

## Guidelines for Communication with God (Prayer):

Scripture indicates our petition is directed to God the Father and not to Jesus. Yet our petition is made in the name of Jesus. (Also refer to Block #3: *No Relationship with God According to Knowledge* for further clarification.)

> **And in that day ye shall ask me nothing. Verily, verily, I say unto you, Whatsoever ye shall ask the Father in my name, he will give *it* you. John 16:23**

Your communication with God should therefore include the following elements:

- Confession of your participation with sin

- Deliverance from the bondage to sin

- Thanksgiving for forgiveness of sin and removal of its curse

An example of such communication with God may be:

*Father God,*

*I come to You in the name of Jesus and I acknowledge the work of sin in my life, as well as in my family tree. I confess to You my own sin and the iniquity of my forefathers. I take responsibility in my life for _____ and I renounce it. I repent for the work of sin in my life.*

*I confess I have allowed bitterness to work through me. I choose not to hold bitterness against _____ anymore. I let go of any bitterness against myself or even You.*

*I ask You to forgive me for participating with this sin.*

*I release myself from this behavior and thought life. I will not allow bitterness in my life again. I ask that the curse of _____ [this disease], which is the fruit of bitterness in my life, be canceled.*

*In the name of Jesus Christ of Nazareth, all bitterness must leave me now.*

*Father, I thank You for forgiveness of my sin and for the restoration of my body in the name of Jesus. Amen.*

### Healing vs. Miracles

It may be appropriate to speak healing to your body as well. If you need healing of some tissue, such as the regrowth of skin or the mending of a broken bone, then speak healing to your body in the name of Jesus. For those tissues that do not have regenerative powers, such as organs and nerve tissue, speak a creative miracle to those tissues in the name of Jesus.

Remember, as a believer, you are given the authority to speak things into being in the name of Jesus!

> **Jesus answered and said unto them, Verily I say unto you, If ye have faith, and doubt not, ye shall not only do this which is done to the fig tree, but also if ye shall say unto this mountain, Be thou removed, and be thou cast into the sea; it shall be done. Matthew 21:21**

"What if I do not get healed?" This is a very valid question.

Once we are delivered from these roots of sin, it becomes our responsibility to renew our minds and change those old patterns of ungodly thinking. We call this process "Walk Out."

Your thought life is **your** responsibility. Do you cast down imaginations or do you keep hitting the replay button? Are you filled with the Word of God or with those bitter words from your earthly father chewing you out? Your walk-out will be a daily exercise. Do not be discouraged—it does get easier!

As we walk out of our ungodly thinking patterns into *a more excellent way*™ of living, let us also consider our brothers and sisters who may be in a similar process. Please extend the same amount of grace to them that you might expect in return.

> **Brethren, if a man be overtaken in a fault, ye which are spiritual, restore such an one in the spirit of meekness; considering thyself, lest thou also be tempted. Galatians 6:1**

## Separation (Romans 7)

I want to take you into Romans 7 and give you a case history of a believer and a leader named Paul. Do you want to go past discernment into freedom? Paul is our example.

In Romans 7:15, Paul is speaking about himself. Paul is a believer. He's not only a believer—he's been an apostle for at least 20 years. He's talking about his life and his challenges in living a Christian life.

> [14]**For we know that the law is spiritual: but I am carnal, sold under sin.** [15]**For that which I do I allow not: for what I would, that do I not; but what I hate, that do I. Romans 7:14–15**

Does that sound familiar? The things that I want to do, I do not do. The things that I hate, that's what I do.

Do you think Paul was sinless? Do you think I'm being disrespectful to him? There is only one man who was sinless, the man Christ Jesus. The rest of us are a bunch of sinners saved by grace, working out our salvation daily with fear and trembling.

> **For he *is* our God; and we *are* the people of his pasture, and the sheep of his hand. To day if ye will hear his voice, Psalm 95:7**

> **(For he saith, I have heard thee in a time accepted, and in the day of salvation have I succoured thee: behold, now *is* the accepted time; behold, now *is* the day of salvation.) 2 Corinthians 6:2**

> **And he said to *them* all, If any *man* will come after me, let him deny himself, and take up his cross daily, and follow me. Luke 9:23**

> **Wherefore, my beloved, as ye have always obeyed, not as in my presence only, but now much more in my absence, work out your own salvation with fear and trembling. Philippians 2:12**

Romans 7:16 goes on to say, if then I do those things that I wish I wouldn't do, I consent unto the law that it is good.

> **If then I do that which I would not, I consent unto the law that *it is* good. Romans 7:16**

Now let me bring you to a point. Paul is saying, If I do those things that are evil, I'm telling the law or the Word that this new law that I'm following (which represents evil) is good and the Word of God is evil. If then I do those things which I would not, I consent unto the Word that this new law that I'm following is the proper law.

Are we following a "different law" in our lives sometimes than the law of God? When the Word says "Forgive your brother," and we do not, are we following a different law, a different gospel, a different way of thinking? Do you ever see Christians who do not forgive people? Have you ever seen any Christians gossip? Have you seen any Christians shun another Christian? Have you ever seen Christians do evil?

In other words, what Paul is saying is that when he does those evil things he wished he would not do, he's consenting unto the law of God, that this thing that he should not be doing is good and that automatically puts him under the authority of another gospel. Do you see what I'm saying? When we hate our brother, we are affirming a new gospel that overthrows the gospel of our God. The gospel of God says to forgive our brother. When instead we hold onto that unforgiveness and bitterness toward our brother, we are in fact following a different law, a different gospel, a different way of thinking from that of God. Do you know any Christians who gossip or have bitterness and unforgiveness toward another?

It's very important that you understand that sin involves the overthrowing of the government, the laws and the precepts of God. By so doing we are establishing another gospel in the earth for mankind to follow to their destruction, not to their benefit. There's not enough emphasis put on this dimension of sin in the Church today. We've become so anti-social around the issue of sin because we do not like to think that we have sin in our lives as Christians. I'm sorry, but it is in the Bible. I try to teach it in such a way that I do not hit you over the head. I hope you do not feel like I'm oppressing you with truth. If I am, I apologize; I'll cut your cabbage for a hundred years.

I want you to understand that when we allow fear to rule our lives, we are affirming the gospel of fear. Fear destroys faith, which is of God. When we are allowing guilt to rule our lives, we're affirming the gospel of guilt to the destruction of forgiveness by God. It's very important that you understand that we are setting up one gospel or another. We're either establishing the law of the kingdom of God or we are establishing the laws of Satan's kingdom. You cannot have your cake and eat it too! You cannot serve two masters; either you are going to love the one or hate the other. That has to be understood in this discussion. It has to be understood with regard to certain diseases before you can be healed. You cannot be healed of *lupus* and hang onto self-hatred. It's just not going to happen.

> **No man can serve two masters: for either he will hate the one, and love the other; or else he will hold to the one, and despise the other. Ye cannot serve God and mammon. Matthew 6:24**

How do you figure that's possible? John says whosoever is born of God cannot sin.

> **Whosoever is born of God doth not commit sin; for his seed remaineth in him: and he cannot sin, because he is born of God. 1 John 3:9**

Does it mean we're not born again? "Whosoever is born of God cannot sin and he that sins is of the devil." How do you reconcile that with the rest of the canon of Scripture dealing with grace and mercy?

This brings us to a place where we are working out our own salvation daily by faith through grace and mercy. Our spots and our blemishes can be dealt with before the living God as the work of *sanctification*. God has taken the absoluteness of His position for us and He has shoved us back under the blood, grace and mercy.

Now we are in a car wash called *sanctification*. Paul is describing himself in the car wash and he's not been cleaned up yet. Neither have you. If you tell me you are sinless, I'm going to tell you that you are a liar. The Word says that whosoever says he has not sinned is a liar.

> **⁵This then is the message which we have heard of him, and declare unto you, that God is light, and in him is no darkness at all. ⁶If we say that we have fellowship with him, and walk in darkness, we lie, and do not the truth: ⁷But if we walk in the light, as he is in the light, we have fellowship one with another, and the blood of Jesus Christ his Son cleanseth us from all sin. ⁸If we say that we have no sin, we deceive ourselves, and the truth is not in us. ⁹If we confess our sins, he is faithful and just to forgive us *our* sins, and to cleanse us from all unrighteousness. ¹⁰If we say that we have not sinned, we make him a liar, and his word is not in us. 1 John 1:5–10**

These Scriptures are not addressed to unbelievers but are addressed to believers who sin after conversion. I heard someone say the other day, that if you sinned after conversion, you were never saved. I guess there are no Christians in the earth today. We all fall short of the glory of God every day, don't we?

> **For all have sinned, and come short of the glory of God; Romans 3:23**

There are many who say this verse only applies to unbelievers, yet I see many of the same sins in believers today as those that can be found in the unbeliever. *In both cases, saved and unsaved have fallen short of the glory of God. Both need to repent.* Let me ask you a question: Why would God require the unsaved to repent for a sin and not require the saved to repent of that sin? That would make God unjust and He would condone evil in the name of salvation. But the Scriptures refute this position.

> **⁶:¹What shall we say then? Shall we continue in sin, that grace may abound? ²God forbid. How shall we, that are dead to sin, live any longer therein? Romans 6:1–2**

Have you ever struggled with any insecurities and fears? Do you ever doubt, have suspicions, even doubt your salvation from time to time? Do you ever get into a place where you wonder if your wife loves you? Ever get to a place where you think your husband doesn't love you? Ever get into those places where you think God is a million miles away? Do you ever go through those valleys of the shadow of death? Do you ever go into those dry places?

I had a cartoon of a guy driving down the highway on the interstate. The sun was shining and then there was a line; there was a shaded area in the rest of the cartoon. It said, "Shaded area next 1460 miles." Have you ever been driving through life and you just drove into those shaded areas? The only thing you had going for you was that the sign said, "This will end some day."

Paul said that when he was doing things that were not right, it was no more he that did it (evil), but sin that dwelled in him.

> **Now then it is no more I that do it, but sin that dwelleth in me. Romans 7:17**

Let's think about this. Paul was an apostle, born again, filled with the Spirit of God, teaching righteousness, and *he's* saying *he* has sin within. *Paul needed ministry.*

If Paul needed help, what is our condition? These thoughts and blemishes, these "yucky-puckies," these "crispy critters," this stuff that I'm dealing with that produces disease involves the issue of sanctification. That is where the minister gets to come in and help you deal with it. It is in this ministry area where we confess our faults one to another that we may be healed.

> **Confess *your* faults one to another, and pray one for another, that ye may be healed. The effectual fervent prayer of a righteous man availeth much. James 5:16**

*We must separate ourselves from the sin that dwells within us and that dwells within our neighbor.* When you look at your neighbor, you are going to have to be able to separate them from their sin, to bring any kind of sanity into your Christian walk before God.

What happens when you see sin in your neighbor is that you make him the same as his sin. He's not sin and if he's a believer, he's the redeemed of God. He may have sin, but he is not sin. He is the one whom God saw from the foundation of the world. He's the one whom the Spirit of God lives within. He's the one who's being redeemed. He's the one whom God loves, but he's got some sin tagging along that needs to go. The sin needs to go; it's interfering with his sonship, interfering with his sanctification, interfering with his position before God and that is the area we need to deal with.

Discernment unto freedom requires separation—seeing sin for what it is. What I am about to teach you right here is the foundation for your freedom—that's discernment and separation. You must be able to separate yourself from the sin that dwells within you. You must be able to separate the sin that dwells within others from who they are as people. The day that I got this insight from Paul, in Romans 7, and saw that I needed to separate myself and my heart from the sin within, that is the day that *sanctification* began in my life: I was on my way to freedom. Our battle is not with flesh and blood but with entities from another kingdom.

> [12]**For we wrestle not against flesh and blood, but against principalities, against powers, against the rulers of the darkness of this world, against spiritual wickedness in high *places.* Ephesians 6:12**

> [12]**For the word of God *is* quick, and powerful, and sharper than any twoedged sword, piercing even to the dividing asunder of soul and spirit, and of the joints and marrow, and *is* a discerner of the thoughts and intents of the heart. [13]Neither is there any creature that is not manifest in his sight: but all things *are* naked and opened unto the eyes of him with whom we have to do. Hebrews 4:12–13**

We hear much quoting of verse 12, but seldom is verse 13 quoted along with it. Notice in verse 13 that the Word of God is making manifest those creatures that are within. That's those "yucky-puckies"/"crispy critters" that Paul is talking about in Romans 7. That's the stuff that I'm dealing with that produces disease. Dealing with this stuff for our healing and deliverance from these "yucky-puckies" that dwell within is the process of *sanctification.* No doctor of the physio can do this and no psychologist of the psyche can do this. This is in the realm of the spirit where the pastor and the Church must deal with the spirit of man with the Word of God.

I cannot forgive my brother unless I do separation. I cannot forgive myself if I do not do separation. Without separation, I have become one with the sin, but that's not who I am. I'm not one with sin. *I am not sin.* I'm Henry, thank you! I reserve the right to deal with sin, get it out of my life and remain Henry without it. When somebody victimizes me, I'm able to see the evil in them that they are now possessed with or under the control of that is now making a victim of me and I see it's not them. It's the sin that lives within them. So I can exchange compassion for bitterness according to the knowledge of God. We must come to the place that we stop making ourselves, our brother, our children, or our neighbor one with the thoughts and blemishes, "yucky-puckies," "crispy critters," and all the sin that manifests within our hearts.

Now in your own life you see that sin that dwells within and you know it yields the fruits of self-hatred, bitterness, unbelief, doubt, fear, jealousy, envy, competition and strife. Do you know that strife is found in the same verses as murder? adultery? fornication?

Romans 1:28–31, Mark 7 and Galatians 5 list many sins, all of which may be found in all Christians at one level or another.

> [28]And even as they did not like to retain God in *their* knowledge, God gave them over to a reprobate mind, to do those things which are not convenient; [29]Being filled with all unrighteousness, fornication, wickedness, covetousness, maliciousness; full of envy, murder, debate, deceit, malignity; whisperers, [30]Backbiters, haters of God, despiteful, proud, boasters, inventors of evil things, disobedient to parents, [31]Without understanding, covenantbreakers, without natural affection, implacable, unmerciful: Romans 1:28–31

> [15]There is nothing from without a man, that entering into him can defile him: but the things which come out of him, those are they that defile the man...[20]And he said, That which cometh out of the man, that defileth the man. [21]For from within, out of the heart of men, proceed evil thoughts, adulteries, fornications, murders, [22]Thefts, covetousness, wickedness, deceit, lasciviousness, an evil eye, blasphemy, pride, foolishness: [23]All these evil things come from within, and defile the man. Mark 7:15, 20–23

> [19]Now the works of the flesh are manifest, which are *these;* Adultery, fornication, uncleanness, lasciviousness, [20]Idolatry, witchcraft, hatred, variance, emulations, wrath, strife, seditions, heresies, [21]Envyings, murders, drunkenness, revellings, and such like: of the which I tell you before, as I have also told *you* in time past, that they which do such things shall not inherit the kingdom of God. Galatians 5:19–21

Why is that? Because we are not sanctified. That is what is causing our biological, spiritual and mental diseases. That is what we are talking about. Paul is pointing the finger right back at himself.

When I get to heaven, I'm going to find brother Paul. I'm going to get hold of that boy. I'm going to hug him and I'm going to say, "Paul, Chapter 7 of Romans saved my life." I could not separate myself from my sin and I felt yucky and pucky every way to Sunday. Then I realized I had an enemy. I really had a heart for God, but I had an enemy that had to go. *The day that I learned to separate myself and my heart from my sin is the day that sanctification in my life began.*

> [17]Now then it is no more I that do it, but sin that dwelleth in me. [18]For I know that in me (that is, in my flesh,) dwelleth no good thing: for to will is present with me; but *how* to perform that which is good I find not. Romans 7:17–18

That is, in my flesh. Now here's a situation where "flesh" does not mean the human body. It's talking about something of the old man, the old nature, the unrenewed part of him; something within him was not of God. The word "flesh" has to do with the carnal nature. Paul is not talking about his human flesh.

Paul goes on to say in verse 18, for I know that in me (that is, in my flesh) dwells no good thing: for to will is present with me but how to perform that which is good I find not.

Have you ever found yourself that way? Have you ever had a wonderful heart toward God and the harder you tried the behinder you got? Have you ever had struggles in your Christian walk where it just didn't come together as fast as you wanted it to?

You see the prototype. You look into the mirror, the perfect law of liberty and when you turn away, you see the sin, don't you? Do not forget what you saw in the perfect law of liberty, but back over here is the real you. That's what Paul is looking at. He's looking at sin with eyes of honesty.

In Romans 7:19, Paul said, the good that I wish I would do, I do not do it and the evil that I wish I wouldn't do, that's what I do.

> For the good that I would I do not: but the evil which I would not, that I do. Romans 7:19

What Paul said in verse 17, he repeats in Romans 7:20, which said, as I do those things that I wish I wouldn't do, it is no more I that do it but sin that dwelleth in me (is doing it).

> **Now if I do that I would not, it is no more I that do it, but sin that dwelleth in me. Romans 7:20**

He was talking about his carnal nature, that unrenewed part of him that didn't match the nature of God within him. He came to the realization that it was not him, for he knew his heart before God was to do good; so he concluded that it was something else that was within him that was doing it, that is, the sin; yet the conclusion of this is that it was sin that dwelt within, causing an action through Paul that became sin to him.

In this discourse of personal transparency in Romans 7, Paul said more than once, his conclusion was the evil he was doing in his life as a Christian and apostle was *not him doing it. He determined it was evil/sin that was dwelling in him, doing it through him.* Do you think he was recognizing his own need for deliverance? I think so. He's looking at himself with eyes of honesty.

Have you ever found yourself that way? You know you have a wonderful heart toward God and you want your nature to match His nature; but the harder you try, the behinder you get. The beginning of understanding is to be able to separate yourself from the sin that dwells within that is acting out its nature through you; thus the full meaning of Hebrews 4:12–13.

> [12]**For the word of God *is* quick, and powerful, and sharper than any twoedged sword, piercing even to the dividing asunder of soul and spirit, and of the joints and marrow, and *is* a discerner of the thoughts and intents of the heart. **[13]**Neither is there any creature that is not manifest in his sight: but all things *are* naked and opened unto the eyes of him with whom we have to do. Hebrews 4:12–13**

### *This is where healing of disease begins.*

This sin that dwells within Paul is identified in Hebrews 4:13 as the creatures that need to be made opened and naked before Him with whom we have to do.

> [21]**I find then a law, that, when I would do good, evil is present with me. **[22]**For I delight in the law of God after the inward man: **[23]**But I see another law in my members, warring against the law of my mind, and bringing me into captivity to the law of sin which is in my members. **[24]**O wretched man that I am! who shall deliver me from the body of this death? Romans 7:21–24**

Paul very clearly stated that evil was present with him and that law (sin/evil) was in his members, warring against the law of his mind and bringing him into captivity against the *law of sin* which was *in* his members. He was asking for deliverance right up front and he told us the answer in verse 25:

> **I thank God through Jesus Christ our Lord. So then with the mind I myself serve the law of God; but with the flesh the law of sin. Romans 7:25**

Romans 8 is a continuation of chapter 7. There should not be a new chapter. Before we go to chapter 8, I want to give you a story of something that happened about 10 years ago.

I had a Christian man call me. He was a businessman who had heard that I was helping people get straightened out in life. He had all kinds of problems in his business and problems in his life and marriage. He called me and I listened to him for a while. I said, "Brother, you've got sin in your life."

He said, "Brother, you err." I said, "How do I err?"

He said, "Have you not heard the Word of God?" I said, "Yes. What do you have in mind?"

He said, "In Romans 8:1, it says there is therefore now no condemnation to them that are in Christ Jesus. So I'm a free man and I'm free of sin and the consequences of it." I said, "Why don't you read the rest of that verse?"

He said, "There isn't any more."

He was reading from the *New International Version* (NIV) text. The NIV says this: "There is therefore now no condemnation to them that are in Christ Jesus." But the Majority Text (King James Version) says it a little differently. I'll read it to you.

Romans 8:1 says that there is therefore no condemnation to them that are in Christ Jesus, who walk not after the flesh but after the Spirit.

> ***There is*** **therefore now no condemnation to them which are in Christ Jesus, who walk not after the flesh, but after the Spirit. Romans 8:1**

I said, "Brother you have blown it. You're on the wrong side of the road. I want you to notice that it says there is condemnation to them who walk after the flesh. Yes, there is no condemnation to them who walk after the Spirit. You're following after the old nature, the old man. You're following after the lust of the flesh in your life, your business and your family. Condemnation is here because the only place that you're free from condemnation under the law is if you're walking after the Spirit of God."

When you step outside those parameters, you are back under the law again and there is a consequence. Your freedom is directly related to your obedience. There is a consequence to sin and disobedience to God's Word

(Deuteronomy 28). That's not legalism; that's simply what Jesus meant when He said, If you love Me, you will keep My commandments.

**If ye love me, keep my commandments. John 14:15**

*Keeping God's commandments is not legalism.*
*Taking God's commandments and forcing them*
*down someone's throat is legalism.*

The letter of the law killeth, but the spirit of the law giveth life.

**Who also hath made us able ministers of the new testament; not of the letter, but of the spirit: for the letter killeth, but the spirit giveth life. 2 Corinthians 3:6**

If I could bring you the spirit of the law and let God the Holy Spirit convict you in your hearts and liberate you, then let you keep your sin if you want to, would that be all right? *No*, it wouldn't be all right.

Paul is dealing with an issue. He's saying, I myself serve the law of God, but I've got a problem. I have a problem in my life. I've got sin that dwells within me. Do you think he was just playing with us, or do you think he really meant that?

*Fear is sin. Unforgiveness is sin. Strife is sin. Self-hatred is sin. Heresy is still sin. Adultery is still sin. Lasciviousness is still sin. Backbiting is still sin. Causing church splits is still sin. Jealousy and envy are still sin.*

The disciples made a very serious mistake. They didn't wash their hands before dinner and the Pharisees caught them. Jesus picked up this discussion in Mark 7:15: There is nothing from without a man that entering into him can defile him, but the things which come out of him, those are they that defile the man.

**There is nothing from without a man, that entering into him can defile him: but the things which come out of him, those are they that defile the man. Mark 7:15**

It's not what goes in your mouth that defiles you; *it's what comes from within you, out of your mouth.*

Mark 7:16–23 says, If any man have ears to hear, let him hear. And when He was entered into the house from the people, His disciples asked Him concerning the parable and He saith unto them, Are you so without understanding also? Do you not perceive that whatsoever thing from without entereth into the man, it cannot defile him because it entereth not into his heart but into the belly and goeth out into the draught purging all meats? Then He said, *That which cometh out of the man, that defileth the man. For from within, out of the heart of men,* proceed evil thoughts, adulteries, fornications, murders, thefts, covetousness, wickedness, deceit, lasciviousness, an evil eye, blasphemy, pride, foolishness: *all these evil things come from within, and defile the man.*

> **20And he said, That which cometh out of the man, that defileth the man. 21For from within, out of the heart of men, proceed evil thoughts, adulteries, fornications, murders, 22Thefts, covetousness, wickedness, deceit, lasciviousness, an evil eye, blasphemy, pride, foolishness: 23All these evil things come from within, and defile the man. Mark 7:20–23**

Jesus was identifying the "yucky-puckies" within the spirit of man that defile the man. Paul recognized this in Romans 7 and then we find Paul developing it as a spiritual principle of sanctification for the *Church* in 2 Corinthians 7:1.

Paul was talking about spiritual defects in the area of the human spirit.

Second Corinthians says that since we have these promises, we should cleanse ourselves from all filthiness of the flesh and spirit, perfecting holiness in the fear of God.

> **Having therefore these promises, dearly beloved, let us cleanse ourselves from all filthiness of the flesh and spirit, perfecting holiness in the fear of God. 2 Corinthians 7:1**

Paul was addressing the believer, not the unbeliever. Very clearly, Paul was setting the stage for something called sanctification subsequent to salvation. In 1 Thessalonians 5:23, Paul again brought emphasis to sanctification as a very important first step to produce wholeness.

> **And the very God of peace sanctify you wholly; and *I pray God* your whole spirit and soul and body be preserved blameless unto the coming of our Lord Jesus Christ. 1 Thessalonians 5:23**

Jesus was talking about what is in the heart of man that needs to be dealt with. Paul also picked up the topic in 2 Corinthians, 1 Thessalonians and in Romans 7 and said that it applied not just to himself but to every one of us.

I'm working out my salvation daily through grace and mercy, applying the love of the Father, the Word of God and the work of the Holy Spirit, so that my heart, my spirit man, can be purged of all evil. My poor head gets the picture finally and I become *one* in my thoughts spiritually (spirit) and psychologically (soul) so I can fulfill the Scriptures. I am in the process of putting on the mind of Christ. From glory to glory, I am being changed into His image.

> **But we all, with open face beholding as in a glass the glory of the Lord, are changed into the same image from glory to glory, *even* as by the Spirit of the Lord. 2 Corinthians 3:18**

This is the process of *sanctification*, starting to remove spiritual, biological and psychological diseases of life, both generationally and personally. When we get before God and take an honest look at ourselves, when we survey our past generations and deal with the sin we find, we then come before God to let Him "work us over."

The Lord is saying to you today, "I'm here knocking. Would you open the door of your heart? Would you let Me come in with the Holy Spirit and cleanse you, sanctify you and remove the things that are separating Me from you? Could I heal you, could I deliver you, could I establish My heart for you? Would you enter into that degree of covenant with Me? Could I be a God to you? Could I be a Savior to you? Could I be a Healer to you? Could I be a Redeemer to you? Could I be a Husband to you? Would you fellowship with Me?

> [19]**As many as I love, I rebuke and chasten: be zealous therefore, and repent.** [20]**Behold, I stand at the door, and knock: if any man hear my voice, and open the door, I will come in to him, and will sup with him, and he with me. Revelation 3:19–20**

This Scripture in Revelation is not addressed to unbelievers. It is addressed to a New Testament church at Laodicea. The Lord is not in their hearts when they think He is, but He is outside. I find this a tragic picture of the Church today. I do not want to hear these words being said to Him, "Yea Lord," and He saying to me, "Depart from Me; I never knew you."

> [20]**Wherefore by their fruits ye shall know them.** [21]**Not every one that saith unto me, Lord, Lord, shall enter into the kingdom of heaven; but he that doeth the will of my Father which is in heaven.** [22]**Many will say to me in that day, Lord, Lord, have we not prophesied in thy name? and in thy name have cast out devils? and in thy name done many wonderful works?** [23]**And then will I profess unto them, I never knew you: depart from me, ye that work iniquity. Matthew 7:20–23**

Romans 6:6 says, Knowing this that our old man is....

"*Is*" is a present tense positional statement. Everyone considers this to be an historical happening, but, in fact, that historical happening is a present tense application in which we daily work out our own salvation with fear and trembling.

> **Wherefore, my beloved, as ye have always obeyed, not as in my presence only, but now much more in my absence, work out your own salvation with fear and trembling. Philippians 2:12**

Because of what Jesus did for us at the cross, according to Romans 6:6, it is now possible that the body of sin might be destroyed today in your life. Because of our positional obedience, we should not be serving sin, although many do and that's not historical, that's present tense.

### *Has the body of sin been destroyed in your life*
### *or are you still serving sin today?*

> **Let not sin therefore reign in your mortal body, that ye should obey it in the lusts thereof. Romans 6:12**

It does not say that sin is **not** reigning in your body today. It says that you **should not** let it reign and you should not obey it.

> **Neither yield ye your members *as* instruments of unrighteousness unto sin: but yield yourselves unto God, as those that are alive from the dead, and your members *as* instruments of righteousness unto God. Romans 6:13**

It does not say you are **not** yielding your members as instruments of unrighteousness. Paul is saying you **should not** be. You should be yielding yourself to God and your members as instruments of righteousness unto God.

In that setting of obedience and application, grace makes it possible for the power of the law to be broken. Sin will not have dominion over you, but in many sectors and teachings, grace has now become a license to sin.

Paul, in verse 15, asks this question: What then? shall we sin because we are not under the law, but under grace? God forbid.

> **For sin shall not have dominion over you: for ye are not under the law, but under grace. What then? shall we sin, because we are not under the law, but under grace? God forbid. Romans 6:14–15**

In conclusion, in verse 16 the big question is this: "Who is your master and what are you a servant to? Sin unto death or obedience unto righteousness?" If you decide to serve sin, then sin becomes your lord and you become its slave.

> **Know ye not, that to whom ye yield yourselves servants to obey, his servants ye are to whom ye obey; whether of sin unto death, or of obedience unto righteousness? Romans 6:16**

## Romans 8:1

Finally, one of the tragedies of the Bible translations is the removal of one half of Romans 8:1. In removing the second part of Romans 8:1, the conditions of not being condemned in Christ Jesus have been removed. In fact, many translations now just say, "There is therefore no condemnation to those who are in Christ Jesus," but Paul conditioned this freedom to those who are walking after the Spirit. Those who continue to walk after the flesh bring themselves back into condemnation and Satan has a legal right to their life until they repent.

> ***There is*** **therefore now no condemnation to them which are in Christ Jesus, who walk not after the flesh, but after the Spirit. Romans 8:1**

Paul identified something within himself and it was called sin. Maybe it's time for us to recognize that it wasn't just in him. It may be in each of us and the fruit of our service to sin is spiritual, psychological and biological disease.

# 7 Steps to Sin

There is a place of rest for the people of God, but they do not rest because of unbelief or because of getting out ahead of God by fighting their own enemies themselves. There's a time to defeat an enemy and there is a time of preparation before you take your enemy on for size.

*Before you can defeat sin,*
*you need to understand what is occurring within you.*

**And he said, "That which cometh out of the man, that defileth the man. For from <u>within</u>, out of the heart of men proceed evil thoughts..."**
**Mark 7:20–21**

So, when have you committed a sin and when haven't you? This is a reality to set you free.

*There are seven steps to a completed sin.*

## 1. TEMPTATION

The first step to sin is temptation.

*Temptation is the thought of evil.*

Temptation comes in the form of thoughts—without exception! No matter what the sin is, it starts as a part of your thinking process. It can be so strong that it feels as if it has already happened. Many people sin simply because they had the thought of sin and they therefore think they have sinned already, so they go ahead and actually sin.

*Temptation is not sin.*

*You do not have to sin just because you feel like doing it.*

With temptation, there is always something within us that has nothing to do with anyone else. There may be temptation or evil in another person that hooks up with the temptation or evil in you and the two start working against each other so both people fall. Especially in relationships between husbands and wives and churches, there may be temptation or evil within you to hook up with the temptation or evil in the other person. Then the two start working against each other and both people fall because of anger or bitterness or strife.

### *Lust is not just a sexual thing.*

Even if temptation involves as simple a thing as having a disagreement with your brother or sister in the Lord, the process of lust is there. Lust includes everything. We have many examples written to us personally from the Old Testament. First Corinthians 10:6 says,

> **Now these things were our examples, to the intent we should not lust after evil things, as they also lusted. 1 Corinthians 10:6**

Lust includes exalting ourselves over another in every area of our existence, whether from jealousy or envy or bitterness or hatred or whatever. Your self-exaltation and self-fulfillment is idolatry. You are king and everything revolves around you.

### *Satan wants to steal your faith because whatever is not of faith is sin.*

> **But without faith it is impossible to please him. Hebrews 11:6**

Every problem and every temptation you have already exists within your spiritual makeup. Satan comes with his kingdom to exploit your weakness. You could have a thousand temptations, but there is one you are going to fall in. Satan will always work on you at your weakest link. Most of your trials and tribulations and temptations are already spiritual problems in your life.

Job was perfect in a lot of ways, yet he had weaknesses. He was full of pride and fear. He tried to be God over his family, making sacrifices for his children. The thing he feared most came upon him.

> **...for Job said, It may be that my sons have sinned, and cursed God in their hearts. Thus did Job continually. Job 1:5b**

> **For the thing which I greatly feared is come upon me, and that which I was afraid of is come unto me. Job 3:25**

There is incorrect teaching that says that when you are tempted, it is God's way of teaching you something.

> **Let no man say when he is tempted, I am tempted of God: for God cannot be tempted with evil, neither tempteth he any man. James 1:13**

Everything that is going on, as a temptation to you, is common in the world.

> **There hath no temptation taken you but such as is common to man: but God is faithful, who will not suffer you to be tempted above that ye**

are able; but will with the temptation also make a way to escape, that ye may be able to bear it. 1 Corinthians 10:13

You can quit praying for God to remove the temptation. He wants you to defeat it. He will make provision for you so you can overcome. It has to be dealt with because it comes from within and is already in place. It is already a problem.

The difference between "defeat" and "resist" is this: "defeat" is permanent; "resist" indicates there is still a battle taking place.

That the trial of your faith, being more precious than of gold that perisheth, though it be tried with fire, might be found unto praise and honor and glory at the appearing of Jesus Christ. 1 Peter 1:7

*God wants you to defeat temptation because,*
*in the day you don't,*
*it becomes your sin*
*and you are fellowshipping with devils.*

But I say, that the things which the Gentiles sacrifice, they sacrifice to devils, and not to God: and I would not that ye should have fellowship with devils. 1 Corinthians 10:20

All evil in mankind comes from within the heart of a man, woman or child.

And he said, "That which cometh out of the man, that defileth the man. For from within, out of the heart of men proceed evil thoughts..." Mark 7:20–21

Jesus was tempted in all points such as we are.

For we have not an high priest which cannot be touched with the feeling of our infirmities; but was in all points tempted like as we are, yet without sin. Hebrews 4:15

Every demon of hell was looking for Him to trip up so they could have a legal right to come into His Spirit and cause Him to become sinful. Satan personally tempted Jesus at the highest level possible—spiritual intellectualism and pride.

### *There is a blessing in the midst of temptation.*

Blessed is the man who endureth temptation: for when he is tried he shall receive the crown of life which the Lord hath promised to them that love him. James 1:12

Every temptation you face is an open door to God's blessing. Every trial you have is a stepping-stone to success.

## 2. BEING DRAWN AWAY

The second step to sin is becoming preoccupied with a thought. To be drawn away is to have a strong imagination about a temptation, to start to view it and to let your mind be drawn to it. At this stage, sin is starting to form a reality in you. It is not just an idle thought; it is starting to take form.

***Being drawn away is still not sin.***

## 3. PERSONAL LUST

The third step is the forming of the sin.

**...when he is drawn away of his own lust... James 1:14b**

You have a strong imagination and you start to take pleasure in watching what is in your mind and in your thoughts. It is no longer an idle thought. First you had the thought and then you had the strong imagination. Next you sit back and turn your mind's TV on and start to take pleasure in watching what is in your mind and your thoughts. This is still not sin. It is an evil spirit integrating itself with you and you are starting to weaken and fall into agreement with it simply because you are entertaining the thoughts.

An evil spirit is like a projector; it projects images in you because of its nature and it wants to fulfill its nature and make you a sinner in that area. You think it is you because you have fallen into agreement and started becoming one with it, which is the process of you becoming ***prepared to sin***.

## 4. ENTICEMENT

The fourth step to sin is enticement. Enticement is the weakening of the will. You can have every feeling and seemingly enjoyment of a lustful thought in any area of your life. The object is to weaken your will because Satan wants you to act it out.

***The ploy is to get you to start weakening,***
***to get you to yield your will to what the temptation is.***

If Satan can break down your will so you are no longer resisting him, then he has you in motion to commit a sin.

**...Resist the devil and he will flee from you. James 4:7b**

## 5. LUST CONCEIVED

The fifth step to sin is "lust conceived." You cannot have sin until you have lust conceived. Lust conceived is the birthing of something not in place yet. The entire weakening of the will is occurring and you are about to come into agreement with it so it can be birthed within you. It is also a yielding.

*Lust conceived is the entrance into the physical of what is spiritual.*

At this stage it is very difficult not to sin because your total will has yielded to what the temptation represents.

## 6. ACTUAL SIN

The sixth step to sin is the actual sin.

*There are many people who say something with their hearts but not with their mouths. They still have a completed sin in their heart because they are one with it and in full agreement with it.*

It is your choice to reject a thought or dwell on it.

**That whosoever looketh on a woman to lust after her hath committed adultery with her already in his heart. Matthew 5:28**

Any person in agreement with a thought in his or her heart will eventually act on that thought.

## 7. THE CONSEQUENCES OF SIN

The seventh step to sin is the actual consequence of sin.

*The result of sin is death.*

**...and sin when it is finished bringeth forth death. James 1:15b**

Sin not repented for brings spiritual death. It also opens the door to curses in your spirit, soul and physical body. It opens the door for sin to rule you, to reign and to destroy and have dominion over you. Unless it is repented for, dealt with and cast out, it will be continually there to tempt you.

*If a person has fasted, prayed, cried out to God and done everything they could to get rid of a sin, but they keep doing it, they need deliverance because it is no longer just temptation, it is an evil spirit.*

When temptation comes, you can see the process. You can find yourself in the seven steps so you will recognize temptation is not sin. You can start dealing with Satan and your adversaries according to knowledge.

**Prayer:** Father, I thank You for Your Word. God, I hope this has set a lot of Your people free to overcome. God, I trust that this word has set things in place to assist them in becoming more mature in their overcoming. God, I do not ask You to deliver them in spite of the evil. I ask You to deliver them in the midst of the evil so they may be victorious and You may be glorified. And all the people said, Amen.

Chapter Five
# The 8 Rs to Freedom

## Pathway to Wholeness and Freedom

1. **Recognize**

*You must recognize what it is.*

2. **Responsibility**

*You must take responsibility for what you recognize.*

3. **Repent**

*You must repent to God for participating with what you recognize.*

4. **Renounce**

*You must make what you recognize your enemy and renounce it.*

5. **Remove**

*You must get rid of it once and for all.*

6. **Resist**

*When it tries to come back, you must resist it when it tries to come back.*

7. **Rejoice**

*Give God thanks for setting you free.*

8. **Restore**

*Help someone else get free.*

## 1. Recognize

### *You must* Recognize *what it is*

Recognize the problem—have discernment. In Isaiah 5:13, God said, My people have gone into captivity because they have no knowledge. They had no discernment. In Hosea 4:6, God said, My people perish for lack of knowledge. They had no discernment. Hebrews 5:14 tells us that strong meat belongs to those that are full aged, even those that by reason of use have their senses exercised to *discern* both good and evil. Not just good—you must be able to discern evil also.

> **Therefore my people are gone into captivity, because *they have* no knowledge: and their honourable men *are* famished, and their multitude dried up with thirst. Isaiah 5:13**

> My people are destroyed for lack of knowledge: because thou hast rejected knowledge, I will also reject thee, that thou shalt be no priest to me: seeing thou hast forgotten the law of thy God, I will also forget thy children. Hosea 4:6

> But strong meat belongeth to them that are of full age, *even* those who by reason of use have their senses exercised to discern both good and evil. Hebrews 5:14

You say, "I'm afraid of evil." Shame on you. Where did you get that from? Watching too much of *The Exorcist*? Why would you be afraid of evil? Are you telling me Satan is greater than God? "Well, something bad might happen to me." Yeah, it might. So what? Why are we afraid of evil?

If I said you had a particular disease because you had a root of bitterness against someone and had not resolved it, what would I have given you? **Discernment**.

If I told you your breast cancer is because you hated your Mama, what would I have given you? **Discernment.**

All right, so what is going on if you have hatred toward Aunt Sally? The principality bringing the hatred into play was bitterness. Hatred is one of the fruits of bitterness.

If you have someone who is angry and hostile, what can you tell them? "You have a root of bitterness." If you find someone who has resentment, what could you tell them? "You have a root of bitterness." When you see bitterness, you can also tell them this: *"If you do not get this under control in your life, the chances of your getting a disease as a bad fruit of this is very likely in your lifetime."*

Now what have you given them? **Wisdom**. Knowledge to put into action.

There are two gifts of the Holy Spirit taught in 1 Corinthians 12. One is the gift of wisdom and the other is the gift of knowledge. What am I giving you now? I am operating in the gift of knowledge and the gift of wisdom in your life right now. I am also operating in the gift of faith, discerning of spirits, knowledge, wisdom, and if need be, I can operate in the gift of healing and the gift of miracles.

Do you know every believer should be participating at some level in this area? 1 Corinthians 12 teaches that *the Church is designed to heal the Church*. Ephesians 4 says pastors are supposed to equip you and bring you to the place where you can do that (regarding the body of Christ healing itself). I first have to be able to demonstrate it.

*Knowledge ties the past to the present,*
*but wisdom takes the present and moves it to the future.*

We are taking your past and bringing it to the present so you can see what in the world is going on in your present state. Then God, through wisdom, can take you into the future to change your circumstances. It's going to take faith and the work of the Holy Spirit to do the rest of it, but we have to be able to teach first because faith comes and hearing by the Word of God (Romans 10:17).

> **So then faith *cometh* by hearing, and hearing by the word of God.**
> **Romans 10:17**

Remember in Jeremiah 3, God said He would give you pastors according to His heart to teach you, lead you and give you understanding.

> **And I will give you pastors according to mine heart, which shall feed**
> **you with knowledge and understanding. Jeremiah 3:15**

I am a pastor; you are the sheep of His pasture and I am an under-shepherd who cares for you just as much as He does. I am not here to fill your head with a bunch of knowledge. I came here to break the power of the devil working in your lives and release you. Your freedom was paid for 2,000 years ago on the cross and the power of God was released into your lives so you can get on with it. He wants you to be free.

I have found many people like being sick because it is the first attention they have received in their life. Do you want to be well? Do you want to be sane? Good! If I come along and put my finger on the stuff making you sick, those creatures from Hebrews 4:13, what are you going to do with them?

You say, "That was a nice time. I'll see you," and you walk out the door taking all those crispy critters with you. It's a lot of work keeping up with a zoo like that!

> **Neither is there any creature that is not manifest in his sight: but all**
> **things *are* naked and opened unto the eyes of him with whom we have to**
> **do. Hebrews 4:13**

## 2. Responsibility

### *You must take* Responsibility *for what you recognize*

After you recognize, the Holy Spirit comes to convict you with discernment. Then the second "R" is to take responsibility. Not everybody wants to take responsibility after discernment. It really bugs me when someone says to me after discernment, "Well, bless God, that's just the way I am." What happened to the Scripture that says, "From glory to glory we are being changed"?

> But we all, with open face beholding as in a glass the glory of the Lord, are changed into the same image from glory to glory, *even* as by the Spirit of the Lord. 2 Corinthians 3:18

"Well that's for someone else. If God wants to change me, He's just going to have to do it."

God couldn't do it if He tried. You won't let Him.

"Bless God, I'm angry; I always have been angry. I am always going to be angry and if you don't like it, I'll eat you for lunch."

Are you going to lock yourself into, "Well, I'll forgive them if they forgive me first"? What are you going to do?

> For I acknowledge my transgressions: and my sin *is* ever before me. Against thee, thee only, have I sinned, and done *this* evil in thy sight: that thou mightest be justified when thou speakest, *and* be clear when thou judgest. Psalm 51:3–4

Someone is going to have to get spiritual. Do you think the other person needs to get spiritual first, or do you need to get spiritual first? Take *responsibility.*

## 3. Repent

### Repent *to God for participating with what you recognize*

*Repent* is the third "R" you need to do in order to be free. Acts 3:19 says:

> Repent ye therefore, and be converted, that your sins may be blotted out, when the times of refreshing shall come from the presence of the Lord; Acts 3:19

Do you want the times of refreshing to come from the Lord in your life? Are you tired of the blistering heat of disease? Are you ready for the oasis? You won't get there unless you go here first: *repent.*

> Therefore I will judge you, O house of Israel, every one according to his ways, saith the Lord GOD. Repent, and turn *yourselves* from all your transgressions; so iniquity shall not be your ruin. Ezekiel 18:30

> If we confess our sins, he is faithful and just to forgive us *our* sins, and to cleanse us from all unrighteousness. 1 John 1:9

> And the seed of Israel separated themselves from all strangers, and stood and confessed their sins, and the iniquities of their fathers. Nehemiah 9:2

Remember from whence thou art fallen and repent and do the first works; or else I will come unto thee quickly:

> Remember therefore from whence thou art fallen, and repent, and do the first works; or else I will come unto thee quickly, and will remove thy candlestick out of his place, except thou repent. Revelation 2:5

Repent or else I will come quickly:

> Repent; or else I will come unto thee quickly, and will fight against them with the sword of my mouth. Revelation 2:16

And I gave her space to repent of her fornication and she repented not.

> And I gave her space to repent of her fornication; and she repented not. Behold, I will cast her into a bed, and them that commit adultery with her into great tribulation, except they repent of their deeds. Revelation 2:21–22

Remember and hold fast and repent:

> Remember therefore how thou hast received and heard, and hold fast, and repent. If therefore thou shalt not watch, I will come on thee as a thief, and thou shalt not know what hour I will come upon thee. Revelation 3:3

As many as I love, I rebuke and chasten. Be zealous therefore and repent.

> As many as I love, I rebuke and chasten: be zealous therefore, and repent. Revelation 3:19

## 4. Renounce

***You must make what you recognize your enemy and* Renounce *it***

After you have repented, which means taking responsibility after recognition and discernment, the next step is to renounce. A lot of people repent, but they do not mean it. A lot of people have remorse, but they do not change on the inside. To repent literally means to "turn away from." There are many Scriptures in the Bible where God told us to get away from idols and heathen practices because they will be our ruin.

> [21]Ye cannot drink the cup of the Lord, and the cup of devils: ye cannot be partakers of the Lord's table, and of the table of devils. [22]Do we provoke the Lord to jealousy? are we stronger than he? 1 Corinthians 10:21–22

Get away from evil—*renounce* it as fast as you can. Develop a perfect hatred for evil in your life. Separate yourself from the evil. Love yourself, but hate the evil. Love your neighbor, but hate the evil he does. Learn to separate yourself and others from their sin.

## 5. Remove It

***Remove* it—get rid of it once and for all**

The fifth "R" to freedom is *remove* what you have renounced. I can bring you to a place of recognition (which is discernment) responsibility, repentance and renouncing openly what evil stands for in your life, but have you removed it? Removing sin is this: not only do I renounce you, but you and I cannot exist at the same place at the same time together. I am removing you; you have to go.

In Ezekiel 18, God's people were complaining that it was not fair for God to bless and forgive the unrighteous who repent yet not forgive them, the chosen ones. After all, they were the children of covenant. They also continued to live in their sin. They were wondering why God did not bless them. God's response to them was very clear.

> **Cast away from you all your transgressions, whereby ye have transgressed; and make you a new heart and a new spirit: for why will ye die, O house of Israel? Ezekiel 18:31**

That is, remove it. Get it out of your face and make yourself a new heart and spirit.

## 6. Resist

### *When it tries to come back,* Resist *it*

Number six of the 8 Rs to freedom is to *resist.* James 4:7 says that we are to submit ourselves therefore to God. Then, *Resist* the devil and he will flee from you.

> **⁷Submit yourselves therefore to God. Resist the devil, and he will flee from you. James 4:7**

What comes first? *Resist* the devil and he will flee, or submit to God? *Submission to God first; then you have power over your enemies, not before.*

Remember, earlier I quoted from 2 Corinthians 10:6: "Having a readiness to avenge all disobedience after your obedience is fulfilled." Do you remember what Samuel told Saul? First Samuel 15:23: "Obedience is better than sacrifice, for rebellion is as the sin of witchcraft and stubbornness is as idolatry." (Self-will, self-exaltation, witchcraft and idolatry.) This is a tough Scripture, isn't it? "Obedience is better than sacrifice."

What you have dealt with will try to come back. That is why we need God and each other.

> **When the unclean spirit is gone out of a man, he walketh through dry places, seeking rest; and finding none, he saith, I will return unto my house whence I came out. Luke 11:24**

## 7. Rejoice

### Rejoice—*give God thanks for setting you free*

The next "R" is *rejoice*. Give God glory for your freedom. Give God thanks that a piece of dust like you could experience grace and mercy from a living God Who loves you. He's worthy of your praise. The greatest song of worship and power and majesty is in Isaiah 35:1–10.

> The wilderness and the solitary place shall be glad for them; and the desert shall rejoice, and blossom as the rose. It shall blossom abundantly, and rejoice even with joy and singing: the glory of Lebanon shall be given unto it, the excellency of Carmel and Sharon, they shall see the glory of the LORD, *and* the excellency of our God. Strengthen ye the weak hands, and confirm the feeble knees. Say to them *that are* of a fearful heart, Be strong, fear not: behold, your God will come *with* vengeance, *even* God *with* a recompence; he will come and save you. Then the eyes of the blind shall be opened, and the ears of the deaf shall be unstopped. Then shall the lame *man* leap as an hart, and the tongue of the dumb sing: for in the wilderness shall waters break out, and streams in the desert. And the parched ground shall become a pool, and the thirsty land springs of water: in the habitation of dragons, where each lay, *shall be* grass with reeds and rushes. And an highway shall be there, and a way, and it shall be called The way of holiness; the unclean shall not pass over it; but it *shall be* for those: the wayfaring men, though fools, shall not err *therein*. No lion shall be there, nor *any* ravenous beast shall go up thereon, it shall not be found there; but the redeemed shall walk *there:* And the ransomed of the LORD shall return, and come to Zion with songs and everlasting joy upon their heads: they shall obtain joy and gladness, and sorrow and sighing shall flee away. Isaiah 35:1–10

Give Him thanks that pieces of dust like us can be redeemed for His glory.

## 8. Restore

### Restore—*help someone else get free*

Isaiah 42 talks about *restoring* others. After you have received the blessings of God, the eighth "R" is the fruit of the gospel. This is you helping others and restoring them.

> But this *is* a people robbed and spoiled; *they are* all of them snared in holes, and they are hid in prison houses: they are for a prey, and none delivereth; for a spoil, and none saith, Restore. Isaiah 42:22

Part of restoring is bringing the gospel to those you love, instructing those sinners who are being separated from the refreshing of the Lord and discipling them.

[12] Restore unto me the joy of thy salvation; and uphold me *with thy free spirit.* [13]*Then* will I teach transgressors thy ways; and sinners shall be converted unto thee. Psalm 51:12–13

## There is a challenge in Isaiah 58:

[58:1]Cry aloud, spare not, lift up thy voice like a trumpet, and shew my people their transgression, and the house of Jacob their sins.

[2]Yet they seek me daily, and delight to know my ways, as a nation that did righteousness, and forsook not the ordinance of their God: they ask of me the ordinances of justice; they take delight in approaching to God.

[3]Wherefore have we fasted, *say they,* and thou seest not? *wherefore* have we afflicted our soul, and thou takest no knowledge? Behold, in the day of your fast ye find pleasure, and exact all your labours.

[4]Behold, ye fast for strife and debate, and to smite with the fist of wickedness: ye shall not fast as *ye do this* day, to make your voice to be heard on high.

## The fast we are called to:

[5]Is it such a fast that I have chosen? a day for a man to afflict his soul? *is it* to bow down his head as a bulrush, and to spread sackcloth and ashes *under him?* wilt thou call this a fast, and an acceptable day to the Lord?

## Reach out to a stranger. Make a difference to your family.

[6]*Is* not this the fast that I have chosen? to loose the bands of wickedness, to undo the heavy burdens, and to let the oppressed go free, and that ye break every yoke?

[7]*Is it* not to deal thy bread to the hungry, and that thou bring the poor that are cast out to thy house? when thou seest the naked, that thou cover him; and that thou hide not thyself from thine own flesh?

## Benefits of restoring others:

[8]Then shall thy light break forth as the morning, and thine health shall spring forth speedily: and thy righteousness shall go before thee; the glory of the Lord shall be thy rereward.

[9]Then shalt thou call, and the Lord shall answer; thou shalt cry, and he shall say, Here I *am.* If thou take away from the midst of thee the yoke, the putting forth of the finger, and speaking vanity;

[10]And *if* thou draw out thy soul to the hungry, and satisfy the afflicted soul; then shall thy light rise in obscurity, and thy darkness *be* as the noonday:

[11]And the Lord shall guide thee continually, and satisfy thy soul in drought, and make fat thy bones: and thou shalt be like a watered garden, and like a spring of water, whose waters fail not.

[12]And *they that shall be* of thee shall build the old waste places: thou shalt raise up the foundations of many generations; and thou shalt be called, The repairer of the breach, The restorer of paths to dwell in. Isaiah 58:1–12

Bear one another's burdens:

Brethren, if a man be overtaken in a fault, ye which are spiritual, restore such an one in the spirit of meekness; considering thyself, lest thou also be tempted. Bear ye one another's burdens, and so fulfil the law of Christ. For if a man think himself to be something, when he is nothing, he deceiveth himself. Galatians 6:1–3

The members should have care one for another:

That there should be no schism in the body; but *that* the members should have the same care one for another. And whether one member suffer, all the members suffer with it; or one member be honoured, all the members rejoice with it. 1 Corinthians 12:25–26

Chapter Six
# The Gifts of the Spirit

Recognizing, taking Responsibility, Repenting, Renouncing and Resisting may not be enough to produce your freedom. What then? You may need ministry. I am looking for ministry teams all over America who can teach. We need teams who can teach churches how to heal the sick and cast out devils. Sometimes people just need a little help. In most churches today, apart from simple prayer, there are no ministry teams to heal disease, cure psychological problems and cast out devils. In fact, lots of churches teach against it. They teach it passed away a couple thousand years ago. I am not here to debate or come into conflict with your theologies. I will tell you this: God has worked many healings, miracles and deliverances at my hand and the hands of my staff. People all over America are suddenly realizing we've been "had." God can and does deliver and heal people today. The evidence is overwhelming that this is true.

## The Fivefold Ministry

Ephesians 4:11–12 teaches the fivefold ministry, of which I am a member, was given by Jesus Christ to equip the saints for service.

> **8Wherefore he saith, When he ascended up on high, he led captivity captive, and gave gifts unto men…11And he gave some, apostles; and some, prophets; and some, evangelists; and some, pastors and teachers; 12For the perfecting of the saints, for the work of the ministry, for the edifying of the body of Christ: Ephesians 4:8, 11–12**

Turn to 1 Corinthians 12; I want to lay a foundation for this teaching.

First Corinthians 12:27–30 says that you are the body of Christ and members in particular. God hath set some in the Church: first apostles, secondarily prophets, thirdly teachers, after that miracles, then gifts of healings, helps, governments and diversities of tongues. Are all apostles? (NO.) Are all prophets? (NO.) Are all teachers? (NO.) Are all workers of miracles? (NO.) Have all the gifts of healing? (NO.) Do all speak with tongues? (NO.) Do all interpret? (NO.)

> **27Now ye are the body of Christ, and members in particular. 28And God hath set some in the church, first apostles, secondarily prophets, thirdly teachers, after that miracles, then gifts of healings, helps, governments, diversities of tongues. 29Are all apostles? are all prophets? are all teachers? are all workers of miracles? 30Have all the gifts of healing? do all speak with tongues? do all interpret? 1 Corinthians 12:27–30**

Because it says that not everyone does these things does not mean there are not some who do these things. Some Christians claim because it says that not everyone does these, then "No one does it anymore." That is not how the Scripture reads. It just says that it's spread out through the body and among specific members in particular. I am a member in particular and you are a member in particular. Also, the Scriptures indicate it is God Who has set these things in the Church. No one has the right or the authority to pick and choose or add or delete anything found in these Scriptures. I am a member in particular and you are a member in particular.

First Corinthians says the manifestation of the Spirit is given to every man to profit withal.

> **But the manifestation of the Spirit is given to every man to profit withal. 1 Corinthians 12:7**

If I come and bring gifts of healing, deliverance, knowledge and discernment, what does this do for you? Does that bring profit to you?

To people who no longer have *lupus,* these gifts were to their profit. To people who no longer have depression, these gifts were to their profit. To people who no longer have fear and anxiety disorders, these gifts were to their profit. They were given to build them up.

Christ in heaven is not sick. His body in earth should not be either. Christ in heaven is not ignorant. His body in earth should not be ignorant.

Chapter 12 of 1 Corinthians identifies the gifts of the Holy Spirit available to the Church today.

> **⁸For to one is given by the Spirit the word of wisdom; to another the word of knowledge by the same Spirit; ⁹To another faith by the same Spirit; to another the gifts of healing by the same Spirit; ¹⁰To another the working of miracles; to another prophecy; to another discerning of spirits; to another *divers* kinds of tongues; to another the interpretation of tongues: 1 Corinthians 12:8–10**

These are gifts of God through the Church, given to bring us to a place of health.

The gift of healing is a gift available from God to stop the forward motion of disease and bring the power of God in so the body will heal.

There are parts of your bodies that do not heal. That is why we have organ transplants. Most nerve tissue does not regenerate. Brain tissue does not regenerate and organs do not regenerate. If God were going to regenerate something that could not be regenerated, then what kind of gift would it take? The gift of miracles.

If an evil spirit had a hold of your life, then you would need what? Discerning of spirits. What good is it to discern a spirit if you cannot get rid of it? Discerning of spirits involves eviction of spirits from God's precious people.

So we have three dimensions of healing: (1) the healing of body tissue, (2) the regeneration of body tissue, and (3) the removal of things alien to us spiritually. Then we can stand before our God and give Him glory because we have just profited from His blessings. *God receives no glory from your disease.*

John 9:1–3 is the Scripture about the blind man the Lord healed. The disciples asked him if this was because of his sin or his parents' sin. Jesus said, "No, this is for the glory of God."

> **⁹:¹And as *Jesus* passed by, he saw a man which was blind from *his* birth. ²And his disciples asked him, saying, Master, who did sin, this man, or his parents, that he was born blind? ³Jesus answered, Neither hath this man sinned, nor his parents: but that the works of God should be made manifest in him. John 9:1–3**

Many people take that Scripture and claim this disease was for the glory of God. *Not at all!*

It was the *healing* of the disease that was for the glory of God. Jesus did not stop and not heal him. If the disease had been for the glory of God, Jesus would have backed off and said, "Sorry, this disease is for the glory of God." He did not say that; He healed him. This miraculous healing by the Lord was for the glory of God. *This healing is something called greater grace.* It was God's absolute mercy. I have seen people take this Scripture and say disease is for the glory of God.

The Word says God receives no glory if we end up in the grave prematurely.

> **For the grave cannot praise thee, death can *not* celebrate thee: they that go down into the pit cannot hope for thy truth. Isaiah 38:18**

The grave cannot praise Him; only you can praise Him in your generation (see the story of Lazarus in John 11).

Why do you think 1 Corinthians 12 says, "God has set some in the Church?" Why? Is it there for a reason? It is because sometimes Recognizing, taking Responsibility, Repenting, Renouncing and Resisting do not produce freedom in itself. It takes someone coming along representing God and using the gifts of God to deal with it in ministry. This is why we need ministers back in the Church and saints ministering one to another under the oversight of the fivefold ministry.

We need people of God, who are anointed by God, raised up by God according to the Word of God, filled with the Spirit of God to do the works of God, to edify the body of Christ and bring them back to health and sanity. This is what our ministry represents. This is our calling.

I am a gift of God to you. I am a gift of God because I am a member of the *fivefold ministry* of Ephesians 4. I am a pastor designed to equip, train and bring to service those in the body so they can start taking care of the body. God intended for you to heal each other through the gifts and through the work of the Holy Spirit and you don't need me to do it. You should be doing it, although the work of the pastor includes more than just equipping, training and bringing to service. It must include the care of those who will be used. *So many times we have directed our attention only to others who are in need at the expense of who we are in need.*

In James, the question is asked and answered: "Is there any sick among you? Call for the elders of the Church."

> **[14]Is any sick among you? let him call for the elders of the church; and let them pray over him, anointing him with oil in the name of the Lord: [15]And the prayer of faith shall save the sick, and the Lord shall raise him up; and if he have committed sins, they shall be forgiven him. [16]Confess *your* faults one to another, and pray one for another, that ye may be healed. The effectual fervent prayer of a righteous man availeth much. James 5:14–16**

First Corinthians 12 teaches us the body is supposed to take care of the body. The references given here in 1 Corinthians 12 to the gifts of the Holy Spirit are not just meant for the church leaders but are also directed to the lay people, the saints. The leadership is directed to set an example so all believers can do the work of the ministry. That means the leadership and the saints are to be equally equipped.

*It is very clear in 1 Corinthians 12
that the body is to take care of the body
in all matters of health and sanity.*

Chapter Seven
# Fear, Stress and Physiology

There are many diseases falling under this category with a spiritual root of fear. One of the diseases is Multiple Chemical Sensitivities/Environmental Illness (MCS/EI).

## Multiple Chemical Sensitivities/Environmental Illness (MCS/EI)

Most people we deal with who have MCS/EI have been devastated for anywhere from 5 to 20 years. Most of them are "universal reactors." I want to give you an idea of just how extensive a healing can be by giving you a couple of personal case histories. As I read these conditions, keep in mind these people are totally healed today.

**Case History One.** This particular person had 17 peripheral diseases and has been well for over 18 years. Prior to intervention by this ministry, her general prognosis was "guarded."

1. Diagnosed with multiple chemical sensitivity as a universal reactor, this individual was allergic to all foods and chemicals which caused an anaphylactic shock reaction including throat closure. She was at one time naked due to the inability to wear any clothing, even white cotton clothing. She was down to only one least reactive food and had to live in foil lined rooms in the mountains or near the ocean. Oxygen and adrenaline were necessary for survival. This condition was ongoing for 10 years.
2. Electromagnetic Field Sensitivity (EMF) was so bad this person would have heart attack type symptoms and at one point could not turn on a 20–watt lightbulb or use heaters during winter months.
3. Diagnosable chemical injury exposure: Exposed for 1½ years to a 40 percent solution of formaldehyde left uncovered in the workplace.
4. Immune Disorders:
   a) Helper/suppressor cells were inverted
   b) Abnormal elevated complement C-3: 212 (normal is 70 to 176)
   c) Complement total Hem lower than 20 (normal is 70 to 150)
   d) Low B cell count of 176
   e) Low T cell count of 700 (normal is 1000 to 2500)
NOTE: This person's immune system has been medically retested and is 100 percent normal.
5. Atypical organic brain syndrome (overall moderate to severe impairment)
   a) Mostly in the right hemisphere, affecting the limbic system/ hypothalamus and right frontal lobe

    b) Dyslogia—short-term memory loss/aphasias

    c) Had a drop of 25 points in IQ for 10 years

    d) Disequilibrium—loss of balance existed; this individual would fall several times a day

Today this person has tested totally normal in all brain functions.

6. Secondary hypoparathyroidism
7. Hypothyroidism since 1957; now medically verified to be "totally well."
8. Primary renal calcium leak (rare kidney disease)
9. Secondary estrogen deficiency due to total hysterectomy, multiple fibroid tumors and pre-cancerous cysts in both ovaries
10. Cervical and lumbar osteoarthritis with narrowing of C5/C6/L5—S1 interspaces—requiring braces, traction, Demerol and hospitalization
11. Leukopenia and neutropenia
12. Secondary kidney dysfunction due to previous renal shutdown and kidney dialysis (in coma for 1 month)
13. Chronic high sedrate (indicative of inflammation in body) for 10 years: 60–80 (0–20 is normal)
14. Positive IgE Rast test for traditional allergies (from childhood). Perennial allergic rhinitis (dust, molds, trees, animal danders, some foods, bee stings).
15. Psychiatric Disease

    a) Schizophrenia/paranoid catatonic episodes (began in 1962)

    b) Manic depressive/circular depressed (began in 1976)

    c) Multiple personalities: 14 (from age 5 to the year 1992)

    d) Had chronic suicidal ideation and attempts (since childhood, age 8)

    e) Anorexia nervosa/bulimia—had to be hospitalized and tube-fed (began in 1964)

(All of the above included obsessive-compulsive behaviors, free-floating anxiety and panic disorders.)

16. Chronic generalized myositis, diffuse arthralgias, tendonitis and bursitis, requiring cortisone injections into joint spaces
17. Chronic severe bladder infections

    **Case History Two.** This person had 21 peripheral diseases brought on by MCS/EI. General prognosis was "guarded." The illnesses started in 1973; the person was healed in 1993.

1. Immune dysregulation deficiency syndrome included chronic fatigue, universal MCS, food allergy, pollen and mold sensitivity
2. Marked allergy hypersensitivity, producing chronic reactive airway disease

    a) Extrinsic asthma

   b)  Obstructive sinusitis/laryngitis

3. Organic brain syndrome with cognitive impairment
   a)  Dyslogia—short-term memory loss/poor concentration and focusing
   b)  Dyslexic dysfunction
   c)  Disequilibrium

4. Diffuse arthralgias/myalgia/fibromyalgia syndrome
5. Marked neuromyasthenia
6. Chemical Injury
   Significant heavy metal toxicity:  Lead 132.6 (normal is below 57)
                                     Mercury 22.65 (normal is 0.63–6.72)
                                     Nickel 131.5 (normal is 18.5–53.8)
   a)  Job-related in manufacturing plant (lead/solders and fluxes, leading to nickel overexposure)
   b)  Deteriorating mercury silver amalgams in multiple dental restorations
   c)  Elevated levels of polychlorinated biphenyls and organo-chlorine pesticide residues
   d)  Heavy exposure to solvent-based marine paint

NOTE: This individual has been retested since healing in 1993. Results: all levels are normal.

7. Epstein-Barr virus
8. Hypothyroidism
9. Marked posterior pituitary dysfunction
10. Chronic blepharitis and lacrimal duct dysfunction (disorders of eyelids and eyes)
11. Electromagnetic fields dysfunction (EMF)
12. Chronic high cholesterol levels (both total and LDL)
13. Bulimia and anorexia (dating back to adolescence)
14. Significant candida antibodies
15. Temporomandibular joint (TMJ)
16. Diminished taste and smell
17. Chronic cervical spine, thoracic spine, as well as lumbosacral connective tissue dysfunction, as a result of several auto accidents
18. Increased susceptibility to viral infections
19. Parasites: entamoeba histolytica, entamoeba coli, entamoeba coli—precysts and trohozoites with inflammatory process
20. Chronic uni-polar depression (free-floating anxiety and hyperirritability)
21. Obsessive/compulsive disorder

     The depth to which God can move in your life is incredibly deep. God is still on the throne. He loves you and He still answers prayer. You need to really let that be part of your heart.

I bumped into MCS/EI in 1990. I received a phone call from a person who said, "I hear God is really using you in people's lives and I believe God can heal me through your ministry."

I said, "What do you have?" They said, "Multiple chemical sensitivity/ environmental illness and I'm allergic to everything. I was exposed to pesticides about 10 years ago. Since that time, my immune system has been damaged and I'm allergic to everything. I'm living in a single room. I cannot be with my family. I'm in a room where the floors are lined with foil. The walls are bare sheet rock; I'm sleeping on the dismantled springs of a box spring wrapped in a material especially conditioned for a year. I can eat hardly anything. I'm on oxygen and respirators. I cannot leave this room or be in the presence of one human being for too long."

I did not know anything about the disease, but I told them I would pray about it. I had some experience in the area of allergies and the healing of allergies. I was praying about it one day and I asked God what He wanted me to do. I had a release to get involved and I followed through. This was a wonderful decision of obedience on my part!

There are hundreds of thousands of people suffering from MCS today. It is one of the most rapidly growing diseases in America along with *chronic fatigue syndrome* and *electromagnetic field sensitivity* (EMF).

I said, "Okay, I'll go." I called the individual and said, "I will give you 10 days of my life." I said, "I will leave the ministry and what I'm doing here and I will fly to where you are. I do not want anything from you." I made arrangements to go to this one person for 10 days.

I was on the plane, flying across America to someone who did not know me and I did not know them. They were expecting to be healed, by God, through me, of a disease I knew nothing about. Would you like this assignment today? I just believed God was in it and He would talk to me and guide me through whatever I was supposed to do.

As I was on the plane with my Bible open, I had a conversation with my "Boss" about what I was supposed to do when I arrived. Now the pressure was building. I would be expected to do something. I knew I could pray, but about what? I was letting my fingers do the walking and the Holy Spirit do the talking. I asked God, "Is there anything in here? Have You said anything about this situation?" I was flipping through my Bible and I bumped into one Scripture. This Scripture had been there since the days of Solomon, approximately 3,000 years ago. It is in Proverbs.

> [22]**A merry heart doeth good** *like* **a medicine: but a broken spirit drieth the bones. Proverbs 17:22**

I began to study that Scripture and right there *I saw a connection between the spirit of man and disease.* There are people who teach there is no connection between the spiritual and the physical. This Scripture blows that concept out of the water for once and for all. I realized a broken spirit or a broken heart could have an impact on our health.

Then I started thinking about what is meant about being "dried up in the bones." It wasn't *osteoporosis* in this case because this individual was too young for it. This person did not have an anemic problem. Drawing back to my college days as a premed student, I started thinking about bones. What is in bones? Stuff. What kind of stuff? Red corpuscles and white corpuscles—the immune system. Part of the immune system is in the marrow of the bones. Another part is in the lymphatic system—the B and T cells. This Scripture was talking about bones. I thought about that and I said, "Wait a minute, it doesn't say that pesticides destroy the immune system."

The Word of God said a broken spirit or broken heart can destroy the immune system. I said, "Is it possible this individual was injured spiritually and emotionally at some point in their life?" I did not know.

I arrived there and went to the house. The individual asked me, "Has God shown you anything about my disease?" I said, "I do not know; I'm not sure. I have to ask you a question. I want to know who broke your heart. I want to know what happened to put this kind of dread within you."

From that point on, we had our hands full. I am happy to tell you that seven days later, this individual was at the Sizzler Steak House eating everything on that smorgasbord, eating everything in sight. We went to the local yogurt shop to eat hamburgers, French fries and yogurt. I talked to this individual recently by phone and asked if MCS/EI had ever come back since that day.

This was the beginning of my journey into MCS/EI. Since 1990, literally had hundreds of people have been healed from this disease all across America. They have been healed from the extremes of being forced by severe allergies to go naked, not able to wear clothes, unable to eat almost every known food, allergic even to water, with multiple allergies from EMF to exhaustion-type symptoms. These people today are living normal, productive lives with no relapse.

This ministry is considered "expert" in the healing of MCS/EI from coast-to-coast. There are people who specialize in the diagnosis, but they are not getting people healed. The environmental ecologist, the allergist with all modalities of Eastern mysticism, alternative modalities, allergy shots, rotation diets, sauna, supplements and other treatments have produced no healings of MCS/EI over the long-term. I have not been able to document any healing during the past twenty years, although there are some reports of people doing better. But again, this is just another form of disease management. I am here to say there are many, many people who are well today because of the involvement of our ministry in their lives. Hallelujah!

I have an article about why females lose the emotional end of marital spats. The guys are over it as soon as it happens; the women do not recover for a long time. The damage to the immune system in a female who comes from strife in the home is incredible. In America, 85 to 90 percent of the people who have MCS/EI are female. The reason why the female is the one who gets sick is because she is more susceptible to the spiritual and emotional damage. God created the female to be a responder to good strong spiritual leadership, not to abuse.

My finding in thousands of cases across America over the years is that MCS or EI is the result of a breakup in the human relationship between the person who has the disease and someone else. The other person is usually a close family member and one or more of four life circumstances is involved. I have found this in every person I have ministered to without exception. Here are the four life circumstances that exist collectively or singly in MCS/EI:

1) Verbal and/or emotional abuse

2) Physical abuse

3) Sexual abuse

4) Drivenness to meet the expectations of a parent in order to receive love

Concurrently, the individuals find themselves living in an atmosphere sterile of love and emotion and it seems like they are in a straight jacket as far as relationships are concerned.

MCS/EI is an *anxiety disorder* compromising the immune system to the degree that allergies, simple and complex, eventually develop. The only way to get MCS/EI healed is to break the anxiety syndrome so the immune system can be healed. Then the allergies will fall away. Many of the accumulated peripheral diseases go away. These include *candida, fibromyalgia, hypothyroidism* and an ongoing list. These peripheral diseases are no big deal once you understand how they gained a foothold to begin with. This is why, once the root has been dealt with behind MCS/EI, these individuals are surprised to find that *candida, fibromyalgia* and *hypothyroidism* no longer exist in their bodies. If you have MCS/EI and you are kind of scattered and smothered because of *candida*, don't worry about it. It'll go away. I do not minister to *candida* in people; I am wasting my time.

If I find *fibromyalgia* in conjunction with MCS/EI, I do not bother to minister to it either. I am wasting my time because it is the by-product of a root problem. *If you start chasing the fruit, then you are going to be just chasing a bunch of fruit. If you go to the root and get the root problem solved, then you will have good fruit one day.* This is ***a more excellent way***™.

I don't start on the outside. The allergist is starting on the outside. The allergist is trying to tell you to avoid everything. God said everything He made was not just good (Genesis 1:31); He said it was *very* good.

In our ministry, the first thing we want to do with people who are coming out of the food allergy profile is to let them get all the foods they ever wanted back into their lives. Do you like banana splits? Let's go for it. Do you want yogurt? Let's go for it. Do you like chocolate chip cookies? Let's go for it. What do you want? God only made good stuff!

This is from the *Dallas Morning News* (November 16, 1996) from an article called "Health and Science."

> **Hormonal reaction to stress is tied to disease, researchers say.** Stress and depression that send emergency hormones flowing into the bloodstream may help cause brittle bones in women, infections, and even cancer, researchers say.
>
> A natural *fight or flight* reflex that once gave ancient humans the speed and endurance to escape primitive dangers is triggered daily in many modern people, keeping the hormones at a constant hyper-readiness, experts say. Even some forms of depression bring on a similar hormonal state.
>
> "In many people, these hormones, such as cortisol, turn on and stay on for a long time," Dr. Philip Gold of the National Institute of Mental Health, one of the National Institutes of Health, said Friday. "If you're in danger, cortisol is good for you...but if it becomes unregulated it can produce disease."
>
> In extreme cases, this hormonal state destroys appetite, cripples the immune system, shuts down processes that repair tissue, blocks sleep and even breaks down bone, Dr. Gold said.
>
> He was among speakers of a two-day conference of the International Society for Neuroimmunomodulation, a group of experts who study the effects of stress and depression on physical disease.
>
> Dr. Gold presented a study of bone density among 26 women, half suffering from depression and half with normal emotional states. The depressed women all had high levels of stress hormones, he said.
>
> Although the women were about 40, he said those with depression uniformly "had bone density like that of 70 year old women. They were clearly at risk of fractures. The magnitude of bone loss was surprising."

What was the root? Fear, stress and anxiety. Continuing in the same article:

> A study at Ohio State University showed that routine marital disagreements can cause the *fight or flight* hormone reaction.

Dr. Janice Kiecolt-Glaser, a psychologist, said a study of 90 newlywed couples showed that marriage arguments were particularly damaging to women.

In the study, the couples were put into a room together with blood sampling needles in their arms. The blood samples could be taken at intervals without the subjects knowing it.

A researcher then interviewed the couples and intentionally promoted a discussion that aroused disagreement and argument.

"The couples were at a point in their marriage when they should be getting along well, when there should be little hostility," said Dr. Kiecolt-Glaser.

Yet, samples taken during the disagreements showed that the women experienced sudden and high levels of stress hormones, just as if they were in a *fight or flight* situation of great danger. The women also had steeper increases than the men.

The test continued through an overnight hospital stay and more blood samples were taken just before discharge. For the men, the blood hormone levels were back to normal, but the women still had high levels.

Remember what Ephesians tells us:

**²⁶Be ye angry, and sin not: let not the sun go down upon your wrath: Ephesians 4:26**

Do you understand why this Scripture is in the Bible now? Do you think God knows what can happen to us because of these spiritual dynamics of our life going wrong? God is saying that if you do not get this thing under your belt by sundown, you have disease beginning to take hold in your body by the morning.

Medical science is telling you the same thing.

Romans tells us,

**¹⁸If it be possible, as much as lieth in you, live peaceably with all men. Romans 12:18**

It is more fun living in peace, don't you think? Isn't it more fun? They tell me it takes only about 17 or so muscles to smile and 30 or 40 to frown. Strife is considered a work of the flesh in the Bible. In fact, the Bible says that where there is strife, there is every evil thing.

**¹⁶For where envying and strife *is,* there *is* confusion and every evil work. James 3:16**

**¹⁹Now the works of the flesh are manifest...strife...of the which I tell you before, as I have also told *you* in time past, that they which do such things shall not inherit the kingdom of God. Galatians 5:19–21**

Would you consider strife to be a sin or a form of recreation? It is dangerous recreation!

Remember what Dr. Kiecolt-Glaser said: The stress hormone levels showed the women were more sensitive to negative behavior than were the men.

> People with such high levels of stress hormones are at a much greater risk of getting sick, said Dr. Ronald Glaser, an Ohio State virologist and the husband of Dr. Kiecolt-Glaser.

> "If the hormone levels stay up longer than they should, there is a real risk of infectious disease," he said.

By the way, there is some evidence that the Gulf War Syndrome may be an *anxiety disorder*. From the *Houston Chronicle*, May 28, 1998, in studies concerning the Gulf War ills, the most common conclusion is that it is a *stress disorder disease*.

Our ministry has been dealing with an individual in another state, a female, who was in the Gulf War with her husband. She came down with a combination of what seemed to be CFS, MCS/EI and Gulf War Syndrome. As we have been plowing into her case history, the evidence indicates it is not bacterial, it is not poison, it is not chemicals. **It is fear** that is the cause of her disease. If I were a female in the Gulf War, I think I too would be afraid. If I were a guy in the Gulf War, I think I would be afraid. It was a fearful (fear-filled) situation for everyone.

I also have an article taken from the World Wide Web about an organization doing research into MCS/EI. They have been tapping into something we have been teaching for almost twenty years. This article has to do with the limbic system. It is basically unfolding the mechanisms of the limbic system involving anxiety, fear, allergies and a compromised immune system involving the hypothalamus. Dr. Iris Bell also has an article printed in support of this insight into MCS/EI.

We are finding that in order to get someone healed of MCS/EI, they have to be freed on two levels: spiritually and psychologically. Mankind is programmed on two levels. You think with your *spirit man and* you think with your *head*. It is your long-term memory. We taught you this already; it involves protein synthesis, the RNA component, genetic component and long-term memory. Your long-term memory locks into your mind the objects of your fears, which are your stressors.

I will never forget the time I was proving this to an individual who came to us for ministry with MCS/EI. I told them, "I want to tell you that your EI reaction is based on the response of the hypothalamus gland, not a chemical." They doubted and did not believe me.

Most people do not believe me because the medical community is telling you just the opposite, especially in the MCS/EI community. We are

180 degrees diametrically opposed to where the medical community is coming from because they are still chasing allergies.

We are chasing what causes allergies and they have not even figured out there is a cause yet! They are calling it "chemical injury" or "chemical sensitivity." I want to tell you that people who have MCS/EI are, in fact, not reacting to any chemical. You have been had! You have been duped and deceived!

When you have a compromised immune system at that magnitude, when your killer cells and your B and T cells are compromised, when your lymphocytes are compromised at that level, you are going to react to everything.

How is it the other 98 percent of our population living in the same environmental setting, going to the same stores, schools, churches and buildings, do not have this problem? If the chemicals are causing the damage at that cellular level, we all would be down with some type of chemical poisoning.

We found that it is not the smell causing the reaction. The smell has programmed a response in you, i.e., fear. The smell is not what you are "allergic to" or "reacting to" and making you ill. The smell is the reinforcement of the mental and spiritual poisoning that keeps you in bondage and makes that smell a stressor. If you are afraid of mice, I will bring you a mouse and you will be on the chair in a split second. If I say there is a mouse, you will still be up on the chair lickety-split. The mass programming of the human mind has fear phobic realities.

I told this person their EI reaction was coming out of a response to their hypothalamus gland, not an exposure to a chemical. They did not agree with me. I bided my time and one day in a ministry session when I had a team with me, I casually walked to the window and said, "Oh! The bug man is here to spray." This individual went into an EI reaction just at the thought of it! They went catatonic and went into a massive EI reaction. They were not exposed to even one single chemical or smell. They came out of the EI reaction in about 10–15 minutes and I looked at this person and said, "There was no bug man." They got mad at me at first. I can handle it. The important thing was that they got the message. The same EI reaction occurred without the chemical or exposure to it and this individual knew they had been had! This same person is totally well today and praising God for their healing.

In a "**Walk Out**" we help a person take back every bit of ground they've lost. Every food, every building, every bit of clothing, everything they ever lost, they are going to take it back.

Well, we took this particular person out to eat at a barbecue restaurant. You know how wood smoke is to some people with EI. It is a major stressor.

We ordered this individual a good meal and the restaurant had just cranked up the barbecue pit with smoke pouring out the chimney. We got in the car and were starting to pull out. This person saw the smoke and, just at the sight of the smoke, was immediately staggering with an EI reaction. I looked at this individual and said, "Do you remember the bug man?" "Uh huh," was the reply. I told this individual, "We're going to park this car and watch barbecue smoke out of a chimney for our dessert."

This individual said, "You can't do that to me." I wheeled that car around with my team and stopped that car at the base of the chimney and we just sat there watching barbecue smoke pile out of the chimney. That day this individual took back wood smoke and never lost it again. Why? This person had been following the limbic system and was following a stressor. This mindset had been built deep in anxiety and fear. This person knew one more time that they had "been had."

**Editor's Note:** The above story was in context of ministry with qualified ministers. I would not want anyone to think this is simply a mind-over-matter situation. This was at a particular stage of **Walk Out** in this person's ministry.

I have an interesting article (from the World Wide Web) confirming what we teach. It says:

> The most vital component of the limbic system, the hypothalamus, governs: (1) body temperature via vasoconstriction, shivering, vasodilation, sweating, fever, and behaviors such as moving to a cooler or warmer environment or putting on or taking off clothing; (2) reproductive physiology and behavior; (3) feeding, drinking, digestive, and metabolic activities, including water balance, addictive eating leading to obesity, complete refusal of food and water leading to death; aggressive behavior, including such physical manifestations of emotion such as increased heart rate, elevated blood pressure, dry mouth, and gastrointestinal responses (Gilman, 1982).

> The hypothalamus is also the locus at which sympathetic and parasympathetic nervous systems converge. Many symptoms experienced by those with food and chemical sensitivities relate to the autonomic (sympathetic and parasympathetic) nervous systems; for example, altered smooth muscle tone produces Raynaud's phenomenon, diarrhea, constipation, and other symptoms reported by these individuals.

> The hypothalamus also appears to influence anaphylaxis and other aspects of immunity (Stein, 1981). Conversely, antigens may affect electrical activity in the hypothalamus (Besedovsky, 19th).

> **It is important to recognize that thoughts arising in the cerebral cortex that have strong emotional overtones also can trigger hypothalamic responses and recreate the physical effects associated with intense anger, fear, and other feelings.** To implement its effects, the hypothalamus not only has a direct electrical output to the nervous system but also produces its own

hormones, many of which stimulate or inhibit the pituitary's production of hormones (Gilman, 1982). Of interest in this regard, is that a disproportionate number of chemically sensitive individuals seem to have been treated for thyroid hormone deficiency at some time in their lives.

This is interesting, isn't it? It goes on and on about the biochemical mechanisms, the vascular mechanisms and so on. This is a secular article coming out of the medical community written by individuals who do research on some of the mechanisms of MCS/EI.

## MCS/EI Reaction Illustrated

Let's say we are up against our stressor. We have touched the "forbidden food"; we're around the "forbidden smell." Someone says the "bug man" is here and we are immediately programmed to think he is the enemy. Instantly, there is a hormone generated by the hypothalamus that goes into the bloodstream. It docks at a receptor cell of the muscles of the heart. The heart and respiratory rates start to increase, rapidity of breathing begins and it can go from slow all the way to panic. It can go so far that you reach a state of anaphylaxis, which is very dangerous because you can die from it. It can go to the extreme of catatonic realities. I have seen this happen in people's lives. *We have been very successful in breaking catatonic episodes, anaphylaxis and panic in every range of occurrence.*

In an EI reaction as we are exposed to our stressor, respiratory rate increases and rapidity of breathing produces something called hyperventilation. In hyperventilation, two things are happening: you have either a reduction of oxygen in the upper level of the brain or you have an increase of carbon dioxide levels. Hyperventilation interferes with getting the proper fuel to your brain cells; that is why, in the case of advanced EI reaction, individuals get fuzziness of thinking. They get "brain fog"; then they are diagnosed with organic brain syndrome. They have fuzzy thinking and as they lose their concentration and brain fog develops, *their fear intensifies*. These people feel like they are literally losing their minds. They cannot figure out what is happening. Fear comes; it increases. More fears develop; more hormones are released, more fears, more hyperventilation. Then they can reach the extreme of catatonic reality or anaphylaxis. It can go from calm to panic just like that, with a massive rush of hormones. Once the stressors and their impact have passed, the fear subsides, the body returns to normal and the EI reaction is over.

An EI reaction does not last forever; however, what does last "forever" is the next stage of this disease—*the resistance stage.*

If a "normal person" is crossing the street in traffic and somebody blows their car's horn, the person would jump. If I were to lay my hand on a hot stove, the alarm stage would come, *fight or flight* would kick in and I would quickly move myself out of the way. I would return back to normal. The parts necessary for homeostasis would kick back in, the parts for *fight or flight* would go away, my respiratory rate would come back to normal, my breathing would return to normal and I would resume a normal life style.

In people with an *anxiety disorder* such as MCS/EI, they never leave *fight or flight*. They move into the second level of this disease, *the resistance stage*. In the *resistance stage*, even though *fight or flight* is not so magnified, homeostasis never comes back to normal because the fear of the "enemy," the "stressor," is always there. That is why you start getting all the various forms of malfunctioning. All the peripheral diseases start to develop.

The first thing affected in the *resistance stage* is the thyroid. That is why most people who are in advanced stages of MCS/EI also have *Hashimoto's disease* and/or *hypothyroidism* which is an under-secretion of thyroxin. Unless someone has messed with the thyroid through radiation or through surgery, most people I have ministered to in the MCS/EI profile have been healed of either *hypothyroidism* or *Hashimoto's disease*, which the medical community would tell you is incurable. I am here to tell you it is curable through the grace of God when His conditions for spiritual healing are met.

Next to be affected is the liver. Right behind it is the adrenal cortex and at the very ionic base of your body, elimination of H+ ions, water retention and sodium retention occurs. All kinds of things start to happen, your body starts to go out of whack because the ionic base, the acidic levels and the alkalinity levels are all messed up.

The next little creature showing up in the marketplace in your life is *candida*. *Candida*, whether it is localized or systemic, is really a very painful disorder. It also does something else: it takes away your self-esteem. *Candida* in a female takes away her self-esteem because her sexual parts are usually affected first. Now we have some more complications because of this.

As the fear intensifies and as it becomes more and more obvious this thing is not going away, then the rudiments and the roots of *fibromyalgia* set in. Pain occurs with no reason behind it. When you have this kind of pain, your faith is under attack. The next thing is hopelessness, despair and more fear, and more and more of you shuts down. When you go to the doctor, I promise you're going to leave with more fear.

This ministry is one of the few in the world where you can come with MCS/EI, chronic fatigue syndrome and fibromyalgia and be told you can have a better day! The medical profession will tell you to avoid this and this and this. You can go to various practitioners, spend $30,000 or more and eventually they will send you either to the desert in Arizona or mountains and oceans *with* your disease to live in isolation for the rest of your life.

Is there anyone here with MCS/EI today? I don't know if you will be healed today, but I will say this: there hasn't been a seminar since I have been in ministry where someone who has had MCS/EI and listened to me teach hasn't experienced release from this disease and total healing within 30 days.

**Editor's Note:** When this seminar was taught in 1998, there was a person in the audience that day who was extremely afflicted with MCS/EI. For three days they laid on the floor in back with a face mask and listened to me teach about the roots of MCS/EI. This person is still well today after years of devastation.

I will say something else to you:

- **Do not be afraid!**

- **Do not look at your symptoms—they are a lie.**

- **You are not alone in this disease anymore!**

**Editor's Note:** Part of our program now involves training churches, pastors and ministries across America to understand these diseases and the roots behind them. If you are a pastor or the head of a ministry or an individual wanting to be trained to minister, please contact us.

The *resistance stage* of the *General Adaptation Syndrome* (GAS) allows the body to continue fighting a stressor long after the effects of the alarm reaction have dissipated. It increases the rate at which life processes occur. It provides the energy, functional proteins and circulatory changes required for meeting emotional crisis, performing strenuous tasks, fighting infection and so on. The *resistance stage* normally should carry you over to the recovery stage. But in MCS/EI there is no recovery. It just gets bigger and bigger. The body stays geared up to fight "the enemy" while the homeostasis needed for the bodily parts are still shut down. *The person is now geared up to fight this invisible threat all the time.*

At some point in this disease it goes to the third and final stage of a fear/anxiety disorder, the *exhaustion stage*. Occasionally the *resistance stage* fails to combat the stressor and the body gives up. In this case, the *General Adaptation Syndrome* moves into the stage of *exhaustion*. A major cause of exhaustion is loss of potassium ions. These are the biological, spiritual and emotional mechanisms that surround MCS/EI.

*I am still convinced that it is a disease of the broken heart.*

²²**A merry heart doeth good** *like* **a medicine: but a broken spirit drieth the bones. Proverbs 17:22**

When you have a broken heart, you have *fear*. When you don't feel safe, you have *fear*. When you have anxiety, you have *fear*. MCS/EI is particularly difficult because it compounds itself upon a foundation of fear that continues to grow.

¹⁸**There is no fear in love; but perfect love casteth out fear: because fear hath torment. He that feareth is not made perfect in love. 1 John 4:18**

From this standpoint of ministry, when dealing with MCS/EI, we bring a person to a place of safety. Safety first before God, secondly with themselves and thirdly with others. *There has to be a reconciliation in their heart at all three levels in order for healing to take place.*

Ultimately the healing of MCS/EI is the removal of the *General Adaptation Syndrome* (GAS) in all three parts of its components. The more fear and anxiety decreases, the more the immune system starts to heal. *Let's say it this way: the more we increase in fear and anxiety, the more the immune system is destroyed. The more the immune system is destroyed, the more we have an increase of allergies.*

As fear, anxiety and stress go away, the reactions go away and a person can take back five or ten foods very quickly. It is amazing to them. Why is it one day they are reacting to a particular food and the next day they find they can eat it—and eat it from that day on? What changed—the food? No, they did! The good news is this: You don't have the reaction but you can eat the food!

> **Audience Question:** I heard a tape on MCS/EI and your profile on the causes did not fit me. My daughter says they don't fit her. I am wondering if it's possible, in dealing with the concept of perfectionism and negativism, that MCS/EI could be the result of what is sometimes called church abuse or legalism rather than an early childhood situation involving a parent?

> **Henry Wright's Response:** Yes, I would say that it probably could be. Again we go back and look at verbal abuse, emotional abuse, physical abuse, sexual abuse and drivenness to meet the expectation of the parent. As we begin to continue to understand this disease, anytime we get trapped in a relationship or we come under the thumb of something taking away our sovereignty and suppresses us, there could be a type of fear that would develop. I have seen a couple of cases where MCS/EI realities have not started in childhood but came out of a marriage. I have seen situations where there has been oppressive legalistic abuse coming out of churches, crushing people's spirits and being very destructive.

This is something that I would be interested in talking further about. I certainly see it has merit and could be a root.

*Anything that takes away our freedom produces fear.*

Anytime we have been humiliated or we have been suppressed, the situation has the potential to produce fear. It is a form of brainwashing. It is a form of oppression and it is a form of abuse. Legalism and church suppression can be abusive and is as dangerous as sexual, physical and verbal abuse. It is a tragedy and it is a horrible sin.

*The elements of healing begin with trust.* Healing of MCS/EI begins with having the ability to trust again, to be vulnerable. I find those with MCS/EI do not want to be vulnerable because they do not want to take the risk of more rejection. They withdraw in a world of protective mechanisms.

One of the things I love to do in ministry is to make these guys and gals vulnerable. They are afraid to be vulnerable because they do not want to get trashed again. Could they dare believe? Could they dare love? Could they dare be vulnerable without being abused? Could I say then, MCS/EI is a total result of some type of victimization? Could I say that so we would not be so black-and-white as we are learning about the disease ourselves?

## Fear, Stress and Physiology Continued

### The Endocrine System

The endocrine system consists of the pituitary gland, the pineal gland, parathyroid glands, thyroid glands, thymus glands, adrenal glands, pancreas, ovaries, testes and hypothalamus. I am going to tell you where the hypothalamus gland is. How many of you have ever struggled with tension? When you have tension, do you ever have the back of your head hurt from tension? You remember which hand goes where? The hypothalamus gland is located in the third ventricle. This is where it starts to hurt. With tension, stress and pressure, you start to rub your neck, don't you? I check people for tension just by checking their neck out. That is the effect of stress and anxiety.

The hypothalamus gland is the "brain" of the endocrine system and it sends out various types of chemical messengers to the endocrine system. There are many types of hormones involved in stress and anxiety. The hypothalamus gland is the facilitator for many things. We will go over this with you.

Hormones travel to receptor sites in muscles or tissues where an action is produced. An EI reaction is a direct result of a combination of hormones being secreted by the hypothalamus and the central nervous system being activated by fear and anxiety and stress. That is an EI reaction.

When you are subjected to your stressor, when you are exposed to the thing you think you are allergic to, sometimes people react. Sometimes they react and do not even know they are around it and this seems to reinforce their belief in their "allergy."

I have learned a lot about an invisible enemy called **"the spirit of fear,"** which can see through walls and can see through you and knows exactly what is going on. You have a very intelligent enemy from the second heaven that may have gained access to your life.

### *FEAR IS NOT JUST AN EMOTION.*
### *The Bible calls fear at this level an evil spirit.*

I will be honest with you: in order to get a person healed of MCS/EI, *the spirit of fear has to be cast out of their life once and for all.* Now I don't know if this is part of your theology. If you can get healed another way, then God bless you! I know when the spirit of fear is gone, people are well. People are so afraid of the terms "demon" or "devil" or "evil spirit." Fear of evil is a national tragedy in the Christian Church.

I am saying this is in a different dimension than the normal *fight or flight* response God created you with. A natural fear is part of your limbic system. *Fight or flight* is part of our creation, *but we have an enemy that would like to take you one step further and make fear a permanent way of life. Yes, I am saying your enemy knows you almost as well as your Creator does. He knows how to manipulate you, to extend his kingdom to destroy you and to manipulate you to bring his kingdom of oppression into your life.*

It is one thing to have *fight or flight* from playing in the traffic or crossing the RR tracks. In MCS/EI, the person is geared up in *fight or flight* all the time. When you gear up to face an invisible unknown enemy, parts of your body that are necessary for homeostasis shut down. Then we have the beginning of *candida, hypothyroidism, fibromyalgia, organic brain syndrome, exhaustion* and all the rest.

The parts of your body necessary for homeostasis are not required for *fight or flight. In fight or flight* you need adrenaline. You are really just shadowboxing the invisible enemy all your life. It does not go away; it becomes progressive. *Like begets like, faith begets faith, fear begets fear, hate begets hate, love begets love, like begets like.* It is a crescendo of programming from the enemy to control our lives.

MCS/EI is rooted in *great insecurity, great mistrust and great fear.* It has one other leg it stands on, which is *occultism.* I like to say, metaphorically, MCS/EI has two legs: one is fear and the other is occultism. **In fact, fear is occultism.** Why? Because it projects into the future something that is not true as it if were true.

Interestingly enough, most people who come to us for help don't come to us first; they come to us last. Pastors aren't supposed to know anything about disease. Yet these people have tried everything, spent all their money and it is not working. They hear there is some success with a pastor and his ministry teams and *then they come to us.*

Before they come to us, they have been to every-which-way doctor for every-which-way treatment known to man trying to become well. They have violated every Scripture against the dark side in trying to get well. They have been to every New Age practitioner and every alternative practitioner. They've used every modality known to man and they are still not well. You need to be careful when you go into that kingdom trying to get well. You open your spirit up to stuff bringing a tremendous consequence and it brings more fear and more torment. I am not trying to convince you at this stage. I am sharing with you what I know. Without seeming presumptuous, with the Lord's help this ministry has had many, many victories in healing disease. We speak with great authority because of what God has done.

You know it is a matter of believing or not believing. I promise if you go into certain modalities of healing for MCS/EI, you can go in with 5 allergies and come out with 50 the first 24 hours you have been there. You can go into an allergist's office with 10 allergies and come out with 15–20 by the time you leave 30 minutes later. I am saying when you go into these modalities of healing, they do not have any solutions.

You try to find a solution, but it produces no fruit. It produces more fear, hopelessness and despair and by the time you come to this ministry, you don't believe us either. **We are the last resort.**

When you are geared up to fight a stressor and that part of you inside is not feeling safe, there are all kinds of weird things happening inside your body and we are going to show them to you.

## Limbic System

Now we are going to take a look at the *limbic system.* Have you ever heard of the mind-body connection? That is what science calls it, but in ministry we call it **the spirit, soul and body connection.**

> [23]**And the very God of peace sanctify you wholly; and** *I pray God* **your whole spirit and soul and body be preserved blameless unto the coming of our Lord Jesus Christ. 1 Thessalonians 5:23**

A principal gland in the limbic system is the hypothalamus. In fact, it is called the brain of the endocrine system. Although it directly answers to the pituitary, which is another gland involved in the limbic system, it is actually the hypothalamus that integrates the autonomic nervous system as well as the endocrine system.

Remember, psychology says the soul is comprised of two compartments: conscious and collective unconscious. I do not find that in Scripture, but I do find *spirit, soul and body* as referenced in 1 Thessalonians 5:23 above. **What psychology is calling the collective unconscious is in fact the "spirit of man."**

Psychology says in the collective unconscious are the *archetypes and dark shadows* of our ancestral heritage. I say in the collective unconscious *(which is the spirit of man) is where the collective garbage of the "crispy critters" of our ancestral heritage resides.*

I am reading now from the textbook *Principles of Anatomy and Physiology* by Gerard J. Tortora and Nicholas P. Anagnostakos, Harper & Row, 2nd edition, 1978:

## Hypothalamus Gland

1. It controls and integrates the autonomic nervous system, which stimulates smooth muscle, regulates the rate of contraction of cardiac muscle, and controls the secretions of many glands. Through the autonomic nervous system, the hypothalamus is the main regulator of visceral activities. It regulates heart rate, movement of food through the digestive tract, and contraction of the urinary bladder.

2. It is involved in the reception of sensory impulses from the viscera.

3. It is the principal intermediary between the nervous system and endocrine system—the two major control systems of the body. The hypothalamus lies just above the pituitary, the main endocrine gland. When the hypothalamus detects certain changes in the body, it releases chemicals called regulating factors that stimulate or inhibit the anterior pituitary gland. The anterior pituitary then releases or holds back hormones that regulate carbohydrates, fats, proteins, certain ions, and sexual functions.

4. It is the center for the mind-over-body phenomenon. When the cerebral cortex interprets strong emotions, it often sends impulses along tracts that connect the cortex with the hypothalamus. The hypothalamus then directs impulses via the autonomic nervous system and also releases chemicals that stimulate the anterior pituitary gland. The result can be a wide range of changes in body activities. For instance, when you panic, impulses leave the hypothalamus to stimulate your heart to beat faster. Likewise, continued psychological stress can produce long-term abnormalities in body function that result in serious illness. These are so-called psychosomatic disorders. Psychosomatic disorders are real.

Let me say this to you: the hypothalamus gland is the facilitator and the originator of the following life circumstances: *all expressions of fear, anxiety, stress, tension, panic, panic attacks, phobia, rage, anger and aggression.* These are all released and facilitated by this one gland. *It only responds to you emotionally and spiritually.* The hypothalamus is called the "brain of the endocrine system," but it is not a brain. It is a gland. *It is a responder to thought. It is a responder to the environment of your life.* It will only produce what is happening deep within the recesses of your *soul and your spirit.*

5.  It is associated with feelings of rage and aggression.

6.  It controls normal body temperature. Certain cells of the hypothalamus serve as a thermostat—a mechanism sensitive to changes in temperature. If blood flowing through the hypothalamus is above normal temperature, the hypothalamus directs impulses along the autonomic nervous system to stimulate activities that promote heat loss. Heat can be lost through relaxation of the smooth muscle in the blood vessels and by sweating. Conversely, if the temperature of the blood is below normal, the hypothalamus generates impulses that promote heat retention. Heat can be retained through the contraction of cutaneous blood vessels, cessation of sweating, and shivering.

7.  It regulates food intake through two centers. The *feeding center* is stimulated by hunger sensations from an empty stomach. When sufficient food has been ingested, the *satiety center* is stimulated and sends out impulses that inhibit the feeding center.

8.  It contains a *thirst center.* Certain cells in the hypothalamus are stimulated when the extracellular fluid volume is reduced. The stimulated cells produce the sensation of thirst in the hypothalamus.

9.  It is one of the centers that maintain the waking state and sleep patterns.[4]

The *limbic system* is the connection between your cerebrum where your brain is, down through to your hypothalamus. *It is the connection between psyche (thought) and physio (the body). It is the connection between soul and body.* Everything concerning thought travels right down this connection. Good thoughts and bad thoughts. All of these parts are connected: the limbic lobe, the hippocampus, the amygdaloid, the hypothalamus and the anterior nucleus of the thalamus. Everything is connected in order to process thought and give it expression in the physiological part of our lives. Just as fear can put you into *fight or flight,* peace can bring you into peace.

Jesus said this: Peace give I unto you but not as the world gives, give I unto you.

> **Peace I leave with you, my peace I give unto you: not as the world giveth, give I unto you. Let not your heart be troubled, neither let it be afraid. John 14:27**

---

[4] Gerard J. Tortora and Nicholas P. Anagnostakos, *Principles of Anatomy & Physiology*, Second Edition, Harper & Row, 1978.

The Bible says in Jeremiah 6:13–14 that the priest and the prophet have erred, saying, "Peace, peace" when there is no peace. In fact, it says the priest and prophet have erred and they have only healed the hurt of the daughter of my people slightly, saying, "Peace, peace" when there is no peace.

> **[13]For from the least of them even unto the greatest of them every one *is* given to covetousness; and from the prophet even unto the priest every one dealeth falsely. [14]They have healed also the hurt *of the daughter* of my people slightly, saying, Peace, peace; when *there is* no peace. Jeremiah 6:13–14**

Who is Jesus called? The Prince of Peace (Isaiah 9:6). He is the architect and He is the designer of our peace. Amen!

> **For unto us a child is born, unto us a son is given: and the government shall be upon his shoulder: and his name shall be called Wonderful, Counsellor, The mighty God, The everlasting Father, The Prince of Peace. Isaiah 9:6**

The Bible says that perfect peace belongs to those whose minds are fixed or stayed on the LORD.

> **Thou wilt keep *him* in perfect peace, *whose* mind *is* stayed *on thee:* because he trusteth in thee. Isaiah 26:3**

*The antidote to fear is fellowship with the Godhead.* Second Timothy 1:7 tells us that God has not given us the spirit of fear but of power, love and a sound mind.

> **For God hath not given us the spirit of fear; but of power, and of love, and of a sound mind. 2 Timothy 1:7**

Power represents the Holy Spirit, love represents the love of the Father and a sound mind represents the Word of God, Jesus. If you are filled with the fellowship of the love of God the Father and of the Son and of the Holy Spirit, fear does not have a shot at you. *If you are listening to fear, you are not listening to God.*

The limbic system functions in the emotional aspects of behavior related to survival. When you do not feel loved, when you have been victimized, when you do not feel secure, you fight for survival. When you have been rejected by a parent or by anyone else, when you do not feel loved, when you feel violated, you are always looking over your shoulder for when the next hit is going to come. You are in *fight or flight.*

The limbic system also functions in memory. Although behavior is a function of the entire nervous system, the limbic system controls most of its *involuntary* aspects. One of the things about Environmental Illness is that it is all invisible (beyond conscious thought). It always involves everything deep within the person and we usually do not understand by our intellectual processes what is going on. That is why it is so difficult to see it. You can only see it if you understand the spiritual aspect from a biblical perspective. You can only see it if you understand the enemy and his methods of attack.

## General Adaptation Syndrome (GAS)

This subject is called **stress and homeostasis.** *Homeostasis may be viewed as a specific response by the body to specific stimuli.* Homeostatic mechanisms "fine tune" the body. If the mechanisms are successful, our internal environment maintains a uniform chemistry, temperature and pressure. Homeostatic mechanisms are geared toward counteracting the everyday stresses of living. This is normal. This is what God created. We are going to show what happens when things aren't fine.

If a stress is extreme or unusual, the normal ways of keeping the body in balance may not be sufficient. In this case the stress triggers a wide-ranging set of bodily changes called *General Adaptation Syndrome* (GAS). Unlike the homeostatic mechanism, *General Adaptation Syndrome* (GAS) does not maintain a constant internal environment. In fact it does just the opposite. For instance, blood pressure and blood sugar levels are raised above normal.

The purpose of these changes in the internal environment is to gear up the body to meet emergencies, known as stressors. The hypothalamus can be called the body's watchdog. It has sensors to detect changes in the chemistry, temperature and pressure of the blood. It is informed of emotions through tracts connecting it with the emotional centers of the cerebral cortex.

When the hypothalamus senses stress, it initiates a chain of reactions that produce *General Adaptation Syndrome* (GAS). The stressors produce the syndrome. A stressor may be almost any disturbance, including strong emotional reactions. When a stressor appears, it stimulates the hypothalamus to stimulate the syndrome through two pathways. The first pathway is stimulation of the sympathetic nervous system and the adrenal medulla. This stimulation produces an immediate set of responses called the alarm reaction. The second pathway, called the resistance reaction, involves the anterior pituitary gland and adrenal cortex. The resistance reaction is slower to start, but its effects last longer.

**The first part of an *anxiety disorder* is called the alarm reaction.** The alarm reaction is *a fight or flight* response and is the body's initial reaction to a stressor. It is actually a complex reaction initiated by hypothalamic stimulation of the sympathetic nervous system and the adrenal medulla. The responses of the visceral effectors are immediate and short-lived. They are designed to counteract the danger by mobilizing the body's resources for immediate physical activity. In essence, the alarm reaction brings tremendous amounts of

# General Adaptation Syndrome of Fear, Anxiety and Stress

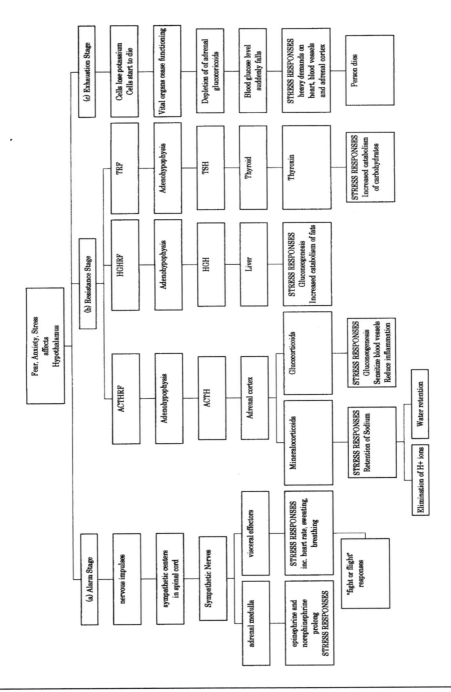

(a) Alarm Stage (called fight or flight); (b) Resistance Stage (being geared up to face the enemy long-term as a way of life); (c) Exhaustion Stage. This is how fear, anxiety and stress affects your body long-term. The final conclusion is all of the above.

glucose and oxygen to the organs most active in warding off danger. These organs are the brain (which must become highly alert), the skeletal muscles (which may have to ward off an attacker) and the heart (which must work furiously to pump enough materials to the brain and to the muscles). Hyperglycemia is associated with sympathetic activity. It is produced by epinephrine and norepinephrine from the adrenal medulla, fat mobilization, glucose sparing and protein mobilization by the glucocorticoids.

The heart rate and strength of cardiac muscle contraction are increased. Blood vessels supplying the skin and the viscera, except for the heart and lungs, undergo constriction. The spleen contracts and discharges stored blood. The liver transforms large amounts of stored glycogen into glucose. Sweat production increases. The rate of breathing increases; the production of saliva, stomach enzymes and intestinal enzymes decrease. This reaction takes place since digestive activity is not essential for counteracting the stress. This is what produces malabsorption. Sympathetic impulses to the adrenal medulla increase its secretion of epinephrine and norepinephrine. These hormones supplement and prolong many sympathetic nervous system realities.

A *fight or flight* stress creates the second stage: the *resistance stage*. The third stage is *exhaustion*. This can be progressive over years. It can come quickly or it can come slowly. What happens is this: when you face the stressor, whether known or unknown, the first thing to be stimulated is the hypothalamus gland. Nervous impulses are generated, the sympathetic centers in the spinal cord are activated, the sympathetic nervous system goes into motion, the adrenal medulla is affected, the production of epinephrine and norepinephrine occurs and then begin the stress responses of an increased heart rate, constriction of blood vessels, contraction of spleen. And on it goes.

**Let's move into the second part of fear, stress and physiology**. I want to begin with an incredible statement from the medical community. This part of the teaching will have to do with **fear and how it affects our lives**. America is plagued by fear. You are afraid of your mother, father, husband, wife, children, boss, disease, death, tomorrow, man, rejection, failure, abandonment, trains, planes, buildings, fear of this and fear of that. It is all over the place, isn't it? Phobias: germ phobias, people phobias, food phobias.

What is the worst thing that can happen to you? Die and go to heaven; so what is your problem? God does not need you in heaven. You are of no earthly good if you go to heaven prematurely. The Lord does not need you there. If you get there too soon, He's going to ask you, "What are you doing here? I wanted you down there in your generation to do something for Me. I don't need you here. I had work for you. Everyone is so much in a hurry to get to heaven. You old lazy thing, you; get a grip!"

*A stressor is anything causing fear in your life.* Let's see what parts of the body one stressor can affect on a long-term basis. First of all, it directly affects the input to the central nervous system, including behavioral adaptations. The hypothalamus integrates the response to the fear. Then things start to happen; we have a releasing factor into the body with a hormone called CRF from the hypothalamus. Directly affected as the fear item begins to grow and progress, the sympathetic nervous system (SNS) becomes involved. The SNS is the part of the nervous system that makes you tick beyond your conscious thought. The voluntary nervous system is what I am using to talk to you. My heart is beating and my good lunch is moving around all over the place. This is happening in spite of my thoughts. It is controlled invisibly within me. This is what God created to make sure that I perk and function without me interfering with it.

So we have the SNS affected immediately in the anterior pituitary, the posterior pituitary, and then out of this, the SNS, the norepinephrine from peripheral nerve endings, starts to get secreted. The adrenal medulla is affected and then we have the epinephrine release.

Because the norepinephrine is being released, we now have fear and anxiety being expressed. We have immune system breakdown effects beginning. We have increased contraction of the arterial smooth muscle; we have increased blood pressure, increased pupil dilation and decreased gastric secretion.

Do you ever wonder sometimes why constipation goes with fear or sometimes diarrhea goes with fear? *Diarrhea and constipation are fruits of fear/anxiety.* What I am teaching you is straight out of the medical community. This is what the medical community has found through years of research.

We have increased force of cardiac action, increased lypolysis of triglycerides and increased circulation of fatty acids. There is a decreased degradation of cholesterol to bile acids. Serum cholesterol is increased. Then as this is beginning and increasing long-term, our liver is affected and so is our pancreas. In the liver we have decreased glycogen synthesis, increased glycogenolysis and increased gluconeogenesis. From the pancreas we have decreased insulin, increased glucagon and increased blood glucose.

The point of all this is fear and anxiety are affecting your body behind the scenes; you do not even see it happening. Is that scary or what? This is just the beginning. It all starts to affect the anterior pituitary and the posterior pituitary. We have vaso-suppression, ACTH being secreted, increased water retention and then the beta-endorphins are affected. ACTH is a tremendous fear hormone. It sets everything in motion and most of the EI advanced reactions are the result of the secretion of ACTH. ACTH, growth hormones, prolactin and the adrenal cortex are affected by an increased release.

## Cortisol

Now we come to cortisol. Cortisol is important in *fight or flight* but, if it is present on a long-term basis, it destroys your immune system. What God created for us to help fight an enemy has now turned on us and has become the destroyer of our lives.

According to medical information, long-term over-secretion of cortisol has direct physiological effects on the following functions (reading from the *Pathophysiology* chart): "Carbohydrate and lipid metabolism, protein metabolism, inflammatory effects, lipid metabolism, immune reserve, digestive function, urinary function, connective tissue function, muscle function, bone function, vascular system and myocardial function and central nervous system function.

"Cortisol directly influences immune responses to antibodies…cortisol inhibits the production of both macrophages and helper T cells. The diminished helper T cells cause a decrease in B cells and antibody production…."

Now begins the destruction of the immune system. What is destroying the immune system? Pesticides? No! According to the medical community it is fear, anxiety and stress. What did Proverbs 17:22 say? A broken spirit drieth up the bones.

**A merry heart doeth good *like* a medicine: but a broken spirit drieth the bones. Proverbs 17:22**

The ongoing over-secretion of cortisol continues immunosuppression, decreased lymphocytes and monocytes, decreased circulating lymphocytes and decreased macrophages. Right here the negative effects begin. Right here we have the breaking down of the immune system. When you have the breaking down of the immune system as we are about to show you, an interesting thing happens with the B cells.

When you have a reduction of B cells at this level, antigen-antibody relationships develop. Your body starts attacking everything. That is what an allergy is. The antigen becomes the enemy, but the antigen is the food you need. Now the body is eliminating what it needs to have in order to stay alive.

Could I say this, *"As the person disappears into fear and disappears into the self-rejection mode, the body takes on a profile of death."* Why? Because the person has been murdered. *Spiritually murdered!* Those are very strong words, aren't they? You say then, "How are they spiritually murdered?" When you deny your existence as God sees you and reject yourself in creation, a spirit of death comes to agree. *Numerous diseases are the result of this spiritual dynamic.*

All I have shown you is what is affected by just *one area* of fear, anxiety and stress. Now let's add 15 dozen different areas at one time. Now we have a compounding of a major spiritual and biological problem.

As fear and anxiety are moving inside you, hormones are released to the α (alpha) and β (beta) receptors and all parts of your body are affected. These are the physiological actions of the alpha and beta receptors: you have muscles affected, blood vessels affected, the urinary tract affected, gastrointestinal tract affected, smooth muscle contraction, some vascular beds, increased insulin secretion, myocardial contraction and you have all smooth muscle relaxation (bronchi, blood vessels, etc.). Everything concerning your entire physiological body is now under attack. Gastrointestinal, cardiovascular, endocrine, neurological systems—everything you are in creation is now taking a hit from fear and anxiety.

Catecholamines include epinephrine, norepinephrine and dopamine. Let's take a look at the physiological effects of the catecholamines now being secreted because of anxiety and fear long-term, not to your benefit but to your harm. Look at the parts of the body affected: the brain, glucose metabolism, blood flow, cardiovascular, pulmonary, muscle, liver, skin, skeleton, gastrointestinal system and lymphoid tissue. All the systems of your body are now being aberrated—are being attacked—and are changing and are being forced to do something they were not designed to do.

Your whole physiological life is now under attack. So I gave you the case histories of those people who had 17–21 different peripheral diseases because this is what comes. When we eliminated the foundational problem or root, then the rest of their body eventually—in a very short time—conformed to health as God intended. The diseases went away and the body snapped back into order: These individuals are well today.

Here is the problem: If you don't know this information and no one tells it to you, then you end up with 15 peripheral diseases and 15 different medical specialists. Not one collaborates with the other and you end up chasing bad fruit with no regard to the originating root of the problem. You might end up on 15 different drugs seeing those 15 different specialists at 15 times the cost with no solution ever in sight because the root problems have never even been discussed.

Continuing to read from *Pathophysiology: The Biologic Basis of Disease in Adults and Children:*

> This is how cortisol affects cell-mediated immunity:
>
> Cortisol inhibits antigen-stimulated production of the peptide interleukin-1 macrophages, decreasing the initial recruitment of T lymphocytes. Cortisol also inhibits production of interleukin-2, reducing secondary proliferation of helper and

suppressor T lymphocytes. Depending in part on the ratio of these two cell populations, production of antibody to the original antigen may be either facilitated or retarded. In some species, large doses of cortisol are lymphocytotoxic, causing cell death.

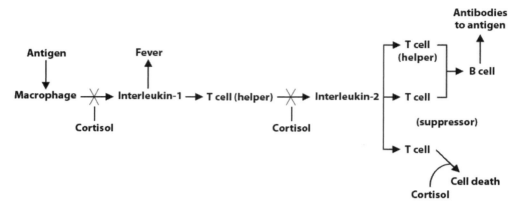

What we are looking at is the antigen and the macrophage and the progression all the way down as cortisol is increased—here are your T cells, here's cortisol and here's cell death. Over here are T cells, helper cells and B cells. When you have this happening, this over here suppressed and these suppressed, you have antibodies to antigen and there is what an allergy is.

When you can get your T cells, your B cells and your killer cells up to normal and get the secretion of cortisol stopped, the immune system will heal itself. When the immune system is healed, the antibody to antigen no longer exists and this is why you can drink milk when before you could not drink it. That is why you can be around certain smells today when before you could not. It is because the foundational material that creates this mess is gone and there is nothing left to stimulate it. *That is exactly where we are in ministry. We want to remove the parts and pieces that allow the foundation of this disease to get a foothold.*

Let's go a little further. What causes the over-secretion of cortisol? *Fear/Anxiety/Stress.*

These are the long-term problems relative to the *resistance* and *the exhaustion stage* of the fear/anxiety disorder. Carbohydrate and lipid metabolism are affected. Protein metabolism is affected. There are inflammatory effects such as lipid metabolism, the immune reserve, digestive function, urinary function, connective tissue function, muscle function, bone function, vascular system, myocardial function and central nervous system function. Concerning the physiologic effects of cortisol, there are many problems; for example, a decreased proliferation of fibroblast connective tissue (which delays healing and decreases bone formation and somehow modulates perceptual and emotional functions).

Let's move away from something like an allergy and see what is said about other diseases caused in the long term by fear, anxiety and stress.

You were throwing diseases at me and I was just saying this is the root and this is the cause. You're going, "Wow, where did he get all that?"

I get it from many sources. I get it from the Word and I get it from studying what the medical community already knows about something. One thing I like about the medical community is that they have done a nice job investigating and documenting our enemy. I want to thank the medical community and the psychiatric industry for their investigation and documentation of our enemy. It has saved me a lot of time and expense. I thank them for defining, showing and demonstrating our enemy.

**These are examples of fear, anxiety and stress-related diseases and conditions as documented in the medical community:**

## Cardiovascular System

*NOTE: Although this section of the teaching concerns cardiovascular disease as a result of fear, anxiety and stress, I am going to cover the full spectrum of cardiovascular disease including three additional root areas and the diseases coming from these root areas so you will have a complete picture of cardiovascular disease regardless of the root.*

### Spiritual Root: Fear/Anxiety/Stress

Angina (Pain)

*Angina*, by definition in the dictionary, is any disease in which spasmodic and painful suffocation or spasms occur. With respect to heart tissue, *angina pectoris* is more commonly known. The word in the Greek language literally means a strangling. The definition includes severe pain in the chest associated with emotional stress and characterized by feelings of suffocation and apprehension. From a physiological standpoint, *angina* occurs as three primary types. First, stable *angina* (or classic *angina*) is caused by luminal narrowing and hardening of the arterial walls. The second type is unstable *angina* and is often caused by a vasospasm, which can cause inadequate oxygen supply. The third type is the variant *angina*, which involves the entire thickness of the myocardial layer. Interestingly, it occurs unpredictably and almost exclusively at rest. Hyperactivity of the sympathetic nervous system, produced by the hypothalamus in relationship to the mind-body connection, is clearly implicated in the medical journals.

The Bible says in the last days men's hearts will fail them for fear.

> **Men's hearts failing them for fear, and for looking after those things which are coming on the earth: for the powers of heaven shall be shaken. Luke 21:26**

In the textbook *Pathophysiology: The Biologic Basis for Disease* under the heading "Examples of Stress-Related Diseases and Conditions," a primary target organ is the heart and/or the cardiovascular system. Diseases such as *angina, hypertension, arrhythmias and mitral valve prolapse* are listed and are considered fear, anxiety and stress diseases by the medical community.

Not only does the medical community say the basis for these diseases is fear, anxiety and stress, but who else said it? In the Scripture we just quoted from Luke 21:26, God said it—in the last days men's hearts will fail them because of fear. What good would it do for God to heal you, for example, of *angina* if you hold onto the spirit of fear and anxiety that is causing the stiffening, hardening, vasospasm or hyperactivity of the cardiovascular system?

Do you think God knows fear and anxiety will produce *angina* pain and other cardiovascular problems? Do you think He knows this? If He knows, don't you think He wants us to know it too? This is why He told us in His Word exactly what would cause certain types of heart disease. He said in the last days men's hearts shall fail them because of fear.

Additional information found in the textbook *Principles of Anatomy and Physiology*, under the section entitled "Blood Supply," states most heart problems result from faulty coronary circulation. *The information continues to state that stress (fear and anxiety), which produces constriction of vessel walls, is a common cause.*

## High Blood Pressure (Hypertension)

What is *hypertension*? It is high blood pressure. High blood pressure is a result of a narrowing of the blood vessels so that there is a resistance to the flow, thus increasing the pressure because of the backup in the coronary vessels. What is the root for high blood pressure? Fear, anxiety and stress. Just as the Bible says in the last days men's hearts shall fail them because of fear, statistics in America indicate one out of every four Americans suffers from high blood pressure.

*What I am teaching is not opposed to medical science.* I am not in opposition to medical science. In fact, what I see in the Bible only proves medical science and medical science only proves the Bible. I find no conflict. It is just that the third dimension of our existence (the spirit of man) is usually not recognized in the scientific and medical community. It is essential to understand man is not just a soul and a body, but he is also a spirit. The problems are spiritual first; thus it is why a pastor needs to understand this information.

### Heart Arrhythmias

Heart *arrhythmias* are disturbances of heart rhythm or such things as arrhythmic problems. Many arrhythmic problems have a root of chronic fear, anxiety and stress. The first target organ for fear, anxiety and stress is the heart. Not only can the heart be stimulated by chemical messengers, but through the involuntary nervous system, it is neurologically sensitive to thought via the mind-body connection.

Because of this reason neurologically, the heartbeat can be interrupted. In the case of the speeding up or slowing down of heartbeat, this can be affected by the autonomic nervous system, which is highly susceptible to thought via the mind-body connection. For example, when a person is startled or traumatized or victimized, the heart rate increases in response to the stressor. To help you understand this mechanism, it would be like cutting the electrical current off to something and then turning it back on.

### Mitral Valve Prolapse (Heart Valve Disease)

*Mitral valve prolapse* can be caused by congenital defect, infections or damage by rheumatic fever. In America today *mitral valve prolapse* is a national epidemic and none of these possible causes can be found. Many people have been healed by God through this ministry of *mitral valve prolapse* over the past few years. We have discovered the mitral valve stays open or closed because of neurological misfiring. It is very similar to arrhythmic problems, the reality of fear, anxiety and stress upstream in the spirit and the soul, which causes a whole sequence of events to go into motion through the mind-body connection so the electrical connection to the valve is interrupted. When the fear, anxiety and stress of a person's life has been dealt with, we have seen *mitral valve prolapse* disappear out of a person's life quickly.

## Self-Bitterness, Self-Rejection and Self-Hatred

### Coronary Artery Disease

*Coronary artery disease* is the number one cause of heart attacks. Primarily, *coronary artery disease* involves blockage so oxygen is prevented from reaching the heart muscle. *Coronary artery disease* involves hardening of the arteries, which effectively leads to a narrowing of the arteries. Recent medical information now indicates that cholesterol is not necessarily the culprit. There are other factors very spiritually rooted in nature that cause this problem in many people, while many other people eating the same foods, living in the same homes and in the same environmental setting, never have a problem.

A recent statement from one of the medical journals gave a sobering insight. Performing triple and quad bypasses does not eliminate *coronary artery disease* or blockage or hardening of the arteries because when they do the triple or the quad bypass, those new arteries will clog also. This indicates something very invisible and very consistent with spiritual roots. In reviewing case histories of people in ministry, we have discovered those suffering from *coronary artery disease* are filled with self-rejection, self-bitterness and self-hatred, and they have never overcome it.

## Strokes

*Strokes* are the result of clogging of blood vessels so the brain tissue is blood-starved. This is known as cerebrovascular insufficiency. In some cases there can be a hemorrhage also interfering with the function by cutting off a part of its blood supply, but do not confuse this hemorrhagic stroke with what an *aneurysm* is. It has been my observation that individuals who have *strokes* also have self-rejection, self-bitterness and self-hatred. I suppose you could say that when you do not like yourself, clogging of the arteries is the immediate fruit physiologically. I guess it might be a good idea not to kill ourselves in our self-esteem because our body might conform to that image very quickly.

## Diseases of Heart Muscle from Inflammation

This type of inflammation is nonbacterial inflammation and is not the result of a bacterial infection. This condition is part of a new disease class we have been observing as a combination of fear, anxiety, stress and self-hatred, and the mechanism that produces this inflammation (this is nonbacterial in nature) has an autoimmune component in which the white corpuscles are congregating in the heart muscle. When white corpuscles congregate, there is nonbacterial inflammation as a by-product. This can be quite serious in heart tissue because the heart can quit beating. It is not quite as serious in other similar diseases of this nature such as prostatitis, interstitial cystitis and asthma, although asthma can be very life-threatening. Whenever I see white corpuscles congregating and/or abnormal white corpuscle activity, I find self-rejection, self-bitterness and self-hatred.

## Anger, Rage and Resentment

### Aneurysms

An *aneurysm* is an abnormal (often balloon-like) swelling on the side of an artery caused by a weakness in the arterial wall. There can be congenital brain *aneurysms* or there can be aortic *aneurysms.* In any event, an *aneurysm* involves either the swelling or the rupturing of blood vessels. Whenever I find exploding blood vessels or bulging blood vessels, I have found anger, rage and resentment in the person. As another observation, this particular disease is highly inherited, not necessarily as a genetic defect disease, but as an inherited spiritual disease. You see, anger, rage and resentment are not genetic; they are spiritual and they are sin.

> **Be ye angry, and sin not: let not the sun go down upon your wrath: <sup>27</sup>Neither give place to the devil. Ephesians 4:26–27**

### Varicose Veins

*Varicose veins* involve a swelling of blood vessel walls. In fact, they are a form of *aneurysm.* Again, the root is anger, rage and resentment. Let me bring forth an important point: this anger, rage and resentment is not always externally explosive against others but can be internalized. Could I say the person is brooding, steaming and deep inside they are filled with anger, rage and resentment? So whether externalized or internalized, it is still sin and the result is the same.

### Hemorrhoids

*Hemorrhoids* are varicose veins. The root is the same.

### Thrombophlebitis (Vein Inflammation)

This type of *vein inflammation* primarily affects the body's superficial veins, those which are easily seen on the surface of the skin, especially in the legs. This condition is very common in persons who also have *varicose veins.* The root follows the rest: anger, rage and resentment.

## Congenital, Inherited or Injury *in utero*

A defect of the heart or major blood vessels can be present at birth. Statistically in America, *congenital heart disease* is found in seven of every 1,000 births. Genetic abnormality can be associated with a heart defect causing the child to be born with a heart disease problem. We would consider this the inherited genetic curse.

Other *congenital heart diseases* can have their origin *in utero* (in the womb). Such things as infections, German measles in the mother during early pregnancy and medications taken during pregnancy also increase the risk. In these cases of *injury in utero*, we minister by simply asking God to do a creative miracle and restore the tissue that has been damaged.

## Muscles

### Tension Headaches

We started this teaching by discussing the hypothalamus. We talked about how you rub the back of your neck when you are under stress and tension. Fear, anxiety and stress produce tension and tension headaches.

### Muscle Contraction Backache

This is connected directly with the central nervous system and to the sympathetic nervous system. It is coming out of *fear, anxiety and stress*.

The next targeted organ system for stress is the connective tissue.

## Connective Tissue Disease

### Rheumatoid Arthritis

I am in a little disagreement with the medical community here. I wonder why the medical community has gone there and I really don't agree with them because I can see where fear, anxiety and stress can play a part in it. Basically, if I were to say it was fear, I would say the person was *afraid of themselves*. They just don't want to face themselves. Out of this comes *self-hatred*, out of that comes the *guilt and* out of that comes the conflict that causes the white corpuscles to attack the connective material of the bones. They then eat at it and produce rheumatoid arthritis.

## Related Inflammatory Diseases of Connective Tissue

### Prostatitis

In related inflammatory diseases of the connective tissue, you have two types of inflammation: bacterial and nonbacterial. In bacterial inflammation, you treat the person with antibiotics. The nonbacterial inflammation is caused by either an over-secretion of histamine (systemic or localized) or by a proliferation of white corpuscles which localize, producing the nonbacterial inflammation. A disease of record is the nonbacterial inflammation of *prostatitis* in men or *interstitial cystitis* in females. These are a couple of diseases that help you understand the roots that are in existence here.

## Interstitial Cystitis

This disease is comparable to *prostatitis* (see definitions above).

## Pulmonary System

### Asthma (Called Hypersensitivity Reaction)

I have been teaching this for a decade and finally the medical community has agreed with me: *asthma* has nothing to do with what you breathe. It has nothing to do with airway obstruction. It has nothing to do with breathing such things as dander, dust, pollen and all the rest of it. Something deep inside the human person is being triggered by something internally. We have known it to be caused by *fear, anxiety and stress* for over a decade.

The Johns Hopkins University Research Team in 1996 confirmed this finding that will change the past 50 years of conventional wisdom concerning *asthma*. Nothing you breathe causes an asthmatic attack. It can be inherited, but it is coming out of *deep-rooted fear, anxiety and stress*. That is right here in this medical information. *Asthma* is now considered an anxiety disorder by the medical community. Now what do you think about that?

**Editor's Note:** Since this seminar was taught, Henry Wright has identified a specific fear issue as a root for *asthma*. That root is fear of abandonment coupled with insecurity.

### Hay Fever

*Hay fever* is also considered a hypersensitivity reaction. *Hay fever* meets the profile of antigen-antibody, as discussed previously, relative to a compromised immune system and is a fear/anxiety/stress disorder.

## Immune System

### Immunosuppression or Deficiency

We just went over what excessive secretion of cortisol produces, what the catecholamines do and how they destroy the immune system resulting in diseases. The autoimmune diseases are not the result of immunosuppression.

The autoimmune diseases are not the result of a lack of white corpuscles. The autoimmune diseases occur when the white corpuscles attack living flesh and destroy it. *Lupus, Crohn's, diabetes, rheumatoid arthritis and MS* are examples and on it goes.

*The body attacks the body because the person is attacking themselves spiritually in self-rejection, self-hatred and self-bitterness.* There is a spiritual dynamic that comes in which the white corpuscles are invisibly redirected to attack living tissue while ignoring the true enemy, which is bacteria and viruses. As the person continues to attack himself or herself spiritually, the body finally agrees and the white corpuscles start attacking the body. That is a high price to pay for not loving yourself.

## Autoimmune Diseases

Even though the medical community now associates autoimmune diseases (including lupus, Crohn's, diabetes [type 1], rheumatoid arthritis, multiple sclerosis) with fear, anxiety and stress, I have come to the conclusion that most autoimmune diseases are primarily the result of an unloving spirit producing feelings of not being loved, not being accepted, self-rejection, self-hatred and self-bitterness coupled with guilt. In fact, it could be said that autoimmune diseases are primarily a self-hatred disease with a fear-anxiety-stress rider attached to them.

## Gastrointestinal System

### Ulcers

I know what you have been reading about bacteria (H-pylori) causing ulcers. For years, we have believed (and the medical community has believed) that fear, anxiety and stress caused a flaring of dendrite activity in the lining of the stomach, producing the irritation and finally the ulceration. Then they came along and said, "Well, we've diagnosed a bacterium, so it is a bacterial problem."

*People who have ulcers also have compromised immune systems.* When you have a compromised immune system, you do not have the firepower to defeat bacteria. The bacterium does not intimidate me about the original assumption of *fear, anxiety and stress.* I am not convinced the bacteria cause ulcers. I am convinced the combination of both is the culprit. *I think the fear, anxiety and stress came first and the bacteria showed up after the immune system was compromised.*

There are a number of gastrointestinal problems caused by fear, anxiety and stress. They include *irritable bowel syndrome (IBS), diarrhea, constipation, nausea, vomiting, ulcerative colitis and malabsorption.* I agree with all these, but there are some more. There's *malabsorption* and *leaky gut,* which I think is probably close to *malabsorption. Much of the malfunctioning of the gastrointestinal tract is caused by not having peace in your heart regarding issues in your life*, with the exception of *Crohn's disease*, which is an autoimmune disease.

## Irritable Bowel Syndrome (IBS)

*Irritable bowel syndrome* (IBS) is a fear, anxiety and stress disorder in which the dendrites are flaring in the lining of the colon, very similar to what is happening in the lining of the stomach which produces ulcers.

## Diarrhea

*Diarrhea* again can be caused by a continual irritation in conjunction with liver malfunctioning as part of the profile of the *General Adaptation Syndrome* of fear, anxiety and stress.

## Constipation

*Constipation* is similar to *diarrhea.* The root is the same, but the mechanisms of the activity of the liver and bowel are different so *constipation* results, rather than *diarrhea.* But fear, anxiety and stress can be a common restrictive reality.

## Nausea and Vomiting

Nausea and vomiting also involve something that could be considered nervous stomach or a result of fear, anxiety and stress. Excessive gastric activity in conjunction with the central nervous system can produce the nausea and in extreme cases result in actual vomiting.

## Ulcerative Colitis

*Ulcerative colitis* is also considered a fear, anxiety and stress disorder in which the lining of the colon is irritated by excessive flaring of dendrites to the degree that the lining ulcerates and bleeds. This is in contrast to *Crohn's disease*, which can ulcerate, not from excessive flaring of dendrites, but because of the attack of the white corpuscles on the lining and in many cases the entire gastrointestinal tract can be affected.

## Malabsorption (Leaky Gut)

*Malabsorption (leaky gut)* has become a national plague in which the food being ingested and the nutrients from it never reach the cellular level through the bloodstream. In fact, a high percentage of the digested food just passes on through, resulting in various stages of malnutrition. The root behind all of this activity is fear, anxiety and stress. The deceptive problem behind *malabsorption* in America is an attempt to compensate by heavy involvement in supplements and other health food products usually at a very high cost, to regain the nutritional loss. *Unfortunately, the expensive health food and supplements pass right on through just like the original food did.* What a deception!

## Genitourinary System

Diuresis, impotence and frigidity are caused by fear, anxiety and stress. Isn't that amazing?

### Diuresis

Diuresis or excessive bladder elimination can be a result of fear, anxiety and stress. Also, incontinence may be found many times in fear, anxiety and stress disorders.

### Impotence

Impotence affects many men in America. A recent statistic indicates as high as 30 to 40 percent of all men in America are impotent. Behind this is a spiritual root of fear, anxiety and stress coming out of self-rejection and lack of self-esteem.

### Frigidity

Frigidity is a female disorder and behind it is fear, anxiety and stress. As a female's value system has been compromised, many times her sexual identity and her uncleanness in it can be implicated.

## Skin

The next system under attack is the skin.

### Eczema

*Eczema* is a skin disorder involving itching, redness, inflammation and occasionally pustules which may or may not ooze. *Eczema* is considered to be a fear, anxiety and stress disorder. There could be some implications of excessive histamine secretion and/or excessive autoimmune activity. This particular disease is clearly identified in Deuteronomy 28 as a curse resulting from disobedience to God and His Word.

Neurodermatitis

*Neurodermatitis* is a chronic inflammation of the skin. The disease may have a strong psychogenic component that is a very definite spiritual root involving anxiety, mental tension and emotional disturbances. It is definitely a result of the mind-body connection and occurs more in women than in men. It is a fear, anxiety and stress disorder.

Acne

*Acne* is a skin disorder usually on the face, neck, back and shoulders. For many years it was considered to be strictly a result of excessive oil in the skin as a result of puberty. However, recent medical research has identified adolescent *acne* as fear, anxiety and stress, which is a result of peer pressure. It is not a genetic, biologic problem by itself, but in most cases the kids are afraid of other kids. This level of fear and anxiety triggers increased histamine secretion behind the skin and also increases the secretion of oil in the epidermis, causing *acne*. Isn't that an amazing discovery? It is the result of fear, anxiety and stress.

**Endocrine System**

Diabetes Mellitus (Type 1)

This is an autoimmune disease like rheumatoid arthritis even though the medical community has grouped these in the fear, anxiety and stress category. I am in agreement partially because in this disease the endocrine system is involved so it interferes with the ability of the pancreas to produce enough insulin or interferes with the ability of the body to use the insulin it has produced. Again, I still consider the root of this disease to be self-hatred and self-rejection coupled with guilt but with a fear, anxiety and stress rider attached to it. As in the case of the autoimmune diseases mentioned above, the medical community does see fear, anxiety and stress as root causes, but they do not see a bigger root cause, which is the unloving spirit allowing self-hatred, self-rejection and guilt to come.

Diabetes Mellitus (Type 2)

Diabetes (Type 2) is not an autoimmune disease but an anxiety disorder where the white corpuscles interfere with the function of the pancreatic tissue, but the tissue is not destroyed. Possible spiritual roots are fear of failing others, fear of failure, fear of man, performance and drivenness. There may also be an inability to receive love, projected rejection, unloving spirits and a spirit of death.

## Amenorrhea

*Amenorrhea* is an interruption or stoppage of the menstrual cycle in females. Behind this is a very powerful root of fear, stress and anxiety. The medical community has defined the root as emotional stress or depression. It has been an incredible observation in this ministry that many females who had complete stoppage of menstrual cycles for years, upon dealing with the fear, anxiety and stress, resumed their menstrual cycle as one of the firstfruits of their healing.

## Central Nervous System

Fatigue and lethargy, Type A behavior, overeating, depression and insomnia are all caused by *fear, anxiety and stress*.

### Fatigue and Lethargy

Fatigue and lethargy can be found as a third stage called *exhaustion* under the *General Adaptation Syndrome of fear, anxiety and stress*. Fear, anxiety and stress are great contributors to fatigue, lethargy and exhaustion.

The number of people struggling with fatigue, exhaustion and lethargy in America today is amazing. The medical community does not attribute this necessarily to a virus, overworking or exposure to chemicals, but in the medical manuals they attribute it to fear, anxiety and stress. In fact, the third stage of *the General Adaptation Syndrome of Fear, anxiety and stress* is *exhaustion*. In the case of *hypoglycemia*, which is a reduction in glucose levels, exhaustion is part of the profile. However, as discussed previously, *hypoglycemia* is primarily a fear, anxiety and stress disorder with an autoimmune rider attached to it of fear, self-hatred and guilt. But again, fatigue, exhaustion and lethargy are by-products of the root problem.

### Type A Behavior

Type A behavior involves drivenness, performance and perfectionism. Many persons are recognizable as workaholics. Many times a root can include fear of poverty and the need to succeed in order to be loved or to be accepted because of a success. Another root cause is the expectation put on someone by a parent or a spouse, which produces a type of anxiety.

### Overeating

Overeating includes an addictive characteristic. Sometimes shades of obsessive/compulsive behavior can be found, but in short, fear of rejection, fear of man, fear of failure and fear of abandonment can be powerful forces driving people and producing long-term fear, anxiety and stress. The overeating aspect is a pacifier to be a false calming reality; in other words, a false comforter. Also, large amounts of fuel supply are burned by a person who is driven, thus producing the chemical need for nutrition replacement beyond the normal scope of life.

## Depression

Depression is many times dealt with by an antidepressant drug such as Prozac, but clinically speaking, depression is a result of a chemical imbalance in the body. It is produced by conflict at the spirit and/or soul level in which the limbic system responds to this stress and the depression is a result of the chemical imbalance produced by the body in response.

## Insomnia

Insomnia or the inability to sleep at night is a recognized fear, anxiety and stress disorder. The hypothalamus gland *(Principles of Anatomy and Physiology,* p. 320) is one of the centers for maintaining the waking state and sleep patterns. Sleep is regulated by the hypothalamus gland. If the hypothalamus gland senses conflict or fear, anxiety and stress in a person's life, it responds by interfering with the peace of the person. A result can be insomnia.

## Scriptural Aspects behind Fear, Anxiety and Stress Disorders

Our teaching continues on fear, stress and physiology, and I think we need to pay attention to 2 Timothy 1:7, which tells us that God has not given the spirit of fear but of power, love and a sound mind.

> **For God hath not given us the spirit of fear; but of power, and of love, and of a sound mind. 2 Timothy 1:7**

Scripture also tells us to love the Lord thy God with all thy heart, with all thy soul, with all thy mind.

> **Jesus said unto him, Thou shalt love the Lord thy God with all thy heart, and with all thy soul, and with all thy mind. Matthew 22:37**

And, you shall love your neighbor as you love yourself.

> **And the second *is* like unto it, Thou shalt love thy neighbour as thyself. Matthew 22:39**

John said it this way, in 1 John 4:11: if God loved us, we ought to love one another.

> **Beloved, if God so loved us, we ought also to love one another. 1 John 4:11**

*First John 4:18 is the foundational Scripture*
*for the healing of many fear, anxiety and stress disorders,*
*including MCS/EI.*

Proverbs 15:13 and 17:22 are the introductory verses for the insight into spiritual roots.

**A merry heart maketh a cheerful countenance: but by sorrow of the heart the spirit is broken. Proverbs 15:13**

**A merry heart doeth good *like* a medicine: but a broken spirit drieth the bones. Proverbs 17:22**

It is quite obvious from these Scriptures that our physiological wellness can be affected by victimization and by rejection by others.

In 1 John 4:18 there are four parts. Each of these four parts must be individually read, recognized and digested to apply it to our lives.

**There is no fear in love; but perfect love casteth out fear: because fear hath torment. He that feareth is not made perfect in love. 1 John 4:18**

Part (a): **"There is no fear in love."** If there is no fear in love, if you are not loved perfectly, *then fear comes.* If I am loving you, are you going to be afraid of me? If I am not loving you, are you going to be a little skittish with me? First John 4:18 says, "There is no fear in love." What is the antidote to fear?

Part (b): **"Perfect love casteth out fear."** If fear comes from not being loved or accepted perfectly and if we have not been loved perfectly or accepted perfectly, then guess what comes into our lives? *Fear.* How is your discernment? Can you tell me? If there is fear in not being loved, if no love is there, there is a fear that comes. That is the fear that causes these diseases. The antidote would be to receive perfect love, or could I say love casts out fear?

All spiritually rooted diseases caused by fear involve a breach in relationship at whatever level. It could be a breach in relationship between you and God. It could be a breach in relationship between you and yourself, because you won't forgive yourself for something you did in 1928. It may be a breach between you and others. Remember what I told you:

*A spiritually rooted disease is a result of separation from God,*
*separation from yourself and separation from others.*

**The beginning of all healing of spiritually rooted diseases is:**

- **Reconciliation with God and His Love, receiving His Love, reconciliation with Him as your Father, and making your peace with Him;**

- **Reconciliation of you with yourself; and**

- **Reconciliation of you and others.**

Many people misunderstand the term "to fear the Lord" and are actually afraid of Him because of that word. They see in the Scriptures, "the fear of the Lord" or "the fear of God." There are 14 different Hebrew words and seven Greek words translated into English as "fear." The one specifically translated "fear" when referring to "fear of God" has to do with *reverential respect* because we honor Him for who He is.

You can respect somebody for who they are, but it does not mean you have to be afraid of them. Let's get the word "fear" out of our Anglo-Saxon mentality and do a word study on the Hebrew and the Greek. Then we will come back into a focus of the correct translation.

From that standpoint, if the breach is between God and ourselves and others, then the beginning of all healing is reconciliation with God, making peace with ourselves and making peace with our brother. First John 4:18 says, "There is no fear in love. Perfect love casts out fear."

Part (c): **"Because fear hath torment."** It is the fear-that-has-torment that produces *paranoid schizophrenia*. It is that fear-that-has-torment that produces DID *(dissociative identity disorder)* [previously referred to as MPD—Multiple Personality Disorder]. It is the fear-that-has-torment that produces many mental and psychological diseases, either through the inherited component of genetics or the inherited familiar spirits coming to produce it. Most of the things happening in our thoughts occur because we are afraid. Psychoses, phobias, panic, fear and anxiety can be a tormenting hell between the ears and in the depth of the heart. How do you get rid of the torment? Part (b) told you. *"Perfect love casts out all fear."*

Part (d): **"He that feareth is not made perfect in love."** This means you have fear because you are in a breach somewhere in your relationships at some level with a parent, boss, teacher, pastor, spouse or your church. This could be anyone you did not feel safe with, who did not cover you with perfect love, did not nurture you, did not forgive you, did not cover you in your weaknesses, drove you and made you attempt to be perfect. It could be someone who put you down, would not kiss you, would not hold you, would not tell you they loved you, would not give you support. Everything happening on that level of "you are not made perfect in love" allows an unloving, unclean spirit to attach itself to you. It will stay there until you are delivered with perfect love. We know this because Scripture says, "Perfect love casts out fear."

*If you are not able to give and receive love, then you have fear.*

Now I want to ask you, "How many people in here have difficulty receiving love and how many people in here have difficulty giving love?" If you are unable to give and receive love, you have the fear we are talking about. This fear produces these diseases, all the way from autoimmune to stress-related diseases.

Again, I think it is important to pay attention to 2 Timothy 1:7—God has not given us the spirit of fear but of power, love and a sound mind. I trust that you have gained insight into the spiritual roots of many diseases that are coming out of fear, anxiety and stress.

**Anti-anxiety drugs and antidepressant drugs are not the answer for fear**. These are neurological blockers and calming agents with extremely dangerous side effects and include *Prozac, Paxil, Xanax, Klonopin and* many more. They are incredibly dangerous drugs and they are given because we in the Church and those who are in the world are not in discernment about the spiritual dynamics and spiritual basis of our lives. Drugs are not the solution. They are a form of disease management and God would have you know with great authority that He wants you to be free of anxiety because He did not give it to you. He would want you to be free to live a life of peace, spiritually, emotionally and physiologically. If you just trust Him and stay away from the rudiments of the world in its thinking, you can come back before Him in simple trust. Drugs are a poor substitute for the peace of God.

There is *a more excellent way*™.

> **Peace I leave with you, my peace I give unto you: not as the world giveth, give I unto you. Let not your heart be troubled, neither let it be afraid. John 14:27**

> **They have healed also the hurt *of the daughter* of my people slightly, saying, Peace, peace; when *there is* no peace. Jeremiah 6:14**

What is the worst thing that can happen to you? You can die and go to heaven. I encourage you to go before God and ask Him to reveal to you the strongholds in your lives.

# Chapter Eight
# Specific Diseases

As we move on to discussing specific diseases, I want you to prayerfully allow God to deal with you. If you need to repent, then repent. If you need to acknowledge in discernment, then acknowledge in discernment. This is a private thing. God knows your heart. He already knows what is in there; you do not have to tell Him. He knows the thoughts of your heart. He knows the stuff causing you trouble. It is no surprise to Him.

## Our Statement Concerning Diagnosis and Success of Diagnosis

The only thing we can do here in any investigation of disease is, first of all, to acknowledge we are dealing with hypotheses. Even from the secular standpoint of ministry, we have to see how many cases in the long-term are healed and stay healed based on the information we have. The more case studies we review, the more we will know. I will tell you, this ministry is on the cutting edge of disease, yet we have a long way to go in getting enough case histories in our research so we can see established, complete patterns. From the standpoint of investigation, I hope, without making this a big issue, that you can hear where I am coming from and where I am going with this.

## Genetically Inherited Disease

The exact cause of manic depression is unknown, but heredity plays a role. There is also evidence of abnormalities in the secretion of the neurotransmitters seratonin and norepinephrine, and psychosocial factors may also be involved.

It was previously thought that abnormalities on the X chromosome contributed to the disease, but more recent evidence shows that there are associations with abnormalities in sequences on several chromosomes. If God created a person's DNA perfect from the foundation of the world, but the devil, because of the generations of sin, was able to interfere, then God can change the DNA back to normal. The devil is not more powerful than God! If Satan can mess with genetics, who do you think can fix them? Would we dare to believe God can change genetics and expect Him to do it?

But what if we don't ask? What if we have withdrawn with unbelief, doubt and fear? Do you think we would get this kind of a healing? No, I want to be just like a kid. "Daddy, I want a lollipop." What does the Bible say? "Except ye be converted, and become as little children, ye shall not enter into the kingdom of heaven" (Matthew 18:3).

> **And said, Verily I say unto you, Except ye be converted, and become as little children, ye shall not enter into the kingdom of heaven. Matthew 18:3**

Have we become so sophisticated in our religiosity we have forgotten how to simply trust the living God for our lives? Have we turned the immortal, invisible God into an intellectual concept? *Do we serve God with our heads or do we serve God with our hearts?*

Jeremiah 32:19 says that He is great in counsel and mighty in works.

> **Great in counsel, and mighty in work: for thine eyes *are* open upon all the ways of the sons of men: to give every one according to his ways, and according to the fruit of his doings: Jeremiah 32:19**

We choose what we shall have daily: blessings or curses, life or death.

> **I call heaven and earth to record this day against you, *that* I have set before you life and death, blessing and cursing: therefore choose life, that both thou and thy seed may live: Deuteronomy 30:19**

As for me and my house, we will serve the LORD.

> **And if it seem evil unto you to serve the LORD, choose you this day whom ye will serve; whether the gods which your fathers served that *were* on the other side of the flood, or the gods of the Amorites, in whose land ye dwell: but as for me and my house, we will serve the LORD. Joshua 24:15**

If I step outside the parameters, I'm going to get back in the parameters.

## Manic Depression

Whereas ten years ago, it was hoped that a single gene for bipolar disorder might be found, it is now clear that many genes are involved. Changes in the levels of the brain neurotransmitters dopamine, serotonin, norepinephrine, and GABA (gamma aminobutyric acid) might be involved in the disorder.

*Prozac* is a serotonin enhancer. It does not increase the secretion of serotonin. It just keeps it out longer on the end of the dendrite in the nerve synapse, which balances the imbalance. It does not solve the problem.

Drugs don't solve problems. In fact, drugs can interfere with the dealing of root problems because they mask the real issues.

I do not tell people to get off their drugs. If you are taking prescription drugs and getting before God and dealing with the issues in your life, then under a doctor's supervision, you can gradually detoxify. Your body will pitch a fit if you try to take away the new chemical reality created by drug therapy. *God created us perfect in Adam. In sin, we have become imperfect.*

I hold out for the removal of depression as a spiritual defect. *Depression is caused by the under-secretion of serotonin.*

There was a wonderful lady in America who called me. Her sister had been helped by our ministry. She said, "I have to have help. I'm a professional and an alcoholic. My marriage is disintegrating. I'm at odds with my family. I'm about to lose my job. I'm on *Prozac and* I'm coming apart."

In two 30-minute sessions over the phone during a two-week period, God delivered her from alcoholism, healed her of a broken heart and delivered her of the depression and anxiety. I saw her years later. She is happy, her marriage has been restored, she has been restored to fellowship with her family, she has never touched alcohol since and she was off *Prozac* by the end of the first week after her healing. She is vibrant, she is going to church, she is active in her church body and she is enthusiastically alive. We sat down together and just rejoiced before the Lord Who had healed her and delivered her.

*A more excellent way*™ is not to be artificially maintained. If God wanted you to be artificially maintained, He would have set in motion artificial maintenance programs for His people. He created you perfect. He created you with an immune system and a body designed to take care of itself for 70 to 80 years and past 70 with some trouble. Moses said in Psalm 90, with some trouble.

> **The days of our years *are* threescore years and ten; and if by reason of strength *they be* fourscore years, yet *is* their strength labour and sorrow; for it is soon cut off, and we fly away. Psalm 90:10**

God established longevity over 3,000 years ago.

The average life expectancy in America is now around 76. We still have not exceeded God's parameters and won't, as an average, until the coming of the Lord and the day of the Lord in the first resurrection. You can try to live to be 120 if you want to! It is appointed to a man once to die and then the judgment.

> **And as it is appointed unto men once to die, but after this the judgment: Hebrews 9:27**

We have our part in the first resurrection. Blessed are they who have part in the first resurrection because they shall not taste of the second death.

> **Blessed and holy *is* he that hath part in the first resurrection: on such the second death hath no power, but they shall be priests of God and of Christ, and shall reign with him a thousand years. Revelation 20:6**

This is good news!

> **We are confident, *I say,* and willing rather to be absent from the body, and to be present with the Lord. 2 Corinthians 5:8**

> **²⁰According to my earnest expectation and *my* hope, that in nothing I shall be ashamed, but *that* with all boldness, as always, *so* now also Christ**

shall be magnified in my body, whether *it be* by life, or by death. ²¹For to me to live *is* Christ, and to die *is* gain. ²²But if I live in the flesh, this *is* the fruit of my labour: yet what I shall choose I wot not. ²³For I am in a strait betwixt two, having a desire to depart, and to be with Christ; which is far better: Philippians 1:20–23

This is a great hope! It takes care of anxiety and fear.

Eye has not seen, ear has not heard nor has it entered into the heart of man what God has prepared for them who love Him.

For since the beginning of the world *men* have not heard, nor perceived by the ear, neither hath the eye seen, O God, beside thee, *what* he hath prepared for him that waiteth for him. Isaiah 64:4

But as it is written, Eye hath not seen, nor ear heard, neither have entered into the heart of man, the things which God hath prepared for them that love him. 1 Corinthians 2:9

I want to be there, how about you? That is my hope: the redemption of my body to what God has prepared for me is the hope I have.

And not only *they,* but ourselves also, which have the firstfruits of the Spirit, even we ourselves groan within ourselves, waiting for the adoption, *to wit,* the redemption of our body. Romans 8:23

I am a happy Henry. I used to be a sad Henry, but now I am a happy Henry because whether I live or whether I die, I know I am the Lord's.

## The Immune System

God created your immune system to maintain your body. God created your body to be able to fight invaders. The average person develops one or two mutant cancer cells at least 200 times in a lifetime. Because you have a healthy immune system, the killer cells are active and in full volume. They recognize the mutant cells or the viruses or the bacterium and they attack and destroy them. God created your immune system to protect you, not to destroy you. In all autoimmune diseases, the white corpuscles decide a part of your body is the invading enemy and needs to be destroyed.

Your spiritual enemy wants to destroy your immune system, which is your marrow. Your blood has its origin in the marrow. The T cells, macrophages, killer cells and white and red corpuscles are found in the marrow.

Here are some ways Satan tries to access your marrow. He wants to:

- control your thoughts,
- make his spirituality your spirituality,
- get you to follow the law of sin,

- create relationship breakups,

- stir up strife and promote conflict,

- promote inappropriate reactions,

- initiate verbal, physical, emotional and sexual abuse, and

- speak to you in the first person, as though it were your own thoughts, so you do not recognize them as from your enemy.

If he can destroy your relationship with God, with others or with yourself, then he has access to your immune system. Relationship is the foundation of the kingdom of God. The breakdown of relationships is *not* the kingdom of God.

> [37]Jesus said unto him, Thou shalt love the Lord thy God with all thy heart, and with all thy soul, and with all thy mind. [38]This is the first and great commandment. [39]And the second *is* like unto it, Thou shalt love thy neighbour as thyself. [40]On these two commandments hang all the law and the prophets. Matthew 22:37–40

So what is the source of your thoughts? From God? From yourself? From Satan's kingdom? Unrighteous thoughts provide the pathway producing the destruction of the immune system.

Fear can cause a compromised immune system because prolonged fear causes excess cortisol drip. Cortisol is a naturally occurring steroid. Cortisol is not the problem, but excessive cortisol is toxic and destroys your immune system. It will destroy Interleukin-1, Interleukin-2 and the T Cells. It is released when you do not feel loved or feel insecure in love. This opens the door to fear.

Cortisol is released in response to fear, or more specifically, anxiety.

By giving in to the fear, you are giving Satan's kingdom permission to weaken your immune system. The more fear you experience, the more cortisol is released into your body. When you have long-term fear, cortisol destroys Interleukin-1 and -2 and the T cells. So any white corpuscles, T cells, macrophages and killer cells left will no longer recognize the invaders. This results in cancer.

Broken relationships can cause toxins to enter the bloodstream. Most cancers come out of loss and conflict, caused by fear and bitterness. Bitterness results in broken relationships. Many cancers are linked to bitterness. The word *bitterness* in the Greek means "poison."

When bitterness and fear separate you from others, cell membrane semi-rigidity sets in and the toxins begin to collect at the cellular level. Once a certain level of toxicity is attained, the immune sentries of your cells, the two anti-oncogenes, are destroyed.

These anti-oncogenes are enzymes protecting you from the mitosis which produces cancer. Cell mitosis is the dividing of cells causing cancer to multiply. Then a tumor is formed. A spirit of death and spirit of infirmity are at work. Bitterness produces a disease unto death because bitterness is a form of murder.

The *Biblical Guide to Alternative Medicine* written in 2003 by Dr. Neil Anderson and Dr. Michael Jacobson documents the story of a pastor's wife with stage IV terminal breast cancer. She had no hope. Because she had bitterness against another female, Interleukin-2 had been devalued so her immune system did not recognize the cancer.

> If you were to ask her, Candice would say that the most powerful physical healing agent available is not a drug; it is a sound (healthy) spiritual heart and mind. As a 50-year-old pastor's wife, Candice was given the devastating diagnosis of metastatic breast cancer. By the time it was discovered, the disease had already spread throughout her body, and she was given only a few months to live. In response to her diagnosis, she and her husband sought the counsel of a Georgia pastor whose ministry orientation is in identifying spiritual factors in the cause of disease. During their conversation, Candice became aware of the possibility that bitterness toward another woman had weakened her immune system and made her more vulnerable to cancer. Shortly thereafter, she sought forgiveness and was reconciled in her relationship with the woman from whom she had been estranged. That was four years ago. As of this writing, her cancer has spontaneously regressed despite the fact that she has never changed her diet, has never had surgery and has not taken any medications. She still has no symptoms and feels great.

When she repented to God and repented to the woman she had bitterness against, she became a doer of the Word and God honored her with healing. She is still healed today, she did not take chemo and no one prayed for her. This testimony reveals that she had a root issue and demonstrates the number one block to healing, which is unforgiveness.

## Crohn's Disease

*Crohn's disease* and *ulcerative colitis* mirror each other, but they are two different classes of diseases. *Ulcerative colitis* is confined to the colon; *Crohn's disease* is usually found in the distal ileum and colon, but it can appear anywhere in the gastrointestinal tract.

*Ulcerative colitis* and *Crohn's* mirror each other as they both involve ulceration of the colon and extreme bleeding. *Ulcerative colitis* is confined to the colon, but *Crohn's disease*, although it is primarily in the colon, can appear in the ileum, the esophagus and at any point of the gastrointestinal tract when in advanced cases of spreading.

*Crohn's disease* is a disease in which the white corpuscles decide it is not virus, bacterium, or mothers-in-law, but it is the lining of the colon that is the enemy of the person. In all autoimmune diseases, the white corpuscles are involved.

In our literature, you will remember, we discuss something we call *"white corpuscle deviate behavior."* It is a term I coined to let you know that something God created, that is supposed to take care of invading enemies, has now decided we are the enemy and is attacking various parts of our body. *The spiritual implications are incredible in that, as we attack ourselves spiritually, the body eventually agrees and starts attacking itself in destruction.*

*Crohn's disease* is believed to be due to an abnormality in the regulation of the proinflammatory response involving the white corpuscles. It is easy to distinguish, in diagnosing from a medical standpoint, the difference between *Crohn's* and *ulcerative colitis*. In *Crohn's disease*, the white corpuscles initially start attacking the lining of the colon, causing ulceration. It is a very serious disease. The root behind *Crohn's* is *extreme self-rejection coupled with guilt. Crohn's* also has a component of hopelessness because the individual does not know how to solve the problem over which they are tribulating. There is a lot of conflict built into it. *Crohn's disease* is a disease coming out of massive rejection, abandonment, lack of self-esteem *and/or drivenness to meet the expectation of another. In fact*, Crohn's disease *involves a great degree of codependency and false burden bearing.*

## Ulcerative Colitis

*Ulcerative colitis* is thought to involve an abnormality in the regulation by dendritic nerve cells of the immune response. Dendrites are fingerlike projections on nerve cells that receive electrical signals from the axon terminals of other nerve cells across a gap, called a synapse. The electrical impulse is received by receptors on dendrites or muscle fibers. The transmitted impulse can then trigger movement of a muscle or chemical response by a nerve cell.

However, stress, anxiety, lack of trust, things bugging you over a long period of time, or even feeling like you don't belong can lead to abnormalities in the function of the dendrites. This results in impaired function and excessive release of inflammatory substances causing ulceration of the mucosal lining of the colon and hemorrhaging from the lining of the colon.

You go to the doctor, and he may give you chemotherapy, prednisone or other steroids or drugs, all of which have incredible side effects.

*Ulcerative colitis* is an anxiety disorder, rooted in extreme fear and anxiety and dread, causing a flaring of dendrites in the lining of the colon, which irritates it in a manner similar to an ulcer. It causes an ulceration of the lining of the colon, producing severe bleeding. This is *ulcerative colitis*. The only way to get *ulcerative colitis* healed is to *deal with the anxiety disorder and the fear behind it.*

## Diabetes (Type 1) (Autoimmune Disease)

I'll tell you what the spiritual root is behind *diabetes (type 1): extreme rejection and self-hatred coupled with guilt.* In the many cases we have ministered to, we have found there was *direct rejection by a father and sometimes a husband or a man in general.* We are not just talking about a little bit of rejection, but bad words like, "You ain't no good," "You ain't never going to amount to a hill o' beans," and then some choice language to go along with it.

We have had tremendous success in seeing *diabetes* healed. There has to be an absolute change in the person allowing them to receive the love of God in order for healing to happen. *Diabetes (type 1)* can be inherited because an unloving spirit can be inherited. A broken spirit (heart) is also implicated.

*Fear can be inherited.* Allergies can be inherited. Many of the things we deal with can either develop in our lifetime or we can inherit them from our family tree. So when I see this happening in a child, I can go back to the father and mother, grandfather and grandmother, on both sides and I'll find some abuse. I'll find some victimization. I'll find rejection. I'll find someone not being nurtured somewhere. This can be inherited, not only from a genetic standpoint, but also from a spiritually inherited standpoint. This is what I would be looking at in that case.

The Bible says in Ezekiel the children do not have to die for the sins of the father, but in Exodus 20:5 it says the curse that is the result of a sin shall be passed on to the third and fourth generation.

> **...he shall not die for the iniquity of his father, he shall surely live. Ezekiel 18:17**

> **Thou shalt not bow down thyself to them, nor serve them: for I the LORD thy God *am* a jealous God, visiting the iniquity of the fathers upon the children unto the third and fourth *generation* of them that hate me; Exodus 20:5**

## Lupus

*Lupus* is an autoimmune disease in which the white corpuscles attack the connective tissue of the organs. I ministered to a beautiful lady in California who has been healed of *lupus*. She was medically diagnosed, documented through her physician's case history and testing and is now healed of *lupus*. Today I can still remember how her voice sounded when calling me on the phone about four years ago. She said, "I just got back from the doctor and he can find no evidence of *lupus* in my body. It is gone." *Lupus is rooted in extreme self-hatred, self-conflict and includes guilt. Performance also may be implicated.*

## Multiple Sclerosis

*Multiple sclerosis* occurs when the white corpuscles decide the myelin sheath of the nerve is the enemy. Recent investigation has shown it is not just the myelin sheath affected by the attack of the white corpuscles, but the nerve itself is damaged. This is recent information I did not know previously. I thought it was just the myelin sheath. The myelin sheath is like the insulation around the nerve, just as rubber insulates the outside of an electrical cord.

*Multiple sclerosis* occurs when the white corpuscles come like a modern day Pac-Man and take a bite out of the coating around the nerve, effectively short-circuiting it. It is not a problem with the muscles; it is the nerve which causes the muscles to become short-circuited during the nerve transmission process. This is called sclerosis and in *multiple sclerosis* there are many of these holes created. It is noted in recent medical information the nerve itself has also been severely damaged in advanced cases of MS.

In a small percentage of cases, the person eventually dies because even the muscles necessary for respiration are no longer functioning. However, 85 percent of these people live a normal lifespan. Generally, nerve tissue does not regenerate; this is why certain parts of your body do not heal. This is why it would take a creative miracle by God and ministry to restore this type of damage.

*MS is rooted in deep, deep self-hatred and guilt* and spiritually it is very close to *diabetes (type 1)* because it involves a father's rejection. I want to say something to you:

> ***The father is responsible for the spiritual welfare of the family.***
> ***The father, not the mother, is responsible***
> ***for his daughter's value system and her self-esteem.***

I don't give men many breaks because I know the tragedy of my own life. I have had to learn this thing the way the Word teaches it, not the way my generation has lived it. I have had to have some paradigm shifts in my thinking as a human being and a man of God. I have to represent God the Father to my children. I have to be to my wife as Christ is to the Church. I do not have a choice.

## Rheumatoid Arthritis

This is an autoimmune disease and affects the joints of the skeleton, the tissues, the cartilage and the connective tissue of the skeleton. It acts on the body like this: your white corpuscles decide the bacteria and the viruses are not the enemy and they attack your joints and cartilage instead.

In *rheumatoid arthritis*, basically there is a proliferation of white corpuscles which congregate in the connective tissue of the skeleton and, like a Pac-Man, they start to eat away and destroy the material. It is degenerative and this is so classic that I end up saying it just the way I am going to say it: *as the person attacks themselves in self-hatred, so the body conforms to this spiritual dynamic and attacks itself in return.*

Lots of people wish they were dead and will say so if you talk to them long enough. They don't believe they belong on this planet. They don't believe God loves them. They don't believe their mother-in-law loves them. They don't believe their father and mother love them. They don't even love themselves and when you get into it, they are attacking themselves spiritually. There is a spirit of infirmity coming to agree with them and to mutate the biogenetic character of the white corpuscles. They then take an assignment from the devil, not from God who created them and they are on a mission of destruction.

*The only way to be healed from rheumatoid arthritis and other autoimmune diseases is to accept yourself once and for all and to get the self-hatred, the guilt, the lack of self-esteem and the junk out of your life.* When you don't accept yourself, you hate yourself and you have called the living God who loved you from the foundation of the world a liar. You have declared He made a mistake in saving you. When you say this you have called God a liar and the devil agrees. He is right there to bless you with the opposite of your Father in heaven's blessing and this is where the *"spirit of death"* comes in.

Can you say this? I want to hear you say it. "I shall live and not die and declare the glories of my God in my generation." What glory is there? Say it: "What glory is there if the grave takes me prematurely?"

> **I shall not die, but live, and declare the works of the LORD. Psalm 118:17**

> **For the grave cannot praise thee, death can *not* celebrate thee: they that go down into the pit cannot hope for thy truth. Isaiah 38:18**

Does God receive any glory out of losing you prematurely off this planet? I want to give you some shocking theology. God does not need you in heaven right now. You are of no earthly good to Him up there and He does not need your help. He has birthed you by His will in the generations of your ancestry and He has called you by His Spirit. He has redeemed you to Himself for His glory in the earth to establish His kingdom, His love, His grace and His mercy through you until you just run into heaven when you have finished all things in your generation. I consider it error to even suggest God needs disease as a vehicle to get you to heaven. There is much evidence to the contrary in Scripture.

*Rheumatoid arthritis is another disease in which the body attacks the body.* As the person is spiritually attacking himself or herself, the body conforms to it spiritually and there you have it. It will be very difficult to be healed of *rheumatoid arthritis* or any other autoimmune disease as long as you are buying that lie and allowing guilt and self-hatred to rule your thoughts and lives. It is not possible to be healed because God is not going to honor it. He says that you are fearfully and wonderfully made (Psalm 139:14–18).

> [14]**I will praise thee; for I am fearfully** *and* **wonderfully made: marvellous** *are* **thy works; and** *that* **my soul knoweth right well.** [15]**My substance was not hid from thee, when I was made in secret,** *and* **curiously wrought in the lowest parts of the earth.** [16]**Thine eyes did see my substance, yet being unperfect; and in thy book all** *my members* **were written,** *which* **in continuance were fashioned, when** *as yet there was* **none of them.** [17]**How precious also are thy thoughts unto me, O God! how great is the sum of them!** [18]*If* **I should count them, they are more in number than the sand: when I awake, I am still with thee. Psalm 139:14–18**

Psalm 139 also says His hand is upon you from the foundation of the world. Before your parts in continuance were fashioned from the dust of the earth, He knew you and He ordained you to be here in your generation. So accept it and get on with it.

Out of darkness, out of bondage, out of the fall of Adam and Eve, He has gathered you to Himself. The Father gathers His children to Himself.

### *You are going to have to accept His love and yourself in it.*

I don't care what your poor head tells you. Let God be true and every man a liar.

> **God forbid: yea, let God be true, but every man a liar... Romans 3:4**

"Yeah, but you don't know what they did to me in 1948." No, but I know what God is doing for you this year! He is going to heal you. Get all your theology straightened out so you can get on the right side of faith and not fear.

## Viruses

I want to tell you about viruses. A virus does not have as its origin its own life. It is a mutation of what is already genetically another life form and then mutates after its aberration. Viruses are an aberration of genetic materials producing various kinds of interference with human flesh. This is a virus. It is a mutant genetic life form which seems to have a mind of its own. It is difficult to destroy and in the case of HIV, it can remanufacture itself in a different form by taking the genetic code of a living organism and using the genetic material of a living organism to produce its own genetic form.

I have finally come to this conclusion and I cannot document it even if I tried. In ministry I have been attacking viruses from this basis and have been getting healing of virally related incurable diseases.

I consider viruses to be *spirits of infirmity* and I consider them to be a physiological expression and work of evil spirits in conjunction with man's flesh and genetics. This is the only thing I have been able to figure out: *A virus has an intelligence behind it that defies imagination.* A bacterium just floating around will duplicate itself and it is still a bacterium. It seems to have a "life form." However, viruses also seem to be very intelligent; so behind a virus there is some type of intelligence and it is not God.

I have been attacking viruses as spirits of infirmity and I got that from the Bible.

> **¹¹And, behold, there was a woman which had a spirit of infirmity eighteen years, and was bowed together, and could in no wise lift up** *herself.* **¹²And when Jesus saw her, he called** *her to him,* **and said unto her, Woman, thou art loosed from thine infirmity. Luke 13:11–12**

Jesus cast out spirits of infirmity with His words. Jesus knew something then that I don't know. I am here, some 2000 years down the road with advanced technology to help me figure it out and I am coming to the same conclusions He did. There is something alien that is an intelligent, invisible being afflicting man's flesh and tissue. You cannot kill it, you cannot destroy it, but you can divert it. So I have tried casting it out and it has worked. Why is it we have a virus sitting around, hanging out, doing no physical harm and then when it is released because of another spiritual problem called fear, anxiety and stress, it does damage to the body? Do you think there's a connection?

Is it possible to make a virus go dormant forever if we deal with other spiritual problems? This is an interesting question and I certainly will be pursuing it to see how much success we have long-term.

## Herpes

When we get into *herpes*, we have more than one kind. We have simplex: whether it be genital herpes or fever blisters and they are viral. Now are you saying *shingles* is viral? This is what the doctors say. When I get into *herpes*, which is viral, I still get into a spiritual problem. There are several cases of *herpes* I have dealt with. It is amazing that *herpes* seem to go into remission, but under stress they erupt. Bacteria can be destroyed easily, but viruses are difficult to destroy because they mutate, change, hide and even go dormant for years. Again, there seems to be an intelligence behind them defying imagination.

## Cancer

Cancer is one of the most feared diseases of this generation, yet there are some cancers we have had some insight into.

Cancer that is the result of metastisizing of cells to other parts of the body is an unfortunate by-product of the disease and may have nothing to do with the root of the original source.

### Colon Cancer

I am coming to the conclusion that it is deeply rooted in bitterness and slander with the tongue. The Bible says life or death is in the power of the tongue. Every evil word we have spoken will be held in judgment against us.

> **Death and life *are* in the power of the tongue: and they that love it shall eat the fruit thereof. Proverbs 18:21**

> **But I say unto you, That every idle word that men shall speak, they shall give account thereof in the day of judgment. Matthew 12:36**

There are a lot of strange things happening between the lips and the anus and in between, all kinds of things can go wrong for many spiritual reasons. If you are verbally abusive to enough people, it comes back to you. I am rapidly looking at colon cancer cases and looking back to past generations because it is clear it can be inherited. I believe colon cancer is an inherited disease. I am looking back to see if we can trace the history of conflict in families. Family conflict, similar to the Hatfields and the McCoys, where unresolved bitterness, unresolved antagonism and words of frustration and anger have occurred, causes damage throughout the successive generations.

Do you know, when you speak evil against someone, it is a curse and what you speak against another returns? Can I give you a Scripture? Jesus said those sins you retain are retained and those sins you remit are remitted.

> **Whose soever sins ye remit, they are remitted unto them; *and* whose soever *sins* ye retain, they are retained. John 20:23**

Do you know when you retain another person's sins and you do not forgive them, you, in fact, have retained the curse yourself? Read the

Scripture—whatever is bound on earth shall be bound in heaven and whatever is bound in heaven shall be bound on earth:

> **And I will give unto thee the keys of the kingdom of heaven: and whatsoever thou shalt bind on earth shall be bound in heaven: and whatsoever thou shalt loose on earth shall be loosed in heaven. Matthew 16:19**

The Lord's prayer says that if you do not forgive your debtors, the Father in heaven will not forgive you yours:

> **⁹After this manner therefore pray ye: Our Father which art in heaven, Hallowed be thy name. ¹⁰Thy kingdom come. Thy will be done in earth, as *it is* in heaven. ¹¹Give us this day our daily bread. ¹²And forgive us our debts, as we forgive our debtors. ¹³And lead us not into temptation, but deliver us from evil: For thine is the kingdom, and the power, and the glory, for ever. Amen. ¹⁴For if ye forgive men their trespasses, your heavenly Father will also forgive you: ¹⁵But if ye forgive not men their trespasses, neither will your Father forgive your trespasses. Matthew 6:9–15**

So the sins you retain are retained. You are holding the other person under the bondage of your judgment. But by the same judgment you judged others, you yourself are judged. This is what the Bible says.

> **¹Judge not, that ye be not judged. ²For with what judgment ye judge, ye shall be judged: and with what measure ye mete, it shall be measured to you again. Matthew 7:1–2**

> **Therefore thou art inexcusable, O man, whosoever thou art that judgest: for wherein thou judgest another, thou condemnest thyself; for thou that judgest doest the same things. Romans 2:1**

When we get into the area of gossip and slander, tale bearing, sedition, anarchy, division making, causing trouble, not promoting peace, being an instrument of division and anarchy, I wonder if these sins may be the cause of colon cancer.

The cancers I am most familiar with are breast, ovarian, Hodgkin's, leukemia and prostate. In one particular case of pancreatic cancer, I never ministered. The person went off into alternative realities and did not stay in touch with me.

## Skin Cancer

I do not know if there is a spiritual root or not; the evidence seems to involve taking care of the temple (your body) and keeping the skin covered properly to protect it from ultraviolet rays.

## Liver Cancer

Information has come to me concerning liver cancer. Since this seminar was taught, an individual e-mailed me the following Scriptures:

> [21]**With her much fair speech she caused him to yield, with the flattering of her lips she forced him. [22]He goeth after her straightway, as an ox goeth to the slaughter, or as a fool to the correction of the stocks; [23]Till a dart strike through his liver; as a bird hasteth to the snare, and knoweth not that it *is* for his life. Proverbs 7:21–23**

There seems to be some indication that these Scriptures have to do with an individual; in this case, a man who was lusting after a female, either in his mind, or actual fornication or adultery following seduction. The individual who e-mailed me indicated a close family member died from liver cancer, and even though it was not known if actual fornication or adultery had occurred, it was known this individual was heavily into pornography. The question I am asking myself is: was this a warning from the Word of God concerning the fruit of being addicted to pornographic material?

## Breast Cancer

Let me say something to really shock you. I don't mean to scare you and every time I say this there are certain ladies who end up being scared; so please do not be scared. I'll tell you: 10 percent of all breast cancer in America is caused by mammograms.

A big uproar happened about a year ago when the AMA said you do not have to have mammograms until at least age 50. The feminist radicals immediately objected and said women must have them throughout adulthood. However, the medical community had come to the startling conclusion that 10 percent of all breast cancer is caused by mammograms. This is why the feminists backed off. Startling, isn't it?

Why 10 percent? Most of the women who fell into this category had what is called a "predisposition to breast cancer." A healthy cell has two enzymes called anti-oncogenes. They are tied directly to the immune system. There are three classes of cells in the human body: healthy, which have two anti-oncogenes present; predisposed, which have one anti-oncogene present; and compromised, with no anti-oncogenes.

A healthy cell will never become cancerous. You cannot develop cancer with both of the anti-oncogenes present. Something has to come and destroy them. In the case of someone who is genetically predisposed, there is only one anti-oncogene present. A compromised cell is where one or two of the anti-oncogenes have been destroyed by some intrusion into the cell, either by toxic chemicals from outside the body or toxic chemicals manufactured by the body internally for some reason, such as a result of bitterness.

The ladies who developed breast cancer from mammograms had an inherited predisposition for cancer with only one anti-oncogene. The X-rays from the mammogram destroyed the one remaining anti-oncogene, the cell became compromised and breast cancer began. I would tell any woman, "If you're going to get a mammogram, it might cost you a little money, but go to an oncologist first and get tested."

I know they are saying the radiation dosage has been reduced and radiation mechanisms have changed so now the mammograms are safe and won't destroy the anti-oncogenes due to an overdose of radiation. This is what they tell you when you ask the questions. My recommendation is for you to check it out first, especially if there is any history of breast cancer in your family tree.

When I talk about healings having taken place with breast cancer, I am talking about an individual who had gone to an oncologist in conjunction with a geneticist and had her breast tissue tested. If the oncologist finds the breast tissue is compromised (no anti-oncogenes are present), then it would be necessary for you to be re-tested after ministry to see if there are any changes. In ministry, we deal with the spiritual roots and come before God and meet the spiritual conditions for healing to take place. In re-testing of this particular case, it was found both anti-oncogenes were present in the cell after ministry, whereas before they were medically proven to be missing. That's a miracle!

One of the first cases of breast cancer I was involved with occurred in 1984. A lady came to me a couple of days before her scheduled surgery for a radical mastectomy. I got involved in her life and it took a while to determine the spiritual roots of her cancer. There had been competition, sibling rivalry, between the females in her family and the girls were competing with their own mother for supremacy. It was a mess. There was a tremendous amount of bitterness and bickering. I got with her before God and helped her forgive her sisters and her mother. She had a strong root of bitterness.

Concerning a root of bitterness, there is an old saying: "It eats at them like a cancer." If you have this type of festering resentment and bitterness on a long-term basis, then your body will produce toxins that will eventually accumulate to the level and volume where they will destroy the anti-oncogenes of the immune system at the cellular level in the breast tissue.

The target cells in females are in the breast tissue because the breasts are the nurturing aspect of a female. When the female is no longer nurturing, or she is being nurtured yet turns into a spiritual alley cat, there is a problem. It is a tragedy. When the resulting toxins develop, they destroy the anti-oncogenes.

In this lady's case, I began ministering to her and we came before God, looked at all the things she was doing and she repented before God for this long-term historical feud. Her mother had a history of the same type of behavior with her own sisters. These females had hated one another for generations. It was a cat fight all the way.

She had the mastectomy surgery and after coming out of the surgery, we were still doing ministry, dealing with spiritual roots and blocks and coming before God. Her doctor said to her, "I'm going to put you on chemotherapy for five years." She came and told me her doctor wanted to put her on chemo for five years.

I said, "Well, if your anti-oncogenes are present and if God has healed you, you are wasting your time." I suggested she get retested. She went back to her doctor and said, "I think I want my cells tested to see if both anti-oncogenes are now present." He said, "Where did you hear that?" He said, "This is new."

She said, "Henry Wright told me." She asked him, "Doctor, if both my anti-oncogenes are present in genetic testing, can I get cancer?" He said, "No." She said, "Then why do I need chemotherapy?" He said, "For our protection." She said, "What if I don't want it?" He said, "You will have to sign a disclaimer relieving us from all responsibility." She said, "I'll do it." So they tested her and both anti-oncogenes were present, whereas before they had not been. **That's a miracle!** I tell you, we are now over a dozen years down the road and she is still alive today. Praise God! There are also many other cases.

*Breast Cancer* is coming out of the sins of conflict and bitterness between the female and either her mother and/or her sisters or mother-in-law. *Breast cysts* are very similar. Many women get *breast cysts* and think it is cancer.

**DISCLAIMER:** This profile represents a large percentage of breast cancer cases, but there are many other causes for breast cancer also.

**NOTE:** Since this teaching was originally done, there is new information on cancer now being documented by doctors globally in case studies. This information is startling even to this writer although I have seen for years that bitterness was commonly found in relation to breast cancer and fibrocystic breast disease.

Case histories are documenting this bitterness through the ministry. The insight is as follows: cysts or tumors appearing in the left breast tissue seem to follow unresolved bitterness and conflict between that female and another female blood relative, such as mother, sister, aunt or grandmother. Tumors or cysts that appear in the right breast seem to be the result of unresolved bitterness and conflict between the female who has the tumors and another female (non-blood relative) such as a mother-in-law, a person in the workplace, a person in the church or possibly her husband. Although there are exceptions, this observation is holding true in over 80 percent of all cancer cases. There are an increasing number of females who are being healed. In fact, breast tumors just disappear when that woman forgives another female.

I am excited because it is possible to have the hope of not "just being healed" of breast cancer, but of preventing breast cancer. Females forgiving each other is critical to preventing breast cancer. In fact, this new insight is so startling that **this writer has the faith to believe families now have the ability to prevent cancer in their generations, not just be healed**.

(This entire subject can be found in the booklet, *Insights Into Cancer*, available from the Be in Health™ bookstore.)

### Ovarian Cancer

*Ovarian cancer* comes out of a woman's hatred for herself and her sexuality. Unclean and unloving spirits accusing her in the cleanness of her sexuality can lead her into self-bitterness and self-loathing concerning her own sexuality.

### Uterine Cancer

*Uterine cancer* may be caused by promiscuity and uncleanness; however, behind the promiscuity and the uncleanness is the need to be loved, but this is another issue.

### Hodgkin's Disease and Leukemia

*Hodgkin's disease* and *leukemia* are very similar. They are similar because the root cause is the same in *Hodgkin's* (lymphatic) and *leukemia* (blood). The factors are the same. I have found that many times, *Hodgkin's disease* and *leukemia* are caused by deep-rooted bitterness coming from unresolved rejection by a father. I have always found a breach between the person who has this disease and their father. I have never found a mother involved in the breach. Abandonment by a father, literally or emotionally, is also implicated.

### Prostate Cancer

*Prostate cancer* comes out of anger, guilt, self-hatred and self-bitterness. All cancer with a spiritual root involves some type of bitterness against someone for some reason. It involves long-term, lingering, festering and damage leading toward death. Hatred is the fifth part of bitterness. You wish someone didn't exist. God says, "If they don't exist, neither do you."

[14]**We know that we have passed from death unto life, because we love the brethren. He that loveth not** *his* **brother abideth in death.** [15]**Whosoever hateth his brother is a murderer: and ye know that no murderer hath eternal life abiding in him. 1 John 3:14–15**

Your enemy has as much of a right to this planet as you do. God loves you and your enemy and He might save both of you! You might be an enemy to someone else. In conclusion, though, the bitterness is more directed toward one's self, although others may be indicated in the profile.

Remember 2 Timothy 2:24–26:

[24]**And the servant of the Lord must not strive; but be gentle unto all** *men,* **apt to teach, patient,** [25]**In meekness instructing those that oppose themselves; if God peradventure will give them repentance to the acknowledging of the truth;** [26]**And** *that* **they may recover themselves out of the snare of the devil, who are taken captive by him at his [the devil's] will. 2 Timothy 2:24–26**

There are a lot of people blaming God for their problems and He is not guilty. Let's get this straight: the Word of God says, in James 1:13, that God does not tempt man with evil, neither can He be tempted with it.

**Let no man say when he is tempted, I am tempted of God: for God cannot be tempted with evil, neither tempteth he any man: James 1:13**

I am going to get Daddy off the hook, if you don't mind and put the deceiver back in the frying pan. I want to make sure I sow seed into your lives the Holy Spirit can use, the Father can use and the Lord Jesus, Who is the Word, can use. Then they might bring you into a place of defeating your enemy and bearing fruit in your generation and your lifetime, not to mention extending your life expectancy without disease.

I have said many times in teaching and in seminars that, since Adam and Eve, mankind has been on probation for almost 6,000 years.

God has been trying the reins of men's hearts to see if there would be any who would seek after Him so He may show Himself strong on their behalf. Your hearts are being tried.

**For the eyes of the LORD run to and fro throughout the whole earth, to shew himself strong in the behalf of** *them* **whose heart** *is* **perfect toward him. Herein thou hast done foolishly: therefore from henceforth thou shalt have wars. 2 Chronicles 16:9**

**Examine me, O LORD, and prove me; try my reins and my heart. Psalm 26:2**

Will you choose the good or will you choose evil? Will you repent? Will you take responsibility or will you go into rebellion? The bottom line, whether we like it or not, is submission to the living God, out of our free will, because we want to and because we are in love with Him. He is in love with us. He tells us this over and over in His Word.

When we step outside the parameters of the covenant, outside the holiness of God, then God gives us over to our enemies.

Read the history of the Jews. When they did not like God, they went out and followed the gods of the Amorites, Moabites, Syrians, Egyptians and all the rest. God would say, "Okay, if you don't want Me as Father, let them be your Father. Let them bless you."

What was the blessing? The curse! When God's people had enough of it and they were sick and dying and in captivity, they would come running back to Daddy and say, "We're sorry. We repent. We repent. We repent." And God would say, "I forgive you."

**When we step outside the commandments of God, we open ourselves up to the "blessing" of the devil.** It is as simple as that. When you start to hate your brother, you receive the recompense of the reward. Through "one man sin entered into the world and death by sin" (Romans 5:12). Through one man's disobedience sin came and through the obedience of another man, Jesus Christ, we are free. We are either obedient sons and daughters of God or we are disobedient sons and daughters of God.

Does the devil have a legal right to you after conversion? I am not sure about this, but I'll tell you what: I sure see evidence of it. Many people struggle with the reality and the question: Can a Christian have an evil spirit? I am not sure I have the answer to this, but I would raise this question: *Can an evil spirit have a Christian?*

Proverbs 26:2 says as a bird by wandering and a swallow by flying, so the curse without a cause does not come.

> **As the bird by wandering, as the swallow by flying, so the curse causeless shall not come. Proverbs 26:2**

Your enemy does not have the right to oppress you just because he is out there. Someone has to open the door and invite him in. Go back to Genesis 3. Satan used the serpent as a medium of expression. He did not have access to this planet until Eve invited him in and Adam agreed. In your life, the evil one does not have the right to oppress you; he only takes that right because you give it to him many times through ignorance or lack of knowledge. Proverbs 26:2 says the curse does not come without cause.

**God has set parameters of protection around mankind against the devil**. The only way the devil can get at you through his kingdom is for you to invite him in at some level. These are called **doorpoints of entrance**. If this were not the case, then the Christian would not have a chance. Satan could have killed us all and it would have been over. However, Satan does not have that ability. God forbade him to bring death in the discourse with Job. But in Job's life there was a spiritual root problem. Job had a hedge of protection and Satan challenged this protection. God had no choice but to let Job be sifted so he could be purified at this level of the testing. When you read Job, especially in chapter 3, Job said the thing he feared greatly had come upon him.

> **For the thing which I greatly feared is come upon me, and that which I was afraid of is come unto me. Job 3:25**

### *Faith and fear are equal in this dimension: both demand to be fulfilled.*

Hebrews teaches us about faith:

> **Now faith is the substance of things hoped for, the evidence of things not seen. Hebrews 11:1**

### *Fear is the substance of things not hoped for and the evidence of things not yet seen. Faith is God's future for you. Fear is Satan's destruction of your faith and ultimately your future.*

> **But without faith *it is* impossible to please *him:* for he that cometh to God must believe that he is, and *that* he is a rewarder of them that diligently seek him. Hebrews 11:6**

This is what the Word says. Job had a root problem as stated in chapter 3, verses 2–5: he was full of fear. In chapters 40–41, in the discourse concerning Behemoth and Leviathan, the great parable of his spiritual condition, we find Job had pride and he had spiritual arrogance. You know this because he took God on for size and discourse. God came back with, Where were you, big boy, when I did this, this and this? God turned the captivity of Job around when Job finally was humbled and he prayed for his friends. He received twice as much as he had when he began and his captivity was turned around. Could God turn around your captivity? Yes, He can!

It must be understood and distinguished that not all growths are cancerous. There are two types of growths: one is fibroid tumor (benign) and the other would be considered cancerous (malignant).

*It is my observation that when a tumor does not become malignant, it involves bitterness against one's self. But when it becomes malignant, it involves bitterness against others.*

# Arthritis

### Arthritis (Involving Inflammation of the Joints)

Basic simple *arthritis* is inflammation of a joint usually accompanied by pain, swelling and frequent changes in structure. It might be noted this differs from *osteoarthritis* and other forms of *arthritis* by the type of manifestation and then there is a different spiritual root behind each of the types.

The spiritual root for simple *arthritis* involves bitterness against others.

To help you understand, it seems when you have bitterness against yourself, it involves degeneration; but when you have bitterness against others, it involves swelling and inflammation. It is the swelling and inflammation which produces the deformity.

### Osteoarthritis

*Osteoarthritis* is progressive cartilage degeneration in joints and vertebrae and usually does not involve inflammation. The cartilage is the other material between the vertebrae. *Osteoarthritis* is the result of *self-bitterness* and *not forgiving one's self*. It is holding a record of wrongs against yourself and can also involve an element of guilt.

# Nonbacterial Inflammation

About three years ago, in ministering with people, we found a new disease just now being recognized by the medical community. It is a combination of two diseases having merged into one. Its root is a combination *of anxiety, fear, guilt and self-hatred* producing something called *nonbacterial inflammation*. Inflammation usually comes from bacterial intrusion. When you have bacterial intrusion, you go to the doctor and he puts you on antibiotics. What if you have inflammation and he puts you on antibiotics but there is no bacterial material intrusion? When you continue taking the antibiotics, you are not going to have any relief and after a while you are going to end up with *candida*. Continuous usage of antibiotics destroys the body flora, which you need to maintain your balance. You do not want to destroy all the bugs! Some are helpful!

### Interstitial Cystitis

*Interstitial cystitis* is a swelling and inflammation of the bladder tissue of females. It is very painful, nonbacterial and the current treatment for it is to give an antibiotic. The antibiotic is prescribed, not because there are bacteria present but because a certain antibiotic has been developed which has anti-inflammatory properties. The purpose of the anti-inflammatory is to bring down the swelling. In *interstitial cystitis,* you have the over-secretion of histamine, producing swelling and the proliferation of white corpuscles, also producing inflammation and swelling. In males, it is called *prostatitis.*

### Prostatitis

*Prostatitis* is a disease involving nonbacterial inflammation in males. Prostatitis can be serious because at some point it can lead to prostate cancer. Again, *prostatitis* involves two dimensions, as does *interstitial cystitis and* those are excessive secretion of histamine and a proliferation of white corpuscles on location.

In these nonbacterial inflammation diseases, the spiritual root, as mentioned, is fear and anxiety, which causes excessive histamine secretion, self-rejection and self-hatred coupled with some guilt to produce the proliferation of white corpuscles.

We ran across an individual in New York City many years ago who was light sensitive, in a highly exhaustive state, had swelling and edema and the doctors couldn't figure out what it was. We recognized the spiritual roots at work. The spiritual roots caused a combination of an over-secretion of histamine and a proliferation of white corpuscles in various parts of his body.

This man talked to a member of my staff and related he had been to a doctor at New York City Hospital who said, "This is a brand new disease we have been studying and we are diagnosing you with it. We do not understand much about it, but it has to do with autoimmune and histamine problems."

He said, "I sat in that office for over 30 minutes and every word they said you had already told me a year before, almost word for word."

## Cell Membrane Rigidity vs. Cell Membrane Permeability

We minister to folks with a class of diseases *involving cell membrane rigidity versus cell membrane permeability.* Classic angina, asthma and retention of toxins in the bloodstream fall into this same category. In normal tissue, when you have cell membrane permeability, it means that in the process of osmosis or diffusion (that material in the bloodstream necessary in the cell enters through the semi-permeable membrane of the cell and the waste by-product is exchanged on the same basis; it leaves the cell through semi-permeable membranes), free flow goes unhindered. When you have cell membrane rigidity, you have stiffening of the cell membranes and osmosis is hindered. Behind this is a very definite spiritual root. In the case of toxic retention at the cellular level, toxins build up in concentration and are retained as the cells lose their ability to dispose of waste products.

## Asthma

In the case of *asthma,* there is stiffening of the cell membranes of the alveoli. This causes an entrapment of carbon dioxide and an exclusion of oxygen. Thus, you have breathing problems and find yourself gasping for air.

The inhalant medication given by a physician is a neurological blocker which basically short-circuits the process and allows a relaxation of those cell membranes. The carbon dioxide is then released and oxygen starts to be absorbed. You begin to breathe normally. These are the mechanisms of what happens when drug therapy is applied to the problem. The process of osmosis or diffusion is normalized.

For many years, we have known *asthma is a fear-anxiety manifestation.* It can be inherited. There can be a genetic component. We have observed in medical journals that the hypothalamus gland, when it senses fear and anxiety, causes a hormone called ACTH to be secreted. This hormone goes into the bloodstream and docks at a receptor cell in the alveoli. This produces the stiffening.

*Asthma* is one of the fastest growing childhood diseases in America. I have known the root problem of *asthma* for over a decade. When I taught it, people would look at me and laugh. "Well, this is not what the medical community says. You are out to lunch." I might be out to lunch, but many people are well. Now the medical community is agreeing with me.

The findings from the Johns Hopkins University Research Team, in the fall of 1996, confirmed our spiritual diagnosis of asthma and this changed the conventional wisdom concerning asthma for the past 50 years. You have been taught that many asthmatic attacks are a response to an exposure to allergens, irritants, pollen, dust and danders, things you take into your respiratory system through breathing.

Johns Hopkins University research has conclusively proven that nothing you breathe causes an asthmatic attack. Something is happening in the lungs, in the alveoli, to cause stiffening, an entrapment of carbon dioxide and an exclusion of oxygen. Thus we see the respiratory difficulty, the gasping for air and all that goes with the drama of the situation.

Usually the type of fear and anxiety which produces *asthma* has to do with *great fear concerning relationships.* We have ministered to many people who no longer have *asthma.* Johns Hopkins University is still trying to figure out what this invisible reality is that triggers the stiffening. I'll tell you what it is: a *spirit of fear and* it is able to control your physiology through the hypothalamus.

**Editor's Note:** Since this seminar was taught, evidence has led me to observe the depth of this spirit of fear. In fact, my conclusion is the fear of abandonment and the resulting insecurities are the key issues behind asthma.

## Angina Pectoris

The word *angina* comes from the Greek word meaning "strangling." *Angina* is a cell membrane rigidity disease but does not involve osmosis or diffusion. *Angina* involves the hardening, stiffening and narrowing of blood vessels and produces faulty circulation. *Angina pectoris* occurs when coronary circulation is reduced for some reason. Stress and anxiety (spiritually speaking, fear) produces a constriction of vessel walls and is a common cause. Also implicated is strenuous exercise or a heavy meal. Apprehension and dread increases the problem. The bottom line is that fear, anxiety and stress are common culprits. Remember what the Word says in Luke 21:26:

> **Men's hearts failing them for fear, and for looking after those things which are coming on the earth: for the powers of heaven shall be shaken. Luke 21:26**

## Hypertension (High Blood Pressure)

Again we have cell membrane rigidity, which produces a vasoconstriction of blood vessels, coupled with an increase of cardiac output which increases the blood pressure. It is again caused by *fear and anxiety*. In chapter 9 of the *Pathophysiology* textbook, on page 305, on the subject called "Stress and Disease," it says one of the physiologic effects of the catacholamines is a peripheral vasoconstriction of blood vessels in the cardiovascular system. Also on page 309, in the section entitled "Examples of Stress-Related Diseases and Conditions," under the target organ or system, the cardiovascular system is listed and one of the corresponding diseases listed as a result of stress is *hypertension* (high blood pressure).

Our position is still the same. God has not given us the spirit of fear, but of power, love and a sound mind.

> **For God hath not given us the spirit of fear; but of power, and of love, and of a sound mind. 2 Timothy 1:7**

We have to go back into a person's life and find out where the open doors are, either inherited or personal. It is these open doors that allow the spirit of fear to come in and take over that person's life, controlling them at this level.

## Toxic Retention

When you have cell membrane rigidity, the body will retain various toxins at the cellular level and will not cleanse itself properly because the process of osmosis, or diffusion, is hindered. We ran into this by accident. When we started to review the case histories of people healed of MCS/EI, we came up with a startling observation. When the doctor rechecked their blood, the toxin levels were normal. They had not used any drug therapies or modalities of cleansing to cause the cells to be cleansed of toxins. As these individuals walked out of their disease spiritually, the toxins went away.

As I started ministering, I realized when the mechanisms producing cell membrane rigidity were gone, full cell membrane permeability now existed. *God designed the body to cleanse itself as part of its creation.* When the spiritual roots are dealt with, this is exactly what happens.

Have you not read the Scripture that says, if you drink any deadly thing, it shall not harm you?

> **...and if they drink any deadly thing, it shall not hurt them...**
> **Mark 16:18**

Do you know why? It is because when you are in a right relationship with God, your body cleanses itself of toxins. I am not talking about doing something presumptuous like drinking poison on purpose. I am talking about a normal lifestyle and things to which you are exposed. God created your body to cleanse itself of impurities. The spiritual root of toxic retention is fear and anxiety.

I am for a clean environment and take a stand that government and industry should be responsible in protecting us from excesses of chemical intrusion. I am also fully aware of the possibility of chemical injury. However the majority of toxic blood cases I have reviewed do not include exposure at this level. In fact, in the many cases of MCS/EI involving diagnosable toxic levels, after ministry and Walk Out, the toxic reality was gone and tissue was normal. This has been an astounding fruit in our investigation of cell membrane rigidity vs. cell membrane permeability.

**NOTE:** Even though many people are well today from MCS/EI and toxic retention, including the corresponding allergies and all that goes with them, it does not mean everyone who started to apply our principles has gotten well. The reasons are many because people's life circumstances can be complicated and not everyone has continued with our program to its conclusion. I am not responsible, nor is any other person who is trying to help someone responsible, for the failure of insight to work when a person withdraws from the insight. This does not make the insight invalid; it just indicates there is breakdown at a different level.

# OTHER DISEASES

## Attention Deficit Disorder

There are three ranges: the lower range, the mid range and the high range. The high range is hyperactivity. We primarily deal with ADD in children. Dealing with ADD in adults is more difficult. ADD comes out of a **dumb and deaf spirit.** There are many classes of psychological diseases falling under the category of dumb and deaf. Jesus cast out a dumb and deaf spirit from a person who could not speak (Matthew 11:5; Mark 7:32, 37; Mark 9:25; Luke 7:22).

> **When Jesus saw that the people came running together, he rebuked the foul spirit, saying unto him, *Thou* dumb and deaf spirit, I charge thee, come out of him, and enter no more into him. Mark 9:25**

We are still learning about ADD, involving the spectrums from the lows to the mediums and the highs. We have more experience in the hyperactive range than the lower range, though we have had some cases in the lower and medium ranges.

We understand ADD to be a neurological interruption. We also understand ADD is or can be familial or inherited. It seems to run in family trees. We have a very strong feeling it is tied to a dumb and deaf spirit putting a person into bondage.

ADD, dyslexia and gender disorientation have something in common. Don't think, because I have merged dyslexia and ADD with gender disorientation, that anyone is at risk of becoming gender disoriented because they have ADD. They do, however, have a common thread. There is a *double mindedness* that comes and this is an inherited family curse. A double minded man is unstable in all his ways.

> **A double minded man *is* unstable in all his ways. James 1:8**

When you find ADD, you will also find it in the parents and grandparents. You won't find it in just one place. You will find it right down the line. It is the same with dyslexia. It involves a type of double mindedness and confusion and the prime root of the confusion is gender disorientation because of an inversion of godly order in the home. The home is ruled by matriarchal control rather than patriarchal authority as God intended.

That home is ruled by the female, not the male. The confusion coming from that is producing ADD, dyslexia and gender disorientation. When the male does not rule the home in love, the female has no choice but to take the reins.

The minute she does, Satan's entire kingdom comes to help her. She was never designed to rule the home; she was designed to follow a patriarch, a godly one, I might add. I am not a chauvinist and I do not send females back into the oppressive rulership of ungodly males in the name of the Lord. When the female is being oppressed, I call for immediate separation and resolution.

I will protect the children and the female first before I'll protect the male. The male should be protecting the female and the children to begin with, so I hold him to a higher level of responsibility.

You see, the female and the children should follow the male as he follows Christ. The head of the woman is to be the man and the head of the man is Christ. But the head of Christ is the Father and nobody quotes the rest of that Scripture. It does not stop with Christ; it stops with the Father.

> **But I would have you know, that the head of every man is Christ;**
> **and the head of the woman *is* the man; and the head of Christ *is* God.**
> **1 Corinthians 11:3**

This brings the male back into the rulership—not just as the husband, but in a similar relationship Christ has with the Church as our Husband. The husband is called to represent God as the father to his family just as if it were God Himself. It is a tough job, but it is the work God has called a man to do.

I also have observed various standpoints of rebellion as part of this profile. Historic family rebellion exists in families who have been involved in occultism and false religions. Historically, it is an interrupter of the thoughts. It interferes with self-esteem. *It involves much self-rejection, self-hatred and guilt*. It often involves dyslexia and other various breakdowns of perception. Many times, you will find color blindness, which is also inherited. You can also have other peripheral problems coming with this family profile.

I'll give you one testimony of success in the healing of ADD. I have been asked about ADD in adults versus ADD in children. The roots are the same. One case in particular is astounding.

A child was brought to me. The child's school said they needed a meeting with the parents because this child was so disruptive he had to be placed in the back of the school room in a chair with his face against the wall. He was totally isolated in the classroom and they still could not contain him.

When the parents received the letter and came to me, it was very obvious the next step the school counselors would recommend would be to put the child on the drug *Ritalin*.

*Ritalin* is a very dangerous drug. This drug is the shame of our school systems in America because it is a lazy way out of a problem. The information

I have on children who are on Ritalin is from a national organization's research concerning children on Ritalin and it shows that 50 percent of them, at some point in their lifetime, end up afoul of the law and in jails. This has been directly related and attributed to the drug, not to ADD. There is a psychotic value that comes with this drug and it's horrific. It is a Pandora's Box and yet it is currently the "drug of choice" for ADD.

I had been doing some pastoral studying, in certain levels and I was aware of an alternative methodology that would satisfy the school system. They don't like it and they do not want to be involved in it because it takes work on their part. It takes effort and cooperation with the parents and teachers. It is a technique called *focusing*.

In the hyper range of ADD, the child is fine as long as he or she is concentrating on an object of interest. The nerve synapses and the flow of focusing are normal, but when the child is not motivated, the neurological flow is interrupted and there is activity called *ranging*, including free-floating thoughts and impulsive realities. The child does whatever comes to mind.

This particular child had straight Fs and antisocial, disruptive, mouthy, rebellious and you-name-it behavior. I went with the parent to the school counselor to propose an alternative. The parent did not want the child on Ritalin because of its psychotic side effects and potentially dangerous implications. With *focusing* and with "counseling" (actually, we were talking about ministry; I am not into counseling, I am into ministry), we explained how we felt this child's ADD could be resolved.

*Focusing* is a treatment at the secular level, but you will hardly ever hear about it because it is so much easier to give your children Ritalin. This is the quick way, but Ritalin does not solve the problem. The Bible says in Proverbs 22:6 to train up a child in the way he should go; and when he is old, he will not depart from it.

> **Train up a child in the way he should go: and when he is old, he will not depart from it. Proverbs 22:6**

That is what focusing does.

We took a particular child and made up a chart. It had a row for every day of the week and every week of the month. We charted the next nine-week period of the school semester. The chart had three columns. The first column had a smiling face. The next column had a face with a straight line for the mouth and the next column had a frowning face.

I brought the child in and said, "This is the deal; if we cannot help you through ministry and focusing, they are going to put you on Ritalin, which is a drug." I explained to the child the ramifications of the drug and the consequences. *This is part of focusing—education—*but this is not threatening to the child. Children understand when you take the time to talk to them. You may not think they do, but they really are listening and you can reason with children if you take the time to meet them on a level they can understand.

We asked the child, "If you could have anything today, what would you like?" He said, "A Sega video game console."

"Of course, you want a Sega!" We told the child, "For every day that you turn your homework in and behave well in the classroom, the teacher is going to evaluate you and she is going to put a smiling face in that column for that day when you have succeeded. If you come home with a smiling face, your parent is going to give you $2.00 toward your goal to purchase the Sega. The day you just barely make it is a straight line and you don't get any dollars. The day you blow it and you really blow it, you get a frowning face and will lose one dollar from one of the days you got a smiling face. At the end of the nine-week period, when you have more smiling faces than you have straight lines and frowning faces, then you will receive your prize. If you don't, the alternative is you will have to take Ritalin, because the school will require it. *This is your choice."*

This is where we began. For the first two weeks, it was kind of rough. Remember, we are establishing new memes—new focusing, new concepts— and this takes time. But things started to shift. With ministry and focusing, in conjunction with the teacher's cooperation as well as the child's and the parents', this worked. In the second nine-week period, the child went from Fs to the A-B honor roll. The third nine-week period, the child maintained a position on the A-B honor roll and by the fourth grading period, the child was still on the A-B honor roll. He became student of the year and for the last nine weeks was the teacher's assistant. He went from the back of the room to the front of the room, all by focusing, prayer and ministry and we did not have to go to drugs. This is significant and this is *a more excellent way*™.

This is not the rest of the story. He felt so good about himself; he was so proud when he walked up in front of the assembly at the end of the school year and was given a certificate for Student of the Year. Something wonderful happened inside of him and he never let go of his achievements.

Part of the profile for ADD is *self-rejection.* This young man started to be a winner and he liked being a winner. He did not want to be a rebel anymore. He liked being the teacher's pet. Suddenly a new life had begun and he knew he wasn't on drugs and did not need to be on drugs. This was very important to him.

The second year they brought him to me again and I said, "Okay, you know how we won this battle last year. This year there'll be no reward. You only get one Sega in a lifetime. You know how God met you and you know how you came through with flying colors last year. This year, do you think you can make it through just by focusing and observing how you feel about yourself? He said, "I think I can do it, but I might blow it every now and then." I said, "Well, I blew it yesterday myself."

We have the mentality that white collar is better than blue collar. This is hogwash. We are so success-oriented that we have forgotten the bigger picture. Our children are paying the price for our drivenness to perform and our demand for perfection. It is time to stop. One of the things I do in ministry is to ask parents to "lay off" their children.

Teach them the ways of the Lord and to be what God wants them to be from the foundation of the world. Pray for your children, instruct them in the ways of the Lord and then release them. Leave them alone. They will hear God in due season. You did.

It is amazing to some of your parents to see you serving God today. They're shocked. You know what? The greatest sinners sometimes make the best pastors, too. It is amazing whom God will save. Those saintly ones you were once compared to are still stuck in the mud!

There is an important distinction needing to be made here. I am not a counselor and the members of my staff are not counselors. We are ministers.

> **Who also hath made us able ministers of the new testament; not of the letter, but of the spirit: for the letter killeth, but the spirit giveth life. 2 Corinthians 3:6**

You can be a minister and not be an ordained pastor or evangelist. The Bible makes a provision for ordinary saints to minister the gospel of reconciliation.

> **14For the love of Christ constraineth us; because we thus judge, that if one died for all, then were all dead: 15And *that* he died for all, that they which live should not henceforth live unto themselves, but unto him which died for them, and rose again. 16Wherefore henceforth know we no man after the flesh: yea, though we have known Christ after the flesh, yet now henceforth know we *him* no more. 17Therefore if any man *be* in Christ, *he is* a new creature: old things are passed away; behold, all things are become new. 18And all things *are* of God, who hath reconciled us to himself by Jesus Christ, and hath given to us the ministry of reconciliation; 19To wit, that God was in Christ, reconciling the world unto himself, not imputing their trespasses unto them; and hath committed unto us the word of reconciliation. 2 Corinthians 5:14–19**

Every saint has been given authority to be a minister of the kingdom of God. The word *counselor* is secular. The word *minister* is scriptural and we make the distinction very clearly. However, this does not exclude proper leadership made up of the members of the fivefold ministry to oversee the ministry of the saints and instruct it.

## Epilepsy

The **dumb and deaf spirit** is also found in *epilepsy*. I have always seen healing in cases of epilepsy in 15 years of ministry. Most epileptics who have come to us have been healed, although there is never any guarantee for healing. These healings I make reference to have been documented through EEG tests in which the Alpha, Beta and Theta brain waves were normal. These individuals have never had another seizure and are not on any medication. But in order to get this healing, we had to go back to the gospels to learn how to do it. In these cases, it was not a spiritual root causing the problem. I had to cast an evil spirit out. I do not make a big deal out of it, but I have cast out legions of them. This is what God wants done. I am well able, as every believer should be, to deal with it when necessary.

Psychologists have been able to document many of our personality characteristics including rage, anger, predisposition to mental disorders and certain diseases found in humans without any genetic component, but it can still be inherited. There is not a genetic or a defective gene that has been isolated, but the condition is still passed on in families. We consider those situations to be *inherited familiar spirits* following families to create various breakdowns in the psyche or the soul.

Dumb and deaf spirits rule over the second heaven and try to control the minds of men. Your mind is the Lord's, your spirit is the Lord's and your body is the temple of the Holy Ghost. You are the Lord's and the enemy of your life, Satan, wants to rule you in your thoughts.

I do not believe the devil can read your mind. This would make him omniscient and he is not. His kingdom can project thoughts into your head out of the realm of the spirit, but what you do with those thoughts is up to you.

Paul said in 2 Corinthians 10:5 that we are to bring every thought into captivity, casting down every imagination and every thought that would exalt itself against the knowledge of God.

> **Casting down imaginations, and every high thing that exalteth itself against the knowledge of God, and bringing into captivity every thought to the obedience of Christ; 2 Corinthians 10:5**

I have to subject my thoughts to higher thoughts all the time. His ways are higher than my ways and His thoughts are greater than my thoughts.

> **For my thoughts *are* not your thoughts, neither *are* your ways my ways, saith the LORD. Isaiah 55:8**

The most man's wisdom could ever be only begins to approach the foolishness of God according to Scripture.

> **Because the foolishness of God is wiser than men; and the weakness of God is stronger than men. 1 Corinthians 1:25**

This means we have a long way to go.

My mind has to be renewed by the washing of the water of the Word (Ephesians 4:23; 5:26) and I have to bring every thought into captivity of the knowledge of God (2 Corinthians 10:5).

It says in 2 Timothy 1:7 that God has not given me the spirit of fear, but of power, love and a sound mind.

> **For God hath not given us the spirit of fear; but of power, and of love, and of a sound mind. 2 Timothy 1:7**

What do you think I am holding out for? Power, love and a sound mind!

In 1985, a young lady came to me. She was about 21 years of age and had been experiencing grand mal epileptic seizures for many years. They heard God was using this ministry, honoring our work and people were being healed.

A member of my staff said, "This situation is like the one that the disciples couldn't cast out. They went back to Jesus and He said this one cometh out but by prayer and fasting" (Matthew 17:14–21). The young lady was supposed to be there by 7:00 that night and it was 10:00 in the morning when my staff member asked me, "Don't you need at least three days of prayer and fasting before you can defeat this?"

I said, "What!?" They replied, "Well, that is what the Bible says." I staggered for a moment and said, "You know what? I live a prayed and fasted life with Christ. This woman could die in 24 hours, let alone three days. Today is the day of salvation; now is the appointed time (2 Corinthians 6:2). She is coming; let's go for the gold." In Matthew 17, Jesus taught that my faith concerning this type of ministry was all that was necessary and so I did as Jesus had taught us to do.

> [14]**And when they were come to the multitude, there came to him a *certain* man, kneeling down to him, and saying, [15]Lord, have mercy on my son: for he is lunatick, and sore vexed: for ofttimes he falleth into the fire, and oft into the water. [16]And I brought him to thy disciples, and they could not cure him. [17]Then Jesus answered and said, O faithless and perverse generation, how long shall I be with you? how long shall I suffer you? bring him hither to me. [18]And Jesus rebuked the devil; and he departed out of him: and the child was cured from that very hour. [19]Then came the disciples to Jesus apart, and said, Why could not we cast him out? [20]And Jesus said unto them, Because of your unbelief: for verily I say unto you, If ye have faith as a grain of mustard seed, ye shall say unto this**

**mountain, Remove hence to yonder place; and it shall remove; and nothing shall be impossible unto you. ²¹Howbeit this kind goeth not out but by prayer and fasting. Matthew 17:14–21**

They brought her to me. She was unsaved and she was living with her boyfriend in sin. She had two abortions and I talked to her about these issues. She decided to accept the Lord because I told her that if she accepted the Lord, the chances of Him healing her would be pretty good. "You have come all this distance. I think He really wants to do this." I took authority over the *dumb and deaf spirit* and cast it out of her and commanded the *spirit of epilepsy* to be gone. I did not know if it had gone or not; I did not see any visible evidence.

I said, "Goodbye." One week later, she went to her doctor in Asheville, North Carolina. He ran an EEG on her and her alpha, beta and theta brain wave tests were all normal. The last time I heard about her, she was serving God internationally with Youth With A Mission (YWAM). She was saved, healed and is now serving God. She never had another epileptic seizure, ever again. This was the first of several encounters with people who had epilepsy. So far, we have had great success in the healing of epilepsy in our ministry, although there is never a guarantee. Everything is in God's hands by faith.

*Everyone who is ministered to does not get well. There are reasons for that.* The reasons why they do not get well is what this ministry is all about in America today. We are picking up in situations where people do not get well after prayer.

My ministry began where prayer and standing on the Word and jumping on it did not work. Then God began to teach me about the spiritual roots of disease and the spiritual blocks to healing.

It is not true that God does not want to heal; it is that He would have to deny Himself and His holiness to do so in our lives when those spiritual roots and/or spiritual blocks exist. He is not going to compromise our heart changes in the name of blessing. He would be an unfaithful Father if He let us keep our sins and blessed us anyway. However, there is evidence in Scripture that God healed and delivered people who did not qualify. It is His sovereignty and must be recognized.

**For he saith to Moses, I will have mercy on whom I will have mercy, and I will have compassion on whom I will have compassion. Romans 9:15**

Sometimes, God heals and delivers people first and straightens them out later. However, it is my observation that God is first interested in our sanctification as a prelude to healing and deliverance.

We would not honor Him and we would not serve Him because He would have condoned evil in our lives. Do you really respect anyone who condones evil in his or her own life? Think about it! When your kids were growing up and mommy and daddy said, "Don't do this and don't do that," did they really appreciate it?

No, but when they became older, did they appreciate it?

Do we have respect for people who try to get us in trouble? Do we have respect for people who uphold evil in our lives and jeopardize our very existence? We would not respect God if He did that, would we? We would not serve Him. *We do expect God to be holy.*

## Paranoid Schizophrenia

*Paranoid schizophrenia* is a disease of the mind or the soul that can be inherited non-genetically. It is a classic example of what Scripture calls double mindedness.

**A double minded man *is* unstable in all his ways. James 1:8**

*Schizo* means split or divided and *paranoid* means split because of fear, delusions and projected delusions. Paranoid schizophrenia is the result of a malfunctioning of at least two of the neurotransmitters in the body. It is the result of an over-secretion of norepinephrine and an over-secretion of dopamine. Now there is some evidence suggesting it is also an over-secretion of serotonin.

God created us to be very chemical in our creation. He created us this way in our homeostasis and in our glandular construction. Our glands add the secretions here and there, so in a normal situation our homeostasis is maintained in a perfect way. When your thinking is interrupted, both on a psychological level and a spiritual level, your body responds to a breakdown in thought, feeling, emotion or perception.

As Scripture says, you are being tossed to and fro.

**That we *henceforth* be no more children, tossed to and fro, and carried about with every wind of doctrine, by the sleight of men, *and* cunning craftiness, whereby they lie in wait to deceive; Ephesians 4:14**

You may be regressing in a shield of veneer, not wanting to become vulnerable or transparent, or you may overextend into assertiveness to hide. You either withdraw or you project up front to hide what is behind. You either withdraw and hold up a shield, or you take the shield away and create a new one called a *fabricated personality*. Bullies are this way. The bully is more afraid of you than you are of him; you just don't know it. The facade he projects is there to protect his inadequacies, his fears and his feelings of rejection.

How many of us find ourselves struggling between either withdrawing in a house of fear or stepping out in fabricated personalities we hide behind?

*How many of us are really who God created us to be from the beginning?*
Psalm 139 says that from the beginning, from the foundation of the world,
God knew you. Before your parts were fashioned from the very dust of the
earth, God knew you:

> [13]**For thou hast possessed my reins: thou hast covered me in my
> mother's womb.** [14]**I will praise thee; for I am fearfully *and* wonderfully
> made: marvellous *are* thy works; and *that* my soul knoweth right well.**
> [15]**My substance was not hid from thee, when I was made in secret, *and*
> curiously wrought in the lowest parts of the earth.** [16]**Thine eyes did see my
> substance, yet being unperfect; and in thy book all *my members* were
> written, *which* in continuance were fashioned, when *as yet there was* none
> of them. Psalm 139:13–16**

*You are not an accident in your generation.* God told Jeremiah that
before he was ever conceived, He ordained him to become a prophet to the
nations.

> [5]**Before I formed thee in the belly I knew thee; and before thou
> camest forth out of the womb I sanctified thee, *and* I ordained thee a
> prophet unto the nations. Jeremiah 1:5**

Paul told us that God ordained him to be an apostle to the Gentiles.

> [15]**But when it pleased God, who separated me from my mother's
> womb, and called *me* by his grace,** [16]**To reveal his Son in me, that I might
> preach him among the heathen; immediately I conferred not with flesh
> and blood: Galatians 1:15–16**

> **According as he hath chosen us in him before the foundation of the
> world, that we should be holy and without blame before him in love:
> Ephesians 1:4**

> **Paul, a servant of Jesus Christ, called *to be* an apostle, separated
> unto the gospel of God, Romans 1:1**

Like Paul, it is clear you are no accident and in your generation, God
has called you, elected you and selected you to be a viable part of His
corporate body in the earth.

> [9]**But ye *are* a chosen generation, a royal priesthood, an holy nation, a
> peculiar people; that ye should shew forth the praises of him who hath
> called you out of darkness into his marvellous light:** [10]**Which in time past
> *were* not a people, but *are* now the people of God: which had not obtained
> mercy, but now have obtained mercy. 1 Peter 2:9–10**

Would you mind getting on with it?

In 1 Corinthians 12, we see everyone is important to the whole picture.
If I could strip the facade off you today, drag you screaming out of your
prison house, plunk you down on this planet and release you by the power of
the Holy Spirit to be what God created you to be in your generation, it would
be a miracle!

I would like to ask you a question. If I strip from you all the veneers of life and all the protective mechanisms—all the defense mechanisms, fear and rejection tragedies of your life coming from victimization, fear of man, fear of rejection, fear of failure, fear of abandonment and unloveliness, guilt, rejection and self-hatred—if I stripped all of this away from you, *who would you be?*

*If I could strip all of this away from you, there is a good chance all your diseases would go away.* All your diseases are the result of what you carry around; I call it the plaque of life. It is like going to the dentist to have the plaque on your teeth removed. It is time to do some spiritual cleaning.

We looked at *fear, stress and physiology* and found just how powerful Satan is. The power of Satan is *fear.* Do you know why? The Scripture says, The devil knows his time is short so he goes about like a roaring lion seeking whom he may devour (1 Peter 5:8; Revelation 12:12).

> **Be sober, be vigilant; because your adversary the devil, as a roaring lion, walketh about, seeking whom he may devour: 1 Peter 5:8**

> **...for the devil is come down unto you, having great wrath, because he knoweth that he hath but a short time. Revelation 12:12**

The devil *knows* his time is short. His days have been numbered. Remember in Daniel:

> **²⁵And this *is* the writing that was written, MENE, MENE, TEKEL, UPHARSIN. ²⁶This *is* the interpretation of the thing: MENE; God hath numbered thy kingdom, and finished it. ²⁷TEKEL; Thou art weighed in the balances, and art found wanting. ²⁸PERES; Thy kingdom is divided, and given to the Medes and Persians. Daniel 5:25–28**

Satan has been numbered and he has been found wanting in the balances. His very soul and spirit person is required for judgment. This is where our archenemy is headed. He knows he is already judged and he knows he has lost, but because he is a sore loser, he is going about trying to convince you, like a bully, that God has lost and he has won.

You can listen to this lie if you want, but it is why the enemy is so powerful. He is in fear. His greatest fear is eternal banishment to the lake of fire and this is where he and all his angels with him are headed. This is their destiny.

In dealing with mental and psychological diseases, we find dumb and deaf spirits can attach themselves to you and control your mind. *Why do you halt between two opinions?*

> **And Elijah came unto all the people, and said, How long halt ye between two opinions? if the LORD *be* God, follow him: but if Baal, *then* follow him. And the people answered him not a word. 1 Kings 18:21**

Choose! Remember, Israel's great challenge; do you want to follow Baal or do you want to follow the God of Israel? What do you want to do?

In this last Scripture, the people did not answer. When asked this question by Moses in the sanctification of Israel in Exodus 24:3, they said, "All the words which the Lord hath said we will do." Did they? No, they lied and went their own way. Such is the case many times today! We hear God's word and say nothing, or we say we will and we don't.

How many of us say we are following God, we are "believers," but in our real life we are following the other kingdom? We come and say, "Yea, Lord," but in real life we forget the Lord and follow the voice of the goat, the enemy.

When you are following fear, you are not following God. Second Corinthians 10:5 says that we should hold every thought in captivity, cast down every vain imagination and hold every thought up against the knowledge of God.

> Casting down imaginations, and every high thing that exalteth itself against the knowledge of God, and bringing into captivity every thought to the obedience of Christ; 2 Corinthians 10:5

Everybody quotes this one. Everyone knows this one. Do you ever quote verse 6?

You know 2 Corinthians 10:5 as well as you know John 3:16 and Hebrews 4:12. But no one quotes Hebrews 4:13 and no one quotes 2 Corinthians 10:6. I want you to defeat the enemy. I am looking for something to happen inside of you.

2 Corinthians 10:6 says that we should also have a readiness to revenge all disobedience after our obedience is fulfilled.

> And having in a readiness to revenge all disobedience, when your obedience is fulfilled. 2 Corinthians 10:6

*You cannot defeat your enemy in disobedience.* You cannot be healed of your disease and continue to be disobedient to God and His Word when He has told you what is causing your disease. You cannot expect to be healed of anxiety and fear disorders if you continue to operate in fear and anxiety and stress and tension. You can quote all the Scriptures about being anxious for nothing,

> Be careful for nothing; but in every thing by prayer and supplication with thanksgiving let your requests be made known unto God. Philippians 4:6

and God has not given us the spirit of fear,

> For God hath not given us the spirit of fear; but of power, and of love, and of a sound mind. 2 Timothy 1:7

but unless you are prepared to make fear your enemy, you are wasting your time quoting the promises.

Are you ready to do a little circumcision? Are you ready to put to death those things that do not come from God? Are you prepared to come before God in trust and in love, not in condemnation and become transparent with Him?

James talks about confessing our faults one to another that we may be healed.

> **Confess *your* faults one to another, and pray one for another, that ye may be healed... James 5:16**

The problem today is that we have become so dysfunctional. We do not trust each other. We do not even trust our own husbands or wives. Husbands do not talk to their wives and wives do not talk to their husbands about the deep torments of their heart.

They believe their spouse already has so many problems that their own burdens are just one more thing to add to the situation: just one more fight on top of the six they already have. *Have we lost our way?*

If my wife cannot talk to me, who in the world do you think I should send her to? If my family cannot live in peace in my home, where do you think I should send them to have peace on this planet? If I cannot love my wife, whom do you think I should send her to, to get love?

We are in prison houses. God has not called you to bondage. He has called you to freedom. If we walk in the light together as He is in the light, then we have fellowship one with another.

> **But if we walk in the light, as he is in the light, we have fellowship one with another, and the blood of Jesus Christ his Son cleanseth us from all sin. 1 John 1:7**

If you confess your sin to me, I am going to love you in it. Galatians 6:1 says that if a brother be overtaken in a fault, those of you who consider yourself spiritual are to restore such an one in the spirit of meekness and consider yourself also, lest you be tempted in like manner and fall away.

> **¹Brethren, if a man be overtaken in a fault, ye which are spiritual, restore such an one in the spirit of meekness; considering thyself, lest thou also be tempted. ²Bear ye one another's burdens, and so fulfil the law of Christ. Galatians 6:1–2**

Verse 2: Bear ye one another's burdens and so ye fulfil the law of Christ.

God forbid that anyone have a problem in most churches. The one way to get the left hand of fellowship is to have a problem. We hide behind our fears because we are supposed to be so "spiritual." Maybe we should go back and take a good look at Jesus' disciples to see the kind of people He had in His ministry: thieves, betrayers, unlearned, ignorant, fearful and the list goes on.

I had a recent meeting with my staff because God is adding people to our staff as our ministry is growing. I asked them, "Are you prepared to be honest with me about every facet of your life? Are you prepared to share with your peers?" I asked this because my staff was saying, "We need ministry, too." I said, "Are you prepared to be ministered to by your peers with my oversight?"

They gulped and said, "Well, I have something in my life I just want to talk to *you* about."

I said, "If a member of my staff over there is going to murder you because of this information, I don't need them. Let's find out. If I cannot trust them with you, I cannot trust them with the masses who are coming. We have a sterling reputation internationally to maintain regarding our confidentiality."

I talked to a beautiful young lady recently who said, "Since I've heard your teaching, I now have the faith to confess the rest of my problems to my husband—things about me he doesn't know."

I asked her husband, "Are you ready to handle it?"

He said, "I'm ready to handle it!"

Do you know what is going to happen in this marriage? God's going to come and they are not going to be hiding in fear from a skeleton in the closet. This stuff is going to come before the altar of God and the cleansing power of God is going to come to bind and to heal.

If we had done these things years ago, we would not have these problems today. If we had done these things years ago, we would not be as sick as we are today. Are you ready to be transparent before God and each other?

I ate at a restaurant a while back and had a little food poisoning. I was really sick and the best thing happening to me was when the stuff came up and I regurgitated. When the poison came up out of my stomach, I was better. Now, it wasn't any fun regurgitating, was it? What could have been worse was to have the stuff stay down there for hours and just tear me apart. When it started to come up, I gave it a little help. Then I began to feel better.

You can also hold every thought in captivity. You can cast all vain imaginations down. You can know the Word of God. You can know truth and you can be an expert in the law of God, *but if you don't live it, it is heresy.* You are able to defeat all evil *when your obedience is fulfilled.*

> **And having in a readiness to revenge all disobedience, when your obedience is fulfilled. 2 Corinthians 10:6**

Fear is an enemy. Self-hatred is an enemy. Guilt is an enemy. Condemnation is an enemy. Denial is an enemy. Bitterness, rage, anger and resentment are all our enemies.

## Autism

*Autism* is a disease I have been asked to get involved with and I am now studying four case histories. Our initial investigation has to do with a neurological breakdown coming out of rejection and rebellion. The entrance points, considering the young ages of autistic children, are some things we are not sure about. I have information coming to me all the time from research.

I had a call from Pennsylvania recently from a lady we have been working with. Her autistic son is now cutting himself. This is self-hatred and brings a new component into this disease. I believe *autism* is a result of rejection. The other components of *autism* involve rebellion and anger. They are almost the same principles eventually producing *schizophrenia.* However, *autism* is not *schizophrenia.* Recent medical research indicates an imbalance in a particular neurotransmitter secretion is implicated.

## Parkinson's Disease

We have enough insight on this disease initially and spiritually to give me the faith to move ahead now in actual ministry. The only way we know we are going to get this one is to be involved and start applying the principles we see. Then, if God will honor this insight, He will give the healing.

In the state of New York, there is a family of three generations with *Parkinson's disease.* Two brothers have already died. In the three generations, they all have Parkinson's.

I am a member of the Parkinson's Foundation of America because I am tapping into what they are doing. Current research is pointing to a deficiency of dopamine as the cause. When we have either under- or over-secretion of various neurotransmitters, I have always found either a genetic or spiritual component behind it. Either way it has a spiritual root. I consider *Alzheimer's, Parkinson's* and *autism* to be spiritually rooted diseases.

In the case of *Parkinson's,* my initial investigation indicates unresolved rejection, massive amounts of abandonment, rejection and hope deferred. As a point to ponder, personal and family involvement may be implicated.

> **Hope deferred maketh the heart sick: but *when* the desire cometh, *it is* a tree of life. Proverbs 13:12**

Parkinson's is the result of lowered levels of dopamine, the pleasure neurotransmitter of the body. Faith is the substance of things hoped for. So when you have hope deferred, that is a state of lack of faith. Therefore dopamine values are lowered resulting in the tremors of Parkinson's.

The beginning of healing and prevention is the second part of this Scripture. But when desire cometh, it is a tree of life. Dopamine values will increase with respect to the renewed desires, which are the foundation of hope. Hopelessness is then defeated and the disease can be healed.

The disease can be prevented by avoiding brooding over past failures and mistakes. Things of the past that did not work out need to be released and new projects planned. I have a saying: "You don't cry over spilled milk…you just find a new cow and milk her." So pick up your failures, leave them in the past and let His mercies and faith be part of your new day in Him.

## Alzheimer's Disease

*Alzheimer's disease*, according to recent research in the medical community, seems to involve a proliferation of white corpuscles congregating at critical nerve junctions in the brain.

Wherever I find white corpuscles congregating and causing trouble, I know the root cause. White corpuscles are either eating at linings of flesh, eating the myelin nerve sheath as in *MS*, eating at the connective tissue of the organs as in *lupus*, eating at the cartilage connective tissue of the skeleton as in *rheumatoid arthritis*, destroying pancreatic function as in *diabetes (type 1)*, eating at the lining of the colon and ulcerating it as in *Crohn's disease*, congregating in a nonbacterial inflammation as in *prostatitis*, or congregating in the brain and producing nonbacterial inflammation with interruption of nerve transmissions as in *Alzheimer's*. Whenever I find white corpuscles attacking the body and not doing what God created them to do, I have, without exception, found various degrees of *self-hatred and guilt*.

If we could stop the white corpuscles from collecting at critical nerve junctions of the brain, then *Alzheimer's* might cease to exist. If we can get dopamine levels back up to where they need to be, then *Parkinson's disease* might cease to exist. This is elementary and God will give us the understanding as to the spiritual roots so healing can happen. I know God wants to heal *Alzheimer's*.

The medical prognosis for many "incurable diseases" is bleak. I held a weekend seminar in New York City in 1997 and a doctor attended. We were discussing the fact that the "best" the medical community can expect to offer is **disease management**, because in my teaching I made a statement that the best allopathic medicine could offer was various forms of disease management. He came up to me and said, "You're being very generous with my profession. The medical profession can only hope to achieve *disease management and* we are a long way from even doing that."

So, if we are not even getting disease management from the medical profession, how will we see cures?

A national magazine discussing the frontiers of medicine for the next millennium included the following observation: In the areas of cancer, disease, aging, strokes, AIDS, fertility, alternative therapies, gene therapies, organ transplants, mental illness and more, the best that we can look forward to, nationally and internationally from the medical community, is either miracle drugs or genetic engineering.

In their mind, there is no other alternative left except for gene therapy or miracle drugs. This is all you have left to look forward to. The rest of it has been exhausted. There is no hope. There are no solutions. This is what the medical community is telling us. I am reminded of the Scripture which says, "Physician, heal thyself" (Luke 4:23). But, they cannot even do it.

> **And he said unto them, Ye will surely say unto me this proverb, Physician, heal thyself: whatsoever we have heard done in Capernaum, do also here in thy country. Luke 4:23**

We are not against doctors; they have their place. But doctors are not equipped to deal with incurable diseases because of the following:

1) 80 percent of diseases are psychosomatic and spiritually rooted.

2) Doctors have not been trained concerning the roots of disease.

3) Doctors do not understand the connection between sin and disease.

4) God did not set up doctors to bypass the penalty of the curse with disease management and drugs.

## Cholesterol

America has been on a yo-yo. You need some cholesterol to grease your veins. The worst thing you can do is remove all of your cholesterol. Having high triglyceride levels and/or high cholesterol levels does not mean it is caused by what you eat. If you are avoiding fatty foods to keep cholesterol down, this is not the issue. Why is it some people eat whatever they want and never develop a problem with high cholesterol? Why do others have a problem?

It is because certain people have a predisposition to high cholesterol and others don't. *There is a spiritual component to high cholesterol.*

I ministered to a lady who had a triglyceride level of 378 and within 48 hours of ministry it had dropped to 178. What changed? Let me give you an example of how this works. Look at the veins: the inside is hollow and blood runs up and down inside like a drinking straw. In people who have a predisposition to high cholesterol, something on the inside is reaching out and grabbing the cholesterol and binding it to the cell membrane. The plaque finally thickens and thickens and thickens until you have the potential closure of the vein or the artery. The mechanisms causing this plaque to form and to collect have a spiritual root.

This is my spiritual diagnosis: ***cholesterol*** *is directly related to people who are very, very angry with themselves*. There is a high degree of self-deprecation; they are against themselves; they are always putting themselves down. It is more than merely putting themselves down; they are very hostile with themselves. They are very angry with themselves.

I dealt with a woman who is totally well today. In fact, she is a member of my staff now; however, she was sick for 55 years. She had 17 different major "incurable" diseases and she has been healed of all 17. She had so much self-hatred and self-anger at one point that she burnt her flesh and carved it with knives. Her flesh was literally mutilated with fire, knives, razor blades and glass.

I have some good news for you: she is a wonderful lady. She is gloriously saved, gloriously healed and she loves herself today. She serves God, working 12–16 hours a day in our ministry. She has been marvelously healed and delivered by God. This *was* a high level of self-hatred, wasn't it? Self-mutilation and self-hatred. Self-mutilation is a national epidemic today, especially among the youth.

It all begins with rejection.

> ***The beginning of all disease is***
> ***the separation from God,***
> ***separation from your own self***
> ***and separation from others.***

## Skin

Skin rashes, itching, hives, blotching, swelling. How many of you have had a rash appear on your arm? It itched, you scratched and you went to the doctor. He prescribed a topical salve for you. Did you ever look at the ingredients of the topical salve? When you look at the small fine print on the tube you squeeze, it is an antihistamine. When you have an over-secretion of histamine in your body, whether it involves your skin, sinus, or an internal organ or tissues, you have swelling. When you have swelling, you have pressure on your nervous system and you have pain, discomfort and irritation. The spiritual root behind this is fear, anxiety and stress over some issue in your life.

## Shingles and Hives

Behind all skin eruptions, which would include many rashes, humps and bumps, hives and *shingles*, you are going to find the over-secretion of histamine and, in conjunction with it, a congregating and a proliferating of white corpuscles. Shingles is an *anxiety and fear* disease coupled with an autoimmune component involving *self-rejection*.

Hives are a direct manifestation of fear and anxiety. Your skin is very responsive. Right behind the epidermal layer of your skin is your immune system, blood vessels, nerves and every facet of your existence just beneath the layers of your skin. Your white corpuscles can congregate and secrete histamine. Systemic histamine can be created anywhere in the body: in localized sinuses, skin, internal connective tissue, etc. Histamine can be over-secreted and when you have an over-secretion of histamine, you have swelling, edema and pain. Hives and *shingles*, in conjunction with dendrite flaring, give you a double problem. You have your nervous system; you have the secretion of histamine. This is the chemical part of you, with the electrical part of you connecting and expressing itself as an extension of your anxiety and stress.

The definition of *shingles*: an acute central nervous system infection involving primarily the dorsal root ganglia and characterized by the vesicular eruption with neuralgic pain in the cutaneous areas, supplied by peripheral sensory nerves arising in the affected root ganglia.

Many latent viruses are often released in conjunction with fear, anxiety and stress. Thus, *shingles* and *hives,* for example, are considered to be anxiety disorders, even though there may be viruses implicated in the profile.

Inflammatory changes occur in the sensory root ganglia and the skin of the associated dermatome. In some instances, the inflammation may involve the posterior and anterior horns of gray matter meninges and the dorsal and ventral roots. There is no specific therapy.

We have had some success with it. I told you it had an autoimmune component attached to it before we began this discussion. I said this one was straight anxiety but also coupled with self-rejection and self-hatred. What does a virus do with that? What triggers these things to come up? What allows a virus to work?

When you look at classes of viruses, you see they are almost like a phylum that has a particular object of its attention. I do not have all the answers to viruses but I certainly am following their persnickety ways around mankind. They are interesting because they seem to be on a highly destructive mission.

They are very calculated and have become a real pain to mankind. Behind viruses, there also seems to be an intelligence that defies imagination.

In conjunction with other factors such as fear, anxiety, stress and lack of self-esteem, there are other problems of a non-viral order. What does a virus do? Why does it attach itself to other spiritual problems? I do not have an answer to this. I would certainly like to know. In the meantime, in ministry, I would say that with all viruses, we have had to minister and do deliverance.

## Rosacea

*Rosacea* has more of an autoimmune component to it, rather than anxiety, which involves self-hatred. Rosacea is a chronic disease of the skin on the face.

## Acne

Recent information on acne is really interesting. In 1997, they came out with a statement in the medical community saying that adolescent acne is the result of peer pressure. It is not just the child being in puberty with their oil glands exploding—and presto—they have acne. What they have discovered for the most part is that adolescent acne is rooted in *anxiety and fear coming out of peer pressure. Simple acne comes from fear of man. It is fear of rejection and fear of man. In puberty and adolescence, it is peer pressure and peer pressure is fear.*

I have six children and four are teenagers. I'll tell you, they are overly concerned about what their buddies think. Do you know what designer labels are? Kids are vicious with each other. Children are vicious and children are more afraid of their peers than they are of their parents.

This is why I try to get the children to know adults. I encourage them to fellowship so they can have alternative peer pressure. Then they are not just stuck with the tunnel vision of kids who maliciously shame them, but with adults who will love them.

There can be an antidote to this problem. This is my position. I want my children to grow up knowing adults, not just other children. I look for spiritual adults I can trust my children with.

## Psoriasis

Psoriasis is an autoimmune disorder in which the white corpuscles are congregating on the skin, creating the scaling, the flaking, the redness and the hardness. Psoriasis is rooted in *self-hatred, lack of self-esteem and conflict with identity.*

## Ovarian Cysts, Breast Cysts and Cystic Acne

*Cystic acne* is different. You will find this occurring mainly on the back and mostly in females; it is like erupting cysts. *Cystic acne, ovarian cysts* and *breast cysts* have something in common as a spiritual root. We have seen great success nationally in our ministry with *breast cysts, ovarian cysts and cysts. Ovarian cysts, breast cysts* and *cystic acne* are taught together because of a common root.

I have found one thing to be true without exception: these conditions come out of the breakup of a relationship between a girl and her mother. Unresolved issues involving a great breach where there is no fellowship. It extends down into the reproductive area. It involves a full issue of femininity. The girl may even begin to question her own femininity or the female part of her creation. The mother has reached it at this level.

Many times there is great bitterness, anger and great resentment toward the mother. I have found it true, coast-to-coast, that the people who have been healed of *ovarian cysts, breast cysts* and *cystic acne* have had to make things right before God concerning their mothers.

## Premenstrual Syndrome (PMS)

PMS and menopause are not the same. Menopause is part of life. I do believe God can make a provision for you in menopause so you don't have a hormonal tragedy. There is much debate about estrogen therapies and I have mixed emotions about them. I would say it is probably best if you could go the more natural route. You would be better off because of the cancer risk.

PMS is another story. PMS basically comes from a tightening of the muscles of the uterus and uterine walls, producing pressure, pain, distress and discomfort. Part of it is tied to fear—*fear of pain*. The first area of ministry in PMS is to pray for peace and ask God to take away the *fear* of pain and discomfort. We ask God to bring the person to full relaxation of the muscles in that area. It is nothing more than muscular tension. Complicating the syndrome can also be feelings of uncleanness around a person's sexuality because of a stigma attached to the monthly cycle.

You can get pills to "treat" PMS. What are they going to do for you? They are a neurological blocker designed to give you muscle relaxation. Personally, I believe the root behind PMS is part of the curse on females. Not all females have PMS, just as some do not have pain in childbirth. They have pressure but not the pain. Most people we have seen who have PMS are fairly introspective females. They are females who are really bound with the stress of *introspection* and *phobic realities* in their minds.

I also found another ingredient in PMS: sometimes females do not like being females. I find some females really get hostile at "that time of the month" because they just don't like going through it. Although I recognize hormonal shifting can be a factor, this can be overamplified by a spiritual and emotional conflict. As a result of the mind-body connection, the hormonal shift is now magnified and complicated by thoughts, thus increasing the problem. On the other hand, when I deal with people who have MCS/EI, many of them have not had a menstrual cycle for years. One of the first signs of healing in females with MCS/EI is they get regular cycles back. One lady called me after eight years of no female cycle. "I had my period!"

I said, "Glory to God."

I had another one say, "Oh no, it is here."

I had one response of rejoicing and one saying, "Oh no." I'll tell you what is worse than PMS: not having your cycle—if this is any consolation!

**Fibromyalgia**

It goes with the MCS/EI profile. When you find MCS/EI, you will find *primary fibromyalgia syndrome* (PFS) almost without exception. PFS is often a misunderstood disease. The first time I ran across someone with PFS, I thought they had the worst thing in the world. It can be very painful. It can be localized, generalized or all over your body. Someone said PFS is what causes MCS/EI. I still hear this or I hear how *candida* causes MCS/EI. But this is not true. They are by-products of a whole different root problem.

I have a *Merck Manual*, which is a physician's desk reference on disease. I also have a *Physician's Desk Reference* (PDR) on disease and drugs, a good college textbook on *Pathophysiology and* many books on anatomy and physiology. We don't have to be in the dark about the enemy. When someone comes to me about disease I want to be able to help them in addition to what their doctor is doing. I have discovered through this ministry, in some cases, I know more about the etiology (cause) of certain diseases than some doctors know.

Your doctor can tell you where it is and what it is doing and how to drug it or cut it out, but he still does not know why you have it. If you go to the doctor's desk reference many times it will say: "etiology unknown." The cause of the disease is unknown.

I believe God knows what causes our diseases and in the case of over 600 different "incurable" diseases, He has revealed why people have those diseases. Doctors consult with us concerning their patients from coast-to-coast. There are doctors who consult with us for their own health and healing. Some doctors refer their patients to us by phone for insight and ministry. The reason I am sharing this with you is because I want to bring you into focus. You do not have to be ignorant about what you don't know. You just need to know where to look it up!

The term *myalgia* indicates muscular pain, in contrast to *myositis,* which is pain due to inflammation of muscle tissues, ligaments, tendons and white connective tissue. *Fibromyalgia* is an appropriate term for pain where inflammation is absent. What does this tell me? PFS is pain without inflammation or swelling as its cause. There is no pressure on the nerve from edema or swelling. Most of the pain we have comes by pressure of swelling or edema on an adjacent nerve. Pressure on the nerve produces pain. I know the pain in PFS is not due to inflammation or swelling or an infection or bacteria. It is true pain in which no inflammation is present.

PFS is a term used to describe pain in fibrous tissues, muscles, tendons, ligaments and other "white" connective tissues. This is a quotation from the *Merck Manual:*

> **Etiology:** Primary Fibromyalgia Syndrome (PFS). The condition occurs mainly in females…is particularly likely to occur in healthy young women who tend to be stressed, tense, depressed, anxious, and striving….[5]

What is the difference in male and female in body parts? There are few differences as far as bone, muscles, tissue and structure. We have the same nervous system. We have the same muscles and ligaments, don't we? Sexually we are different, but basically from a nerve standpoint we are the same. Then why do you think this condition is basically a female condition?

In MCS/EI, 85–90 percent of the individuals who suffer this disease are female and only 10–15 percent are male. Why is this? It is the same reason nearly 100 percent of all PFS patients are female.

The Bible says in 1 Corinthians that man was not made for woman, but woman was made for man.

> [3]**But I would have you know, that the head of every man is Christ; and the head of the woman *is* the man; and the head of Christ *is* God…**[8]**For the man is not of the woman; but the woman of the man.** [9]**Neither was the man created for the woman; but the woman for the man.** 1 Corinthians 11:3, 8–9

Now, this does not mean the man has the right to be chauvinistic or oppressive; this has to do with God's order in creation.

I want to tell you something: I have not found one woman during my ministry who does not want to follow a spiritual man, unless she has a hatred

---

[5] *Merck Manual*, 16th edition (Rahway, NJ: Merck & Co.), 1992, pages 1369–1370.

of men or a distrust of men. God created her to follow an example of nurturing. When the woman is not nurtured, when she has no one to follow and is made the spiritual head of the home by default, she goes down in stress and anxiety.

Someone has to take care of the family. Someone has to represent God. Someone has to be nurturing. Someone has to communicate. Someone has to spout off somewhere. Someone is going to be emotional. Most female disorders are the result of a lack of nurturing and protection (covering) by a male and the female is then saddled with the problems of life without any help, emotionally or spiritually. Occasionally, drivenness and perfectionism may be implicated. If it is, it is an attempt to receive love and feel complete through works.

The reason anxiety, stress and fear come upon a woman under those circumstances is that she was not made to be the stronger vessel. The Bible says she has been created to be the weaker vessel:

> **Likewise, ye husbands, dwell with *them* according to knowledge, giving honour unto the wife, as unto the weaker vessel, and as being heirs together of the grace of life; that your prayers be not hindered. 1 Peter 3:7**

This does not mean she is weak mentally. It does not mean she is weak before God. It means that in the God-ordained order of things, she is designed to respond and be a "helpmeet" to her husband. The husband was designed to lead in all things and to establish the kingdom of God in righteousness, in justice and in love in their home. The woman in Proverbs 31 was no slouch, but her husband was known and did sit in the gates with the elders of the city. Also, "the heart of her husband doth safely trust in her...she will do him good and not evil all the days of her life" (Proverbs 31:11–12). This reality is only possible *if* the man takes his rightful place in the home, in love.

> **¹¹The heart of her husband doth safely trust in her, so that he shall have no need of spoil. ¹²She will do him good and not evil all the days of her life. Proverbs 31:11–12**

When a man molests his daughter or beats his wife or when he won't listen to his children, he violates the protection mechanism and his family does not know where to turn. Fear and anxiety is the result. Then disease comes.

Men, we need to take the time to get our priorities reestablished. If you want your wife to love you, you better get hot toward God first. *Let God teach you how to represent the Godhead in your family.*

*Also, according to the* Merck Manual, *PFS is "likely to occur in healthy young women who tend to be stressed, tense, depressed, anxious...striving,"* driven, perfectionists who are moving all the pieces around. *"Symptoms can be exacerbated by environmental or emotional stress, or by a physician who does not give proper credence to the patient's concerns and discharges the matter as "all in the head."* You want to get a flurry of PFS? Let somebody be insensitive to your problem. What comes in? More hopelessness, despair, anxiety and stress. The root behind *fibromyalgia* is fear, anxiety, stress, drivenness and perfectionism for the most part, unless there is a specific organic reason.

*Fibromyalgia* works like this: let's pretend my arm is a nerve and around my arm is tissue, but there is no inflammation so there's no contact. At the end of your nerves are things called dendrites. They are called dendrites because the word *dendrite* translated means "digit" or "fingerlike." When I want my hand to move, my thought process causes a nerve impulse to be sent. The impulse runs down the nerve to the dendrites, arcs over a nerve synapse to a receptor cell on the corresponding muscle and hooks up with the nerve and the whole process causes my hand to move. The short version is, I think about it and it happens.

In *fibromyalgia*, the nerve impulse is initiated without conscious thought. There is no intended corresponding muscular reaction required. It is triggered by *the spirit of fear in the realm beyond consciousness.* Even if you know it is there, you try to ignore it. It is there and it initiates nerve impulses through the hypothalamus, which is sensing the problem upstream in the soul and the spirit. All of a sudden you have something happening. What happens in PFS, beyond conscious thought, is the nerve impulse runs down the nerve into the dendrites and pulsates. It then dead-ends. This is what causes the pain. You cannot do anything with it.

The only way you can get rid of it is to allow God to deliver you from anxiety, fear and stress. The Bible says to be anxious for nothing.

> **Be careful for nothing; but in every thing by prayer and supplication with thanksgiving let your requests be made known unto God. Philippians 4:6**

God has not given you the spirit of fear, but of power, love and a sound mind.

> **For God hath not given us the spirit of fear; but of power, and of love, and of a sound mind. 2 Timothy 1:7**

This is the mechanism of PFS. The spiritual root can be found in females who don't feel covered, protected, nurtured, don't feel safe, are always looking over their shoulder, are driven, anxious, moving the pieces of their life around and are insecure.

### Endometriosis

You know I have had some success in the area of *endometriosis. I have found self-rejection and self-hatred to be the cause.*

> *(Audience comment on endometriosis: I've done a lot of studying on this because I've been very concerned about abortion. Apparently one of the factors, or results, of abortion is endometriosis because it has to do with the hormonal interruption. Abortion is not a normal miscarriage, so there are a lot of factors that come into play. It seems a lot of women who have had an abortion, whether chemical or otherwise, wind up with endometriosis.)*

### Osteoporosis

The root for *osteoporosis* is envy and jealousy, which matches the Word. (Remember the testimony in the early part of this teaching about the lady from New Jersey who was healed of osteoporosis?) The Word says envy and jealousy result in rottenness of the bones.

> **A sound heart *is* the life of the flesh: but envy the rottenness of the bones. Proverbs 14:30**

The fruit of the root of envy and jealousy is rottenness of the bones. This is not only a physical problem but a spiritual problem. The healing and prevention of *osteoporosis* begins in eliminating envy and jealousy from your life. Envy and jealousy are sins.

### Scoliosis

I have done a lot of research with *scoliosis and* we have seen many healings of curvature of the spine. I did not see all the implications until recently when I was reviewing some medical information and research. I noted something called *proprioception.* Proprioception is tied to the emotional cortex of your brain, down through the thalamus gland and keeps you balanced. It also is tied to the centers of feel, touch and the five physical senses. It allows you to be coordinated. In *scoliosis*, it has been discovered, in 50 percent to 60 percent of all cases, proprioception malfunction is involved.

There is a neurological misfiring. One muscle stiffens and one remains normal. The normal one is now considered weak. If this happens in an adult, there is no cure. In children, if they are treated while they are young enough, they can be put in special body braces and it slows down or stops the process. *Scoliosis* progresses from childhood at the rate of one degree of spine curvature per year. The normal side is now considered weak in one side of the back muscles and the stiffened one is now considered strong and pulls. The weak side is unable to maintain the balance and the spine starts to bend.

Most *scoliosis* cases are an "S" curve. But I dealt with a case of inverted *scoliosis* years ago. When I was first starting in ministry, a young man was brought to me with an inverted spine. His spine was actually out to a place even with his stomach. You could take a basketball and put it on his back and it would fit right into the curvature of his spine.

I'll tell you and I pray you can receive it, that *scoliosis*, like *epilepsy*, is the presence and the fruit of an *evil spirit. You will not get* epilepsy *healed and you will not get* scoliosis *healed, unless you cast out the evil spirit.* I had to cast the evil spirit of *scoliosis* out of this young man in the name of Jesus.

## Sciatica

There is another disease for which an evil spirit has to be cast out. It is called *sciatica* and is an inflammation of the sciatic nerve accounting for 50 percent of lower back pain in most people. Medical observation indicates the left side is most usually affected, but it is occasionally the right side.

If so many people had not received healing over the years, you probably would think I just got off a spaceship. Casting out evil spirits is found in Matthew, Mark, Luke, John and the book of Acts. I thought one day I would just trust God and try it. I thought I would just speak to an evil spirit and cast it out. It obeyed me and left. This was interesting and exciting.

Matthew 10:1 explains how Jesus empowered the disciples in this matter:

> **10:1And when he had called unto *him* his twelve disciples, he gave them power *against* unclean spirits, to cast them out, and to heal all manner of sickness and all manner of disease. Matthew 10:1**

In Luke we read that the seventy were given the same power and they weren't even disciples:

> **17And the seventy returned again with joy, saying, Lord, even the devils are subject unto us through thy name. 18And he said unto them, I beheld Satan as lightning fall from heaven. 19Behold, I give unto you power to tread on serpents and scorpions, and over all the power of the enemy: and nothing shall by any means hurt you. 20Notwithstanding in this rejoice not, that the spirits are subject unto you; but rather rejoice, because your names are written in heaven. Luke 10:17–20**

I believe this is for today and I have seen the results of this belief. *If you don't believe it is for today, then for you, it is not.* Matthew 9:27–38 is another scriptural teaching about healing we must examine.

> **27And when Jesus departed thence, two blind men followed him, crying, and saying, *Thou* Son of David, have mercy on us. 28And when he was come into the house, the blind men came to him: and Jesus saith unto them, Believe ye that I am able to do this? They said unto him, Yea, Lord. 29Then touched he their eyes, saying, According to your faith be it unto you. 30And their eyes were opened; and Jesus straitly charged them, saying, See *that* no man know *it.* 31But they, when they were departed, spread abroad his fame in all that country. 32As they went out, behold, they**

brought to him a dumb man possessed with a devil. ³³And when the devil was cast out, the dumb spake: and the multitudes marvelled, saying, It was never so seen in Israel. ³⁴But the Pharisees said, He casteth out devils through the prince of the devils. ³⁵And Jesus went about all the cities and villages, teaching in their synagogues, and preaching the gospel of the kingdom, and healing every sickness and every disease among the people. ³⁶But when he saw the multitudes, he was moved with compassion on them, because they fainted, and were scattered abroad, as sheep having no shepherd. ³⁷Then saith he unto his disciples, The harvest truly *is* plenteous, but the labourers *are* few; ³⁸Pray ye therefore the Lord of the harvest, that he will send forth labourers into his harvest. Matthew 9:27–38

If we are to pattern who we are after Christ, then these Scriptures include some very important elements relevant for today:

1. Belief that the Lord is able to do it.

2. According to your faith be it unto you.

3. A person had a devil that would not allow him to speak.

4. Jesus cast the devil out and then he could speak.

5. The religious leaders of the day accused him of casting a devil out by the power of the devil. (This is what blasphemy of the Holy Spirit is.)

6. Jesus set the pattern of ministry, which was to teach and preach, heal every sickness and disease and cast out evil spirits.

7. Jesus was moved with compassion for others.

8. God's people are scattered as sheep with no shepherd.

9. The fields are ready for harvest and the laborers are few.

10. Will you help?

Mark 6:7–13 teaches us that Jesus gave the power necessary for dealing with unclean spirits and healing to His disciples.

⁷And he called *unto him* the twelve, and began to send them forth by two and two; and gave them power over unclean spirits; ⁸And commanded them that they should take nothing for *their* journey, save a staff only; no scrip, no bread, no money in *their* purse: ⁹But *be* shod with sandals; and not put on two coats. ¹⁰And he said unto them, In what place soever ye enter into an house, there abide till ye depart from that place. ¹¹And whosoever shall not receive you, nor hear you, when ye depart thence, shake off the dust under your feet for a testimony against them. Verily I say unto you, It shall be more tolerable for Sodom and Gomorrha in the day of judgment, than for that city. ¹²And they went out, and preached that men should repent. ¹³And they cast out many devils, and anointed with oil many that were sick, and healed *them.* Mark 6:7–13

There are many, many people literally running around these days who no longer have *epilepsy, scoliosis* or *sciatica* problems because this ministry dared to believe Matthew 10:1 and Luke 10:17–20 are true for today.

I am not exactly sure what the spiritual root for *scoliosis* is, but I have known for decades that you have to minister deliverance in order for *scoliosis* to be healed. In the case of the young man with the inverted spine, I knew it was an evil spirit. I did not deal with spiritual roots; I just said, "In the name of Jesus, you spirit of *scoliosis* come out of him. I take authority over you." Then I laid hands on him and commanded the spine to straighten.

I will never forget, as long as I live, the tears of rejoicing in his mother's and father's eyes and the looks on their faces as he snapped and his spine became straight as an arrow. They all left rejoicing. He was 14 years old. I will never forget that day. **In that day, I knew of a certainty that God was still on the throne and He still answers prayer.**

## Spondylolysis

*Spondylolysis* is progressive degeneration of the vertebra of the spine. The entire scenario is rooted in self-hatred. *Spondylolysis* is the degeneration of the vertebra caused by *self-hatred*.

## Degenerative Disc Disease

*Degenerative disc disease* is usually caused by anything dealing with the disc, apart from accidents and injury, as degenerative in nature. Inherited or degenerative disc disease is *usually tied to an addictive personality* involving drugs, both legal and illegal, and may be included in the inherited profile. Somewhere in your past, there may have been someone who was a drug runner, a drug user, or someone who put drugs or alcohol to someone else's lips to make them drunk.

> ¹⁵**Woe unto him that giveth his neighbour drink, that puttest thy bottle to *him,* and makest *him* drunken also, that thou mayest look on their nakedness! ¹⁶Thou art filled with shame for glory: drink thou also, and let thy foreskin be uncovered: the cup of the LORD'S right hand shall be turned unto thee, and shameful spewing *shall be* on thy glory. Habakkuk 2:15–16**

These Scriptures are not just about getting someone else drunk or contributing to their demise. It is very clear there is a "woe" (curse) which comes upon someone because he or she has not contributed to a person's welfare. I would not want to be a bar owner for too long.

I have dealt with many cultures and nationalities in ministry and I have observed another characteristic. Have you ever noticed people coming out of the "hippie" days? Many of them have back problems. I have observed degenerative disc disease and back problems coming out of drug addiction and in profiles of families who were addicted to various drugs. It is an observation. I have dealt with some of these people regarding their addictions and have had some success; with others I have not. The first place I look when ministering to someone with degenerative disc disease, apart from injury, is into the drug profile. This is where I have had more success.

## Sinus Infections

*Sinusitis* involves the over-secretion of histamine. We deal with histamine disorders from a standpoint of sinus, skin and systemic. Systemic would be internal. When histamine is over-secreted, it produces swelling, edema and runny noses. When you have sinus problems and you go to the doctor, you are given an antihistamine, which is a drug. The side effects of antihistamine can include a personality change for a minimum of 24 hours. Second, it can also include feelings of rage and anger. Antihistamines are extremely addictive. Many people have stopped using antihistamines before I could get to the root problems of their *sinusitis*.

What happens in *sinusitis*, and the result of taking antihistamines, is you become chemically addicted to the drug. When the drug initially prescribed to combat the over-secretion of histamine wears off, the initial problem no longer exists, but your body is now craving the drug. Your body mirrors the sinusitis symptoms—runny nose, watering eyes, etc.—just to get the drug. Now you have a double problem. The exception is if you have a nasal obstruction from a birth defect preventing proper drainage.

The root behind sinus infection and *sinusitis* is *fear and anxiety*. All histamine, whether involving skin, sinus or systemic, is over-secreted in conjunction with *stress, anxiety and tension*. That whole area of *insecurity* produces an excessive histamine secretion in the human body.

## Sleep Disorders

Proverbs says your sleep shall be sweet.

> **I will both lay me down in peace, and sleep: for thou, Lord, only makest me dwell in safety. Psalm 4:8**

> **…yea, thou shalt lie down, and thy sleep shall be sweet. Proverbs 3:24**

> **Thou shalt not be afraid for the terror by night…. Psalm 91:5**

I claim this. I claim sweet, peaceable sleep without fear at night. If you are not able to sleep, there might be a physical reason, but many times there is a spiritual reason.

The hypothalamus gland is the brain of the endocrine system. The hypothalamus gland is very important because it will make or break you in all areas of disease. The hypothalamus gland controls many things in your body. **It is one of the centers that maintain the waking state and sleep patterns.**[6]

In the book on anatomy and physiology, you find where the problem begins. When you have problems in your mind, the hypothalamus is going to respond to what you are thinking about.

*Sleep disorders can be caused by the hypothalamus responding to your spiritual and emotional state.* Torment can interrupt and perplex you and can stimulate your hypothalamus to keep you awake. I'll tell you why. The hypothalamus is the main gland involved in *fight or flight*, the first stage of the General Adaptation Syndrome in the fear profile.

We taught on fear and anxiety disorders (fear, stress, anxiety and physiology). Remember, there are three stages of an anxiety disorder in the General Adaptation Syndrome: (1) the *fight or flight* stage; (2) the *resistance* stage; and (3) the *exhaustion* stage.

You will find when you are tormented inside, deep in the spiritual or in the emotional part of your soul, it can be beyond your conscious thought in *fight or flight.* Life's circumstances, which include tragedy, torment, victimization, fears, phobias, unrest, uncertainty and all the other vicissitudes of life, come to project themselves into the future and threaten your existence. This is enough to keep you awake all night.

The Bible tells you to take no thought for tomorrow (Matthew 6:34).

**Take therefore no thought for the morrow: for the morrow shall take thought for the things of itself. Sufficient unto the day *is* the evil thereof. Matthew 6:34**

When you are not worried about tomorrow, you will sleep tonight.

When you are worried about tomorrow, you will not sleep tonight. What is the worst thing that can happen to you? You can die and go to heaven, for to be absent from the body is to be present with the Lord.

**⁶Therefore *we are* always confident, knowing that, whilst we are at home in the body, we are absent from the Lord: ⁷(For we walk by faith, not by sight:) ⁸We are confident, *I say,* and willing rather to be absent from the body, and to be present with the Lord. 2 Corinthians 5:6–8**

---

[6] Gerard J. Tortora and Nicholas P. Anagnostakos. *Principles of Anatomy & Physiology*, Second Edition, Harper & Row, 1978.

So what if you lose everything tomorrow? The same God who helped you this far can start over again and probably do better. The Bible says,

> For whosoever will save his life shall lose it: and whosoever will lose his life for my sake shall find it. Matthew 16:25

I think we have been majoring in minors and minoring in majors. I think it is time to get rid of the rudiments of the world's way of thinking and get back into line with the thinking of God.

> 6Be careful for nothing; but in every thing by prayer and supplication with thanksgiving let your requests be made known unto God. 7And the peace of God, which passeth all understanding, shall keep your hearts and minds through Christ Jesus. Philippians 4:6–7

You say, "Well, I don't like what is happening to my life." Maybe you are under the chastening of the Lord, and if you don't go through it you are never going to get through it!

I want to tell you something about problems. How many of you like problems? How many of you like stress in your life? I have learned something about problems. They are always going to be there. The second thing I have learned about problems is when I have a problem and I lose my cool and lose my peace, *I still have that same problem to deal with.* If I still have to solve the problem, then I might as well just be cool. It is much easier to solve the problem when you have not lost your cool and you have your peace. You are going to have to solve it anyway. You can run from it, but it will follow you.

> *What I am saying to you is this: if you have a problem,*
> *it may not just be the enemy trying to oppress you.*
> *It may be God trying to lead you*
> *into the next stage of His will for your life.*

You may never get there if you do not face the issue. You might as well have a good night's sleep before you do. The problem will still exist tomorrow just as well as tonight. If it is going to be there tomorrow, why don't you have your peace tonight and get your rest?

It is the stuff upstream destroying your peace and your sleep. Then your hypothalamus is agreeing with you. The Bible says,

> Many *are* the afflictions of the righteous: but the LORD delivereth him out of them all. Psalm 34:19

Certain sleep disorders can occur from two sources: fear and anxiety or torment from victimization. Of course, it could be from fear after you watched *The Exorcist*. You have been down to that place renting movies for $3 and you have been watching horror films. You have opened your spirit up to the spirits of fear, anxiety, torment, tragedy and horror and you wonder why the stuff is coursing through your spiritual dynamics. You have a responsibility to guard your heart in order to receive protection from God in regard to torment.

Isaiah 33:13–16 says,

> [13]**Hear, ye** *that are* **far off, what I have done; and, ye** *that are* **near, acknowledge my might.** [14]**The sinners in Zion are afraid; fearfulness hath surprised the hypocrites. Who among us shall dwell with the devouring fire? who among us shall dwell with everlasting burnings?** [15]**He that walketh righteously, and speaketh uprightly; he that despiseth the gain of oppressions, that shaketh his hands from holding of bribes**, *that stoppeth his ears from hearing of blood, and shutteth his eyes from seeing evil;* [16]**He shall dwell on high: his place of defence** *shall be* **the munitions of rocks: bread shall be given him; his waters** *shall be* **sure. Isaiah 33:13–16** (emphasis added)

Scripture is telling us there is no protection from God if you don't hide your eyes from seeing the shedding of blood and hold your ears from what is happening in evil. When you watch junk on your video machine and your television with movies about mutilation, horror and murder, there is no protection from God for you from the sleeplessness and the projection of tragedy. You have brought it upon yourself.

I guard my heart as to what I look at. I won't watch anything to make me condone evil. I do not watch rapes on television. I do not watch violence on television. I will get away from it, turn it off and I have taught my children to do their own censorship, too. When you open your eyes and your heart to evil garbage, you are desensitizing yourself to the Spirit of God and condoning evil in your heart. You say, "Well, I'm not doing it. I'm just watching it." God says you are wrong! You are an accessory to evil. What you condone is what you establish!

Isaiah 33:13–16 tells us very specifically what God thinks; God does not pull any punches.

The television button goes off! We are very careful. I won't watch anything having to do with murder or evil and this includes sexual issues and pornography. I won't do it. I am supposed to be saving lives, not destroying them. I am supposed to be establishing righteousness in the earth, not enthroning evil.

If you have a fear of evil, you are a sitting duck for everything invisible traveling in the second heaven. Remember, Job said what he feared most came upon him.

> **For the thing which I greatly feared is come upon me, and that which I was afraid of is come unto me. Job 3:25**

You need to take an assessment of your fears because fear demands to be fulfilled.

> *Fear and faith are equal in this dimension:*
> *both demand to be fulfilled.*

Sometimes in ministry I have had people sitting in and observing, especially in the area of dealing with evil spiritual powers. If I sense people are afraid of the devil or afraid of principalities and powers, I ask them to leave the room. Why? They are on the wrong side of this battle.

Remember when Jesus went back to His hometown? He did very few miracles. He only healed a few sick folks. Do you know why? Great was their unbelief and doubt. If you are receiving this teaching in unbelief, I am wasting my time. In fact, you could stifle the Spirit of God by unbelief and doubt. This is why I ask some to leave the room. Do you understand what I am saying? If you don't believe, I cannot help you any more than Jesus could when He went back to His hometown.

## Dissociative Identity Disorder (formerly Multiple Personality Disorder)

Biblically, there seems to be evidence that DID (Dissociative Identity Disorder) is actually the kingdom called Legion. "We are many" is called Legion.

> **And he asked him, What *is* thy name? And he answered, saying, My**
> **name *is* Legion: for we are many. Mark 5:9**

When Legion was removed, the person was restored to his right mind.

I have a testimony of DID from a woman who had 14 multiples documented a few years ago by a clinical psychologist in a major city in America. She had been in therapy for 14 years to accomplish what is called *integration and fusion*. Integration and fusion is when the therapist tries to get all the personalities to agree to hang out with each other and agree with each other. In Christian therapy, it is to get them saved. That's what it is.

When I read the Bible, it tells me that type of therapy would make a person more double minded.

> **A double minded man *is* unstable in all his ways. James 1:8**

I want what God wants; for the person to be single-minded. I think what God intended in creation was for us to be an extension of who He created us to be from the foundation of the world, not a unified combination of personalities from life circumstances.

> **According as he hath chosen us in him before the foundation of the world, that we should be holy and without blame before him in love: Ephesians 1:4**

This individual, after 14 years of integration and fusion therapy with the clinical psychologist, was still a mess. The amount of time it took to get her free through our ministry was one sentence long. It was over!

I had all 14 personalities talking to me. I listened to these characters talking to me out of this woman and I said to myself at 8:45 that night, *Let's see, there are 14 of them; maybe I can get one out every hour. That's 14 hours. This is not going to fly too well. Maybe I can do one every 30 minutes. That would make it 5:00 in the morning by the time we're done.*

The Spirit of God dropped down in my heart and prompted me to say this: "Listen guys, if you think I am going to mess with you all night long, you have another thought coming. Here's the deal: you're going to join your little demon hands together inside this woman and go 'boogie, boogie.' Book it in the name of Jesus!" One of them spoke out of her. A voice came out of her and said, "We know we have to obey you." They were gone and it was over just like that.

Do you remember Jesus cast out seven devils from Mary Magdalene? Do you *believe* it really happened? Do you *believe* it really happened or is it just there to give us a story to tell?

> **And certain women, which had been healed of evil spirits and infirmities, Mary called Magdalene, out of whom went seven devils, Luke 8:2**

Could you accept the fact that I cast 14 devils out of this woman?

I'll tell you what the Lord said. The things He did we shall do and greater things than He did we would do, because He went to the Father and He sent the Holy Spirit to come and allow us to get this job done. Are you listening to me?

> [12]**Verily, verily, I say unto you, He that believeth on me, the works that I do shall he do also; and greater *works* than these shall he do; because I go unto my Father. [13]And whatsoever ye shall ask in my name, that will I do, that the Father may be glorified in the Son. [14]If ye shall ask any thing in my name, I will do *it.* John 14:12–14**

## Migraines

We have known the spiritual root for *migraines* for quite some time. But we did not know the whole picture until recently when I started to do some research on the drug of choice given to America today for migraines: *Imitrex.* In my study about *Imitrex* and its mechanisms in the human body, I have found "the rest of the story." *Imitrex* is prescribed 70 to 80 percent of the time for migraines.

A migraine is a type of headache pain known as psychogenic pain. Psychogenic means it is not caused by any known organic reason. It is not pain because of injury. It is not pain because of any organic reason. It comes and it goes and it is incredibly painful. It brings with it nausea, flashing lights and a complete shutting down of one's ability to cope with life.

*I think our success with migraines, without drugs, is second to none in America.* Let me explain to you its mechanisms and let me give you the root. In order to show you how this works, I'll give you the mechanism of the drug *Imitrex.*

There are two parts to migraines. First, there is a reduction in the secretion of serotonin and second, there is an increase in histamine secretion. This is triggered by *guilt resulting from conflict in your life in conjunction with fear.* It is not the conflict itself triggering your migraine. It is the conflict you have with yourself over the conflict that triggers the migraine; whether it is either real or imagined.

You might have guilt because you think you spent too much money and you had a little argument with your husband over how much you spent. The argument about this little infringement in finances is not what causes the migraine. It is the guilt you have with yourself producing the migraine.

Migraines are triggered in people who have conflict with themselves about conflict in life or conflict with others. It is rooted in guilt. *All migraines are rooted in guilt.* Out of guilt comes fear and it is always in this order. *It is guilt first and then fear.*

Here is the mechanism. As you enter into guilt over some issue, the hypothalamus gland senses you are in conflict with yourself. A mechanism of *self-hatred* sets in causing the pineal gland to slow down the secretion level of serotonin. This causes a lowered serotonin level. The conflict develops in the realm of the soul and the spirit and fear starts to move. Anxiety concerning the issue starts and histamine begins to be over-secreted in the cranial region.

Serotonin is a *vasoconstrictor*. When your serotonin levels are normal, they maintain the diameter of your blood vessels just the way God intended and they carry your blood supply into each region of your body.

Histamine is a *vasodilator*. As the serotonin levels are decreased and histamine is increased, you have a resulting dilation of the blood vessels. A swelling of the blood vessels puts pressure on sensitive nerves and this is what produces the migraine.

*Imitrex* is a compound drug designed to be an antihistamine and a serotonin enhancer. Serotonin and histamine are antagonistic to each other when they are in opposition to each other in body functions. They repel each other. They do not coexist. When serotonin levels are reduced because of the guilt, then histamine levels are allowed to increase because of the fear. Histamine and serotonin are incompatible with each other in the human body. What happens when the drug *Imitrex* is given is this: first histamine is reduced and then serotonin is enhanced. Vasodilation reduces, vasoconstriction is broken, the blood vessels return to normal and the migraine is over. This is the mechanism behind migraines and this is the mechanism of *Imitrex* drug therapy.

In ministry, our desire is for you not to take *Imitrex*. First of all, it costs a lot of money. Second, it is a form of *pharmakeia*/sorcery. Third, it does not solve the root problem. There has to be *a more excellent way*™.

Let's look at Scriptures defining drugs in the Word. These Scriptures have to do with works of the flesh and are considered to be sin by God.

> [19]**Now the works of the flesh are manifest, which are** *these;* **Adultery, fornication, uncleanness, lasciviousness,** [20]**Idolatry, witchcraft, hatred, variance, emulations, wrath, strife, seditions, heresies, Galatians 5:19–20**

> pharmakeia, Greek *5331*, Strong's, *far-mak-i'-ah*; from Greek *5332* (pharmakeus); *medication* ("pharmacy"), i.e. (by extension) *magic* (literal or figurative) :- sorcery, witchcraft.

> pharmakeus, Greek *5332*, Strong's, *far-mak-yoos'*; from pharmakon (a *drug*, i.e. spell-giving *potion*); a *druggist* ("pharmacist") or *poisoner*, i.e. (by extension) a *magician* :- sorcerer.

In *Strong's Concordance*, the word *witchcraft* is *pharmakeia* (*#5331*) in the Greek. It is from the root word numbered *#5332*. This word, *#5332*, is the Greek word *pharmakeus*, which means a drug, i.e., spell-giving potion; a druggist ("pharmacist") or poisoner, i.e., a magician :- sorcerer. Going back to the main word *#5331*, it literally means, as defined in the *Strong's*, a medication (pharmacy).

If you were God, would you want to maintain your child on the earth through a drug or do better by dealing with the spiritual problem so your child would not have a migraine to begin with? If you were God, what would you do? You would solve the root problem, wouldn't you? This is *a more excellent way*™.

In ministry, we come to people and start dealing with the guilt and the self-conflict. We address the spiritual dynamics tormenting them. We take the situation before the Lord, get them delivered and fixed so when they are faced with conflict and failure, they can have God's peace. They are no longer bound by guilt and conflict. They have been delivered; they have been healed. They no longer have lowered serotonin levels. Fear is not there because anxiety is gone. Histamine is not secreted and migraines do not develop. Our ministry helps people recognize these dynamics. Then, in the Walk Out stage of ministry, on their journey to total freedom, many of them are able to quickly stop a migraine before it gets a foothold. This is *a more excellent way*™. This is true discernment and spiritual warfare producing long-term freedom.

Learning to deal with migraines, as with allergies, can take time. However, now you know the cause and the process and you have the knowledge and the power of God to help you.

### Allergies

An *allergy* is a hypersensitive reaction to any antigen (any substance producing a reaction). This is a strong area where our ministry sees victory with much success over *allergies*. I'll tell you how it works.

**DEFINITIONS:**

- Antigen—any substance that, when introduced into the body, stimulates the production of an antibody.

- Allergen—a substance causing an allergy.

- Allergy—a hypersensitive reaction to environmental factors or substances such as pollens, foods, dust or micro-organisms in amounts that do not affect most people.

So an *allergy* is an acquired, abnormal immune response to a substance (allergen) and does not normally cause a reaction.

- Antibody—any of the complex proteins produced by B lymphocytes in response to the presence of an antigen.

Thus an antigen (allergen) is a substance that induces a state of sensitivity when it comes in contact with body tissues. A reaction called an *allergy* is produced.

This stage of teaching concerns allergies as the result of a compromised immune system. The body produces cortisol to suppress the inflammatory response to the attack. Cortisol (a steroid hormone secreted by the adrenal cortex) is over-secreted long-term and you have destruction of white corpuscles and macrophage and killer cells. Too much cortisol over a long term produces cell death at this level.

Many times you have antibodies to antigens occurring in your body in relationship to a compromised immune system. Fear, anxiety and stress compromise your immune system. This is exactly what we are learning from the medical textbooks: long-term fear, anxiety and stress can destroy your immune system and, when this happens, you have antigen to antibody. This is exactly what an allergy is—a hypersensitive reaction.

Your body was not designed to be allergic to anything. In creation, God created you to be compatible with everything you are exposed to. You have been misled about what really causes allergies. An allergic reaction is actually a byproduct biologically of a compromised immune system. You're experiencing antibodies being formed because of excessive B cell activity, which is a side effect of your compromised immune system. The allergy is an illusion. We've seen 100 allergies leave a person within 24 hours when their immune system was healed.

What the devil did to you through his kingdom was to destroy or compromise your immune system and set up this sequence of events because of fear, anxiety and stress. Why don't you take your life back by the Lord once and for all and tell your friends and your neighbors and your family you've been had?

How often have you heard your friends say, "Well, I'm allergic to peanut butter, I'm allergic to chocolate, I'm allergic to dairy products, I'm allergic to this, I'm allergic to that?"

Tell them they've been had! Get involved in their lives. Ask them what is bugging them. What are they afraid of? What is their stressor? Where is their conflict? What is unresolved? This is the work of the enemy in the human spirit and the human soul. Are you with me? Oh my, it is powerful, isn't it?

Look! Here is something else happening when you experience long-term fear, anxiety and stress. This is also incredible. This is how it affects you. I know this is kind of technical, but I just wanted to show you because this is coming directly out of the medical community and their research. These are some physiological effects of long-term over-secretion of cortisol as a result of fear, anxiety and stress and as a result, the destruction of the immune system. Look what is affected. These functions are affected by cortisol: *carbohydrate and lipid metabolism, protein metabolism, inflammatory effects, lipid metabolism, the immune reserve, digestive function, urinary function, connective tissue function, muscle function, bone function, vascular system, myocardial function and central nervous system function.*

Every bit of this is affected long-term by fear, anxiety and stress and we wonder why we have so many diseases coming out of fear, anxiety and stress.

Now you understand why the Lord needs to deliver you of all your fears. Let me show you something else. Let's talk about the mind-body connection. I know this is not overly spiritual, but you need to know what your doctor is *not* telling you. You need to know what the medical community is *not* telling you.

I'll tell you why the medical community is not telling you this: because they would not know what to do with it if they did tell you about it. They do not know what to tell you, so they don't tell you anything.

Your homeostasis (equilibrium in the body with respect to various functions and chemical composition of fluids and tissues) is controlled by the release of various hormones. You are very chemical in your creation. You are very nuclear, you are very sexual, you are very spiritual, but you are also very chemical. You have a number of organs and glands, particularly in the endocrine system, which secrete a particular chemical. It goes like this: a squirt here, a squirt there, here a squirt, there a squirt, squirt, squirt, everywhere a squirt, squirt.

And your enemy knows he can control the rate of your squirts by your thoughts and by your soul and by your spirit. Your enemy knows things like bitterness and guilt and fear, if allowed to remain within your consciousness, can be used to control you. When your spiritual dynamics are compromised by the enemy in a manner in which he can control your body and your chemistry, then he can put depression or any other psychological or biological malfunction on you when he feels like it.

He can do this because depression, by definition, is no more and no less than a chemical imbalance in the body induced externally or internally.

Your enemy knows that if he can get you "unspiritual" and he can manipulate you in areas of lack of sanctification, then he can control your very thought process.

When Satan can control your thought process, he can also control your chemistry. When you have *serotonin* deficiencies, you do not feel good about yourself because there is a deficiency of the chemical God created in you to make you feel good chemically. For every thought you have, conscious or unconscious, there is a nerve transmission, a secretion of a hormone or neurotransmitter somewhere in your body to react to it.

When you start listening to fear, you start listening to self-hatred, you start listening to guilt, you start listening to rejection, then your body secrets chemicals in response to those spiritual attacks that are counterproductive to your peace.

Your enemy knows this very well. *It is about time you know what your enemy knows about you so you can defeat him at the pass.* You do not have to be a victim nor do you have to be ignorant nor do you have to die of a disease and go to heaven to find out why you died.

## Gastroesophageal Reflux

*Gastroesophageal reflux* and *mitral valve prolapse* (see below for more information) are identical in their spiritual root cause and manifestation. The root problem behind both is *anxiety*.

In the case of *gastroesophageal reflux*, there is a sphincter muscle at the top of your stomach (lower end of your esophagus) and, when it does not stay closed, you reflux stomach acid up into the esophagus. This action creates heartburn and even esophageal ulcers.

## Mitral Valve Prolapse

In the case of *mitral valve prolapse*, the mitral valve in the heart does not open and shut correctly. This allows blood to flow backward into the atrium causing the heart to work harder. This is why it is called mitral valve prolapse. The root problem behind both *reflux* and *mitral valve prolapse* is *anxiety*.

When you have anxiety, the hypothalamus sets into motion not only an imbalance of the endocrine system, but anxiety and fear immediately affect the sympathetic nervous system, which is part of the involuntary, or autonomic, nervous system and the central nervous system.

Both the mitral valve and the gastroesophageal sphincter muscles have a nerve supply. If the nerve malfunctions, neither the valve nor the sphincter muscle will do what it was designed to do. Neurological misfirings can contribute to *mitral valve prolapse* and *gastroesophageal reflux*. The root behind it is *fear and anxiety*. Many people have been healed of *mitral valve prolapse* and *gastroesophageal reflux* through our ministry.

## CFS (Chronic Fatigue Syndrome)

a.k.a. CFIDS (Chronic Fatigue Immune Dysfunction Syndrome)

*Chronic fatigue syndrome* is not Epstein-Barr virus. Epstein-Barr virus is mononucleosis, the old college disease. Epstein-Barr virus is just a new name for it. It used to be called "mono." Now it is called EBV. Epstein-Barr virus is not CFS or CFIDS.

CFS, almost without exception (and this has also been verified by the CFS National Organization in Charlotte, NC, and others who have become "specialists" in CFS), involves a diagnosis *of hypoglycemia/low blood sugar.* You will find that CFS and *hypoglycemia* are often linked together in the diagnosis. Hypoglycemia has an autoimmune component. It is not considered an autoimmune disease proper; however, it has an autoimmune component. This indicates it would have a similar spiritual root to other autoimmune diseases we need to address.

Whenever we minister to someone with an autoimmune disease, we find without exception a degree of *lacking self-esteem and/or guilt.* A person has conflict with himself over his identity, drivenness, performance, conflict and guilt, at some level causing an autoimmune disease. *CFIDS (or CFS) is an anxiety disorder coupled with an autoimmune override* which triggers *hypoglycemia.* The problem with CFS is that the *hypoglycemia* is a disease all by itself.

Some people are going to have *hypoglycemia* and not be diagnosed with CFS. It makes it tough because with *hypoglycemia* you have a neurological triggering in the bloodstream keeping the manufactured glucose from getting to the brain. Glucose provides the energy for the firing of the brain cells which creates in you the ability to process thought; it makes your brain work. Complicating the diagnosis is that there is evidence of people who have been diagnosed with CFS but do not have *hypoglycemia.* It is my position in ministry that if fatigue and exhaustion show up in a person without the corresponding diagnosis of *hypoglycemia,* then the person does not have CFS but is in the third and final stage of the General Adaptation Syndrome of the anxiety profile, which is *exhaustion.*

Now in the case of *environmental illness,* we have "brain fog," but it may not include *hypoglycemia.* The reasons for brain fog with *environmental illness* are different than the reasons for brain fog in CFS. In the case of MCS/EI, we have a combination of less oxygen or too much carbon dioxide coming out of *anxiety,* specifically hyperventilation, because in MCS/EI when we have stress our heart starts to race, we have repetitive breathing and the respiratory rate increases. We also have potassium levels depleted and the third stage of an anxiety disorder called the *exhaustion stage* sets in. The long-term effect of a decrease in potassium ions is *fatigue.*

In CFS we do not have a lower potassium level; we have a lowered level of glucose. You do not have the glucose necessary to fuel the firing of the brain cells. This is part of it. *Chronic fatigue* is the first part of the name of the disease. The symptoms are exhaustion, lethargy, lack of motivation and lack of energy flow. The word "syndrome" basically means they do not know what causes it. *When you hear the words incurable, etiology unknown, or syndrome, you usually have a spiritually rooted disease.*

I have had to look at the many CFS cases I have dealt with, and up until a couple of years ago, it looked like one member of the family tree was primarily responsible for them. I have run across people in the past few years, as we have had more CFS cases surfacing and it has not held true. I have had to modify a black and white statement to what I consider to be a majority statement. I'll give you my insight into CFS.

When we minister to people with CFS, we do ministry in what is called blood sugar profile. We minister against hypoglycemia first because the *hypoglycemia* comes to hide the real problem.

Many others doing diagnosis of CFS do not include the insight of *hypoglycemia* as the primary problem. I am shocked! It is like a form of disease occultism. Do you know what occultism is? It is when the real thing is hidden. Something comes before it that hides it. It is like the real root problem for CFS is here, and as the profile of the syndrome develops, then *hypoglycemia* comes and gets a foothold. There are such a myriad of physiological problems hidden by the real enemy. We have learned this slowly and surely in ministry.

The first thing we do in ministering to CFS these days is to get rid of the impostor hiding the real root problem. Behind the *hypoglycemia* is the real problem. CFS is an anxiety disorder coupled with hypoglycemia override (which would be the autoimmune rider) clouding a *very major fear/anxiety disorder and is the result of drivenness to meet the expectation of a parent in order to receive love. The love is usually sought from a mother*, but not always.

CFS is a result of drivenness to meet the expectation of a parent in order to receive love and acceptance. In most cases, the man or woman who comes down with CFS is not doing in life what they wanted to do but instead is trying to meet the expectations of a parent. Many times you will find behind the scenes a parent who is very controlling regarding what the child is going to be in life. It is easy to better understand CFS if you first eliminate the MCS/EI diagnosis.

I consider CFS to be a *performance disorder*. It is called "yuppie disease" or a white-collar disease. It usually hits professionals at the height of their careers. After they have achieved what they were supposed to achieve to meet the expectations of others, they crash. As they crash, the guilt and the self-hatred come and the autoimmune components set in. Then we have hypoglycemia, which clouds the whole issue. We are now chasing this imaginary problem.

I have many medical books on this subject in my library. I have read them all and no one knows the "cause" of CFS. *It is not the result of chemical exposure. The only way I can tell you our etiology and our diagnosis of the spiritual roots are correct is because so many people are now well!* **This is *a more excellent way***™. It is kind of a reversed thing. Rather than trying to get a diagnosis, let's go and get involved in somebody's life and see what is going on and come back through the mess to see what we have. In doing this reverse process, we have seen healing. From this standpoint we have unraveled this mystery by getting involved with people at their spiritual and emotional levels and helping them come to grips with their innermost thoughts and innermost fears.

*I consider CFS to be a fear and anxiety disorder producing drivenness to meet the expectation of someone in order to "measure up" and receive love.*

There are people in the secular world who consider MCS/EI and CFS as one and the same disease. I don't agree because they have two different components. The person who has CFS has not usually been victimized at the level we see in those with MCS/EI, because in most MCS/EI cases we have seen a breakup in human relationships, usually concerning a close family member and usually going back to childhood. One or more of these four life circumstances is usually involved:

- emotional and verbal abuse,

- physical abuse,

- sexual abuse, including molestation, and

- drivenness to meet the expectation of the parent in order to receive love in a sterile, loveless environment.

This is heavy stuff for a child to deal with while they are in the process of growing up.

## Parasites

You don't usually see parasites unless somebody has a compromised immune system. People often come to me, especially with MCS/EI, and they say, "I have parasites."

I say, "Oh well, no big deal." I don't even bother ministering to the parasite issues. I am wasting my time. If you want to get rid of parasites, let's go ahead and get the fear and anxiety dealt with because it may cause a weakened immune system.

When your immune system is healed, parasites don't stand a chance. I have had call after call in this ministry where people have said, "I just went to the doctor and there are no more parasites." Parasites usually get a long-term foothold because of a compromised immune system. You can have a compromised immune system because of *fear, anxiety and stress*.

## Irritable Bowel Syndrome

*Irritable bowel syndrome* (IBS) is caused by the misfiring of nerve dendrites in the lining of the intestine. IBS comes directly out of *anxiety, fear and insecurities.*

## Colic

Colic can be from an *inherited spirit of fear.* Colic is a neurological manifestation in the child as a direct result of a spirit of fear coming in at conception, in utero or at birth. It is easy to deal with. Many times it is inherited from the mother.

## Flu

The Bible seems to indicate there are certain things "common to man." There is no spiritual root behind the flu necessarily. There are things common to man, but the Lord delivers us out of them all.

> **Many *are* the afflictions of the righteous: but the LORD delivereth him out of them all. Psalm 34:19**

There is another Scripture I've been thinking about. The Bible talks about something called our "often infirmities" in 1 Timothy 5:23. Often infirmities are things common to man in the earth because of bacterium and other aspects of Adam's fall. They do not necessarily have a spiritual root as such, but are a part of the fall of man.

The exception: not taking care of your body, not getting enough rest and enough good nutrition. You did not take care of the temple and have compromised your immune system and thus you are more open to viruses and flu.

## Sjögren's Syndrome

*Sjögren's syndrome* has an autoimmune mechanism attached to it. It is a chronic systemic inflammatory disorder of unknown etiology characterized by dryness of the mouth, eyes and other mucus membranes. It is often associated with rheumatic disorders. *Sjögren's* shares certain autoimmune features with *scleroderma.* I am familiar with *scleroderma.* If *Sjögren's* is related to *scleroderma,* we have very obvious *extreme self-rejection and self-hatred coupled with much guilt.* The autoimmune component gives us the key. The inflammation indicates there is a proliferation of white corpuscles, so we know we are dealing with a person *in conflict with self.*

When you have classes of disease, you find the spiritual roots to be the same. The faces and the names may change and the open doors may change. You have to get involved in the person's life to find out where exactly the curse came in, as well as how and why. This is part of our ministry and investigation. We find out where the devil came in, why he has a right to be in someone's life, where the curse came from and what the cause was. This is all part of ministry.

## Panic Attacks

Panic attacks are a phobic, fear and anxiety disorder. Panic attack is an aggressive stage of a fear and anxiety disorder. The hypothalamus gland is the originating point and facilitator of the following life circumstances: *fear, anxiety, stress, phobia, phobic realities, panic attacks, rage, anger and aggression.* All of these expressions in mankind are set into motion by one gland, the hypothalamus. In an anxiety attack there would be a rush of the hormone ACTH into the bloodstream. In a panic attack it goes directly to the receptor cells in the muscles of the heart causing an immediate respiratory rate increase, a pounding of the heart, automatic immediate hyperventilation and over involvement of carbon dioxide retention in the brain. It causes fuzziness of thinking, a shutting down and can even produce anaphylaxis and catatonic reality. It can go a full range just like that. It is caused by *the spirit of fear.*

## Phobias

*Phobias are a little different. Phobias* are associative; panic is not associative. Panic can come out of nowhere. When you study what *phobias* are, you will find that someplace in the person's life, they have associated a geographical location or situation with a fear or unpleasant feeling. They immediately come to associate the location or situation and a feeling with the presence of a problem. *Agoraphobia (fear of leaving a familiar setting)* and *claustrophobia (fear of closed spaces)* are examples.

Phobic realities involve two mechanisms, projection and displacement, which constitute avoidance. It is a preconditioning of a phobic stressor that will reinforce itself by feelings of discomfort. To go near the stressor or even to think about it will send a hormone into the bloodstream via the hypothalamus and produce the beginning stages of a panic attack in relationship to the phobia. It is nothing more than a *spirit of fear* and that's the first way you have to deal with it. How many times do we project things, then avoid them out of fear? *The battle is won or lost in the mind.*

## Hypoglycemia (Low Blood Sugar)

*Hypoglycemia* is low blood sugar. It is rooted in *anxiety and fear coupled with self-hatred and self-rejection coupled with guilt.* There is a neurological misfiring not allowing the glucose to reach the brain. Glucose is the fuel to fire the brain cells. *Hypoglycemia* also involves an autoimmune component attached to it as a rider. In effect, *hypoglycemia* can be the result of anxiety coupled with self-hatred and guilt. It is deeply rooted in lack of identity and insecurity. Performance orientation may also be implicated.

### Hyperglycemia (Diabetes (Type 1))

This involves high blood sugar and there is much evidence of an autoimmune component attached to it. *Hyperglycemia* is an autoimmune disease with an anxiety rider. In the case of *hyperglycemia,* which is *diabetes (type 1),* the white corpuscles attack the pancreas itself and interfere with its performance. On the other hand, in *hypoglycemia* there is a neurological misfiring and it interferes with the glucose reaching the brain after it has been produced. Whenever your tissue is being attacked by white corpuscles, you have an autoimmune disease. Whenever you have neurological misfirings that interfere with the processes, you have stress, fear and anxiety. They are similar, but there are two different spiritual roots behind it. (See diabetes.)

### Hypothyroidism (Hashimoto's Disease)

*Hypothyroidism* in its advanced stages is called *Hashimoto's disease,* which is the manifestation of lowered levels of thyroxin being secreted by the thyroid. In the second stage of the General Adaptation Syndrome of the fear, anxiety and stress profile, the thyroid is directly affected by stress causing an under-secretion of thyroxin. The treatment programs provide for synthetic or animal derivatives of thyroxin to replace the deficiency. Many people have been healed through this ministry of anxiety disorders that included *Hashimoto's disease* as part of the profile. Today, the majority of these people who have been healed of fear, anxiety and stress no longer have *Hashimoto's disease. This disease is considered incurable in the medical community, but I am here to tell you that's not so.*

Just as the thyroid malfunctioned because of fear, anxiety and stress, when fear, anxiety and stress are eliminated through ministry, the thyroid kicks back into balance and begins to secrete thyroxin correctly again.

In *hypothyroidism,* which is the result of fear, anxiety and stress, there is an autoimmune component which kicks in involving white corpuscles which collect at the thyroid location and cause nonbacterial inflammation and swelling. This advanced stage is called *Hashimoto's disease.* In this case, self-hatred, self-rejection and guilt become the major root with fear, anxiety and stress becoming a rider component. In either case, many, many people are well today because of our ministry programs for them concerning it in both of these manifestations. **This is *a more excellent way*™.**

### Hyperthyroidism (Graves' Disease)

*Hyperthyroidism*, which is an over-secretion of thyroxin, is called *Graves' disease* in many of its forms, and it can produce goiters and swelling of the eyes, as well as palpitations and tremors. There is an autoimmune rider attached to *Graves' disease*, but I consider it to be primarily an anxiety disorder initially. Then with the autoimmune component which would produce *Graves'*, as opposed to *Hashimoto's*, and is primarily an autoimmune disease with an anxiety rider. The root behind both these diseases is *anxiety, fear and/or self-hatred, self-rejection and guilt.*

I had a call from an individual who had just been diagnosed with *Graves' disease.* Their doctor, who happened to be a member of their church, suggested the immediate destruction of the thyroid through radioactive iodine. This was a pretty drastic solution, although *Graves' disease* left unattended is life threatening. The doctor's solution was to permanently erase the problem by destroying the thyroid. However, what the doctor did not tell this individual is that removing the thyroid will produce permanent *Hashimoto's disease.* So they would have been exchanging one disease for another.

I want to tell you this insight I had while on the phone that is really incredible. This individual wanted to know what I had to say. So when I reviewed the medical information on *Graves'*, I discovered something. The primary triggering point for *Graves'* can be the result of emotional shock or a prolonged period of anxiety. In my study, I also read that *Graves' disease* can have an autoimmune component attached to it.

Additionally, when I looked at the therapy suggested in lieu of radioactive iodine, there was a drug that could be given for a period of 18 months. This drug immediately arrests the forward motion of the disease and gives a measure of time to try to solve the problem. With this information in hand, I asked this individual, "Did your doctor tell you that by destroying your thyroid, you would have permanent *Hashimoto's disease?"*

His patient said, "No, it was never discussed."

I said, "Did your doctor tell you the findings of the medical community indicate emotional stress could be a cause?"

The individual said, "No."

I asked, "Did your doctor tell you a drug could be taken over a period of 18 months and this time would allow the resolving of the issues?"

I was told, "Yes, but why go this route when we can solve the problem once and for all?"

I said, "Don't you think it would be God's will to go to Him and find out what your emotional conflict is? Then, if there is a conflict, it would be a spiritual issue and God would be able to resolve it in your life."

In our conversation, we discussed many areas of emotional conflict and the guilt and self-rejection coming out of those areas. Those two scenarios are enough to produce *Graves' disease.* The final decision of this individual was to temporarily go on the drug and seek God to resolve the spiritual and emotional conflict. I am happy to say that this person still has their thyroid and is doing well. Don't you think keeping your thyroid and dealing with spiritual and emotional issues to produce healing is *a more excellent way*™?

Sometimes you need help to get well. If you could get well yourself by confession, then you could also get well yourself by responsibility, recognition, renouncing and resisting. Then why would we need the ministry gifts in 1 Corinthians 12? Why would we need to pray one for another? If you could do this all by yourself, why would we need to pray one for another? Why would we need ministry?

I have identified over 40 different statements in Scripture to show how God can be prevented from moving in His people's lives. Knowing the problem is not always the solution. *You are still going to have to line up with God all the way.* We cannot have our cake and eat it too.

**God is a loving Father and He is *not* going to share you with the enemy.** You may want to cohabit with your enemy, but God does not like it and He is not going to compromise His position. Just because you are looking for a way out or *a way to bypass the penalty of the curse* without going the extra mile does not mean that God will allow it to happen.

I don't want God to leave me stranded. I want God to take me all the way into His promises so all the enemies of my land are defeated and I can stand before Him and know we have done a wonderful thing in life. I am still under construction. God is still working me over every single day and I love it. I love the convicting work of the Holy Spirit in my life. I love God molding me and making me into a vessel of honor. I cannot think of any greater honor than to think God would care about me. I submit to Him as my Father; I submit to the Word He sent for me and I submit to the Holy Spirit.

**Editor's Note:** Do not be confused with *Graves'* and *Hashimoto's disease* at this level, because each represents a complete reality in its own right as being taught. However, as part of the profile of these two diseases, *hypothyroidism* and *hyperthyroidism* can exist in their own right and not be either *Graves' disease* or *Hashimoto's disease.* In these stages, both in *hypothyroidism* and *hyperthyroidism,* the sympathetic nervous system is implicated as the result of activity in the second level of the General Adaptation Syndrome of fear, anxiety and stress, which would cause an over- or under-secretion of thyroxin.

## Addictive Personality

### Addictions

We have had some success with healing dopamine reductions in addictions. In dealing with addictions, dopamine is very important to pay attention to because dopamine is the pleasure neurotransmitter of the human body. The body produces it very slowly while serotonin can be replaced very quickly. In fact, cocaine is a very unusual drug because cocaine is not chemically addictive. *Cocaine is psychologically and spiritually addictive.* I'll tell you why.

When a person takes a hit of cocaine, the mechanisms of cocaine release dopamine in mass. It is equivalent to a massive orgasm. Such a huge release of dopamine can never be duplicated a second time. This is why, once users have had their first hit, they will never have the same rush again. They try and try, but what they don't understand is they will never have it because the high is coming from the release of dopamine. It is not the drug giving them the fix; it is dopamine being released to give them the biological fix. This is why people on cocaine are so tormented.

***All addictions are rooted in the need to be loved.***

### Masturbation

Masturbation is a big issue. Masturbation usually begins in childhood, not necessarily because of lust but coming out of families who are full of strife. You see, a child learns this when a house is filled with argument and strife and the tension is building; an orgasm will give him or her a type of physical release from this tension. There is also a release of dopamine because when you have an orgasm, dopamine is the neurotransmitter; when released, it gives you a fulfilled feeling. It is a neurotransmitter and it gives you a neurological-biological "fix."

A child growing up in an atmosphere full of tension and strife will get temporary relief by masturbating, but what comes in behind it are feelings of uncleanness and guilt. It is the same thing with cocaine. Right after it come feelings of uncleanness and guilt. There is a vicious cycle of release and condemnation. Masturbation and cocaine are very similar in their spiritual implications. It is a release and fulfillment and then guilt. Your enemy certainly knows how to work you over!

Those are some of the mechanisms of dopamine and cocaine, but what does this have to do with *Parkinson's Disease?* I am not sure, but we are going to find out.

I do not like losing. I have had so many victories in fighting disease I just figure we'll just win them all one of these days. I think if we get an army here in the body of Christ, we might defeat the devil at some level. But if we do not start, it just isn't going to happen!

Those of you hearing this are experiencing a new frontier. This is a new frontier where God is moving in mankind. I am learning more every day. I do not have all the answers, but what I do know and what has been proven to be true, I'll share with you.

## Alcoholism

Have you ever wondered why some people can drink and are not alcoholics while others drink and are alcoholics? First of all, alcoholism is not a genetically inherited disease. However, there is a genetic component to be paid attention to in an alcoholic family. Did you know alcoholism runs in families because *there is a curse in the family to produce it?* Molestation runs in families. Victimization runs in families. *There are familiar spirits traveling in families.*

A national statistic states 35 percent of all females in America have been molested at some time or another and 25 percent of all males have been molested at some time in their life. This is a national statistic in America. It brings a rollover. The possibility a person who has been molested will molest someone else in their lifetime is very, very high unless they are saved by the blood of Jesus Christ and delivered.

When a child is born into an alcoholic family, he has what is called a *deficient chemical* in the basal ganglia. The basal ganglia is at the top part of your spinal cord where your brain sits. In here are various neurotransmitters connected directly to your central nervous system via the cerebral processes.

There are four major classes of neurotransmitters found in this area.

One has to do with painkillers. When a person is born with an inherited predisposition for alcoholism, there is a defective chemical coming out of the birth. It is not normal. It is like it needs something to give it completeness as a chemical. Alcohol is a chemical; it is a drug. When this defective chemical comes in contact with alcohol, there is a chemical reaction and a brand new chemical is formed. This new chemical stays permanently in the basal ganglia; it is called THIQ. This new neurotransmitter produces a permanent craving for alcohol.

A person who is an alcoholic is considered to be allergic to alcohol by the medical community. This is the reason it only takes one drink to start the thing moving.

I have had some success with alcoholism and some failures. The success with alcoholism comes first of all from the Lord delivering the person, in conjunction with them just having had enough. There has to come a time in the person's life where they make a quality decision to just say, "No." I know God meets us and honors us in this decision.

I have seen unsaved people get free of alcohol. I am not necessarily in agreement with the 12-step program in its present form and I'll tell you why. They teach, "Once an alcoholic, always an alcoholic," and I disagree. The people who have been delivered and healed through our ministry concerning alcoholism need no support groups and they are not drawn to alcohol ever again. I think when you say, "Once an alcoholic, always an alcoholic," you have just told God He cannot deliver you and He cannot save you to the uttermost. I cannot go this route. Although 12-step programs have done some good, there has to be *a more excellent way*™, a greater grace, and it is to be free.

## Weight

There is both a genetic and a spiritual component to weight problems. The rate of your metabolism can be determined by how you think about yourself. The hypothalamus controls sleep, thirst, eating and many other functions of our bodies. When you have lack of self-esteem, when you are in conflict with yourself and others, your hypothalamus gland, in conjunction with your mind through the limbic system, senses the presence of spiritual and emotional problems.

One of the first things the hypothalamus does in relationship to self-conflict is to reduce *serotonin* levels. Whenever you have a reduction in *serotonin* you do not feel good about yourself. When you do not feel good about yourself, you go into insecurity. When you are insecure, you start "sucking your thumb." *The mouth is a contact place for love and security.*

People who smoke cigarettes have exchanged the thumb for something else. *All addictions are rooted in lack of self-esteem and insecurity and the need to be loved.* The mouth and whatever you put in it is designed to try to bring you to emotional security. Excessive eating is a direct result of not feeling good about yourself.

When people do not feel good about themselves, they will usually become involved in either *obsessive compulsive behavior* (OCD) or an addictive behavior of some kind.

OCD is something we have dealt with and we have seen great success. OCD always, without exception, involves a reduction in *serotonin* levels.

I did research involving the work of Dr. Sachs some years ago on *OCD, anorexia* and *bulimia.* In reviewing his material and his conclusions, it was shocking to learn the medical community had no real help. The best they could offer was a 12-step program and synthetic *serotonin* derivatives to take as a supplement and/or anti-anxiety drugs. This is the best they have available in America. As far as I am concerned, this is a form of disease management.

*I am not into disease management; I am into disease eradication and prevention at all times, if at all possible, so help me God.* If you are being managed in your diseases, then God bless you. I don't represent your management; I represent your freedom. The God that I serve does not represent your management; He represents your freedom.

I minister the gospel of Jesus Christ and the gospel of the Father who sent Him and I must hold out for *a more excellent way*™. I will not teach a leavened gospel because of unbelief, doubts, fears and the practices of mankind and hold people in bondage. I will be gracious and loving wherever and whenever I teach, but I am going to help you confront your issues.

Recently the drug *Fen Phen* was taken off the market. *Fen Phen* is an "upper." It was designed to build self-esteem. When you get so high you have to take "downers," then you have to take more *Fen Phen* to come back up. In these peaks and valleys, depression sets in. Depression, by definition, is the result of a chemical imbalance in the body. God created us chemically perfect.

An article in *Time* magazine on July 21, 1997 said,

> It was the latest in a series of setbacks for the new generation of diet pills. They were initially seen as an improvement over the old "speed"-based pills because they were nonaddictive and worked more subtly, stimulating production of the brain chemical serotonin, which is associated with the feelings of satisfaction and satiety.

The problem with the drug *Fen Phen* is the incredible side effects dangerous to health, involving heart attacks, heart problems, depression, mood swings and other aberrations of thought. *Fen Phen* boosts serotonin levels, which would make folks feel better about themselves. When you feel better about yourself, you do not put your thumb in your mouth. You do not put food in your mouth. This is the best that medical science has had to offer!

As we have discussed, *weight gain involves a lack of self-esteem.* This problem tends to grow every time the person looks in the mirror. When it does not tell you that you are the fairest of them all, your self-esteem suffers further. We are into comparing ourselves with others. You have taken your eyes off the living God who has created you and you have set your eyes on others. Others have become your standard of acceptance and they have become your false god or idol.

Scripture says to judge no man; know no man after the flesh.

> **Ye judge after the flesh; I judge no man. John 8:15**

> **Wherefore henceforth know we no man after the flesh: yea, though we have known Christ after the flesh, yet now henceforth know we *him* no more. 2 Corinthians 5:16**

I do not judge you by what your house looks like. I judge you by your spirit. I want to know who you are on the inside. God looks at the inner man. Sometimes we major in minors and minor in majors. I think relationships are important. If you are basing relationships on whether you smell good or not, we have a problem. We all have our moments of odor.

I want to cut through the facade of hypocrisy because we are so busy being rejected and in fear of rejection that we cannot be ourselves. The problem is society has made everything anorexic to be desirable. In Russia, they have banned the Barbie doll. They have more spiritual sense than we do in America.

You know why they banned the Barbie doll in Russia? It did not represent the average Russian woman. There is nothing wrong, ladies, with a little meat with your potatoes. There is nothing wrong with being corn-fed. We accept what Hollywood has presented to us as "normal," and we think we must all be like anorexic Barbie dolls. There is something wrong with this picture.

One of the great blessings promised by God to His people is flesh to their bones. Flesh on our bones is a sign of health. Ladies, there is nothing wrong with you looking like a female should look.

If you have weight increase and would be beyond the parameters of good health, there could be genetic, biological or spiritual problems. The number one psychiatric disease producing death in America is *anorexia*. There are more people who die of *anorexia* in America than suicide.

If there has been an addiction to alcohol, another problem can develop. Alcoholics like sugar, carbohydrates and desserts. Do you know why? Because the body converts the sugars and the carbohydrates into alcohol and you get your fix anyway. If we have a combination of OCD and addictive personality, not only do we have the satisfaction of putting something in our mouth, but we also get the alcohol fix. Alcohol, to the basal ganglia, is a painkiller for emotional turmoil. It is an upper, so now you are getting a fix both ways.

These are the dynamics of addiction in OCD. If you are putting on weight there could be a genetic component, but most weight increase I deal with in ministry comes out of *fear of man, fear of failure, fear of abandonment, fear of rejection, lack of self-esteem, or introspection, where you look inside yourself and you don't like what you see.*

Shoplifting is the same thing as bingeing. Kleptomania is the result of *self-hatred, self-rejection and guilt.* People who take the credit card and spend thousands of dollars on a *spending binge* are exhibiting the same behavior as those who are bingeing on food. They are trying to increase the serotonin deficiency artificially and dopamine, which is the pleasure neurotransmitter, is also being secreted because of the rush they get to fill the void.

### Anorexia and Bulimia

*Anorexia* and *bulimia* have the same profile but a different manifestation. In anorexia the person refuses to eat. In *bulimia* the person eats but purges themselves of the food just consumed. *Bulimia* also includes excessive eating in exchange for the void of not feeling loved. The roots are the same: self-hatred, self-rejection and guilt, which effectively cause the *serotonin* levels to become deficient. Again, when you have lowered *serotonin* levels, the spiritual and emotional feelings of unloveliness are now reinforced by the chemical deficiency.

## Teaching on Nutrition

If you really want to work on excessive weight gain, first of all, I would say you need to begin in your *nutrition.* I think you need to eat meals three times a day. America does not eat breakfast. Too much going on; you are either sleeping in, running off to work or something else. It is the morning meal that sets metabolism into motion for the rest of the day and burns the calories. If you eat lunch and you have not had breakfast, lunch becomes fat because the metabolism is overloaded when it should have been set in motion at breakfast. Eat something nutritious in the morning and drink plenty of water throughout the day. This is important for weight loss and metabolism. Remember, one of the nine fruits of the Holy Spirit is temperance, which is moderation.

If you are concerned about the source of nutrition in today's society, I want to take you away from fear and put you back into wisdom. I tell people this in ministry: a one-a-day vitamin is all you need. All of this teaching on nutrition is not going to work if you are negating what nutrition represents by yielding to fear, anxiety and stress. These will cancel the benefits by producing such diseases as malabsorption (leaky gut syndrome).

People are motivated by fear and are trying to jump-start themselves into better health. If you feel like you need a little vitamin C, don't take 20,000 units of it at one swallow; rather, eat fruit or get it in a one-a-day supplement. I find people who think more is better. They think if a little vitamin C is what they need, then a whole bunch more is better. Wrong! You can risk going into levels of toxic poisonings. You need to understand that when they tell you the daily required amounts you need to exist as a human being, this is what you need. If you continue to put three, four, or ten times what you need into your body out of fear, you will risk throwing your body into chemical imbalance, injuring it and ending up doing just the opposite of what you were hoping to do.

In high school, my best friend's father became obsessed with health. He became obsessed with nutrition and what was "clean" and what was "unclean." He thought carrots and carrot juice were what he needed to be able to defeat all the problems of life. He became so obsessed that he drank carrot juice by the gallon until his flesh started to change colors. He literally died of acute carrot juice poisoning.

In our ministry, proper nutrition is a valid consideration and we help people assess where they are in nutrition. I am not "out in left field." I am in balance. Whatever you eat, if it is not of faith, it is sin. This is what Romans says about food:

> ...for whatsoever *is* not of faith is sin. Romans 14:23

In fact, in the area of vegetarianism and meat, I believe the Bible teaches in Romans 14 that those who are vegetarians are weak in the faith and those who are strong in the faith eat meat. However, if a person is a vegetarian and this is their conscience, then they eat vegetarian style unto the Lord and we are to leave them alone. If I eat meat unto the Lord, the meat is unto the Lord and you are to leave me alone.

> ¹Him that is weak in the faith receive ye, *but* not to doubtful disputations. ²For one believeth that he may eat all things: another, who is weak, eateth herbs. ³Let not him that eateth despise him that eateth not; and let not him which eateth not judge him that eateth: for God hath received him. Romans 14:1–3

The Bible talks about the doctrines of devils: forbidding to marry and forbidding the eating of meat.

> ⁴:¹Now the Spirit speaketh expressly, that in the latter times some shall depart from the faith, giving heed to seducing spirits, and doctrines of devils; ²Speaking lies in hypocrisy; having their conscience seared with a hot iron; ³Forbidding to marry, *and commanding* to abstain from meats,

**which God hath created to be received with thanksgiving of them which believe and know the truth. ⁴For every creature of God *is* good, and nothing to be refused, if it be received with thanksgiving: ⁵For it is sanctified by the word of God and prayer. 1 Timothy 4:1–5**

I am not going to tell you not to eat meat because the Word says it is a doctrine of devils. If you refrain from meat out of conscience or out of your application, then God bless you. I honor you because you do it unto the Lord. I sanctify it with you.

Now you may not be in agreement with this. However, as a student and teacher of the Word, I have to find my place in the midst of mankind without being a bull in a china closet. I have the right to teach truth as it is written; what you do with it is up to you according to your own conscience.

Paul even dealt with long hair for a man. Although Scripture says in 1 Corinthians 11:14: "Doth not even nature itself teach you that if a man have long hair, it is a shame unto him?" Paul, in dealing with the hair issue, came to a conclusion in verse 16 and said that he couldn't tell the Holy Spirit to be quiet in him, so let him prophesy before God and let his shame be his shame.

In essence, Paul established that long hair on a man, according to Scripture, would be a shame, but it would not be a basis for contention or strife and he seems to indicate anyone's hair (male or female) can be different from someone else's and is to be left alone. I guess Paul was saying that what an individual is doing for the kingdom of God is more important than the physical appearance of a saint. Paul did not get into it, so why should you and I get into it?

**But if any man seem to be contentious, we have no such custom, neither the churches of God. 1 Corinthians 11:16**

I want to release you to faith because in the New Testament it says there is nothing evil in itself, but all things, if taken with thanksgiving, are profitable because they are sanctified by the Word of God and by prayer.

**I know, and am persuaded by the Lord Jesus, that *there is* nothing unclean of itself... Romans 14:14**

**³Forbidding to marry, *and commanding* to abstain from meats, which God hath created to be received with thanksgiving of them which believe and know the truth. ⁴For every creature of God *is* good, and nothing to be refused, if it be received with thanksgiving: ⁵For it is sanctified by the word of God and prayer. 1 Timothy 4:3–5**

So, when we sit down to eat, we bless the food before God and then sanctify it so it will be made meet to our bodies. We do this because the Word tells us to do it so when there is anything unclean, we are protected. In faith and with wisdom we eat it, sanctify it, receive it and ask God to bless it, and I believe He does.

*Whatever God has created is for you in moderation, without guilt and without self-rejection. You belong here just the way you are.* There are ways to lose weight and I'll be very honest with you: I believe most diet programs are of the devil. I believe they are evil, rooted in fear and self-hatred. I do believe you can come before God and manage your lifestyle regarding food; and in ministry, deal with *unloving spirits, self-hatred, guilt and lack of self-esteem.* You can come to a place where you will be comfortable with your body.

## Chapter Nine
# Spiritual Blocks to Healing

The next subject we will cover is spiritual blocks to healing. We will look at spiritual blocks as taught in the Word that will keep you from being healed by God, even if you know the spiritual roots of disease. Just because you now have discernment doesn't mean you have lined up with Him to receive healing.

Sometimes people are not healed. If He doesn't heal you, I am going to ask Him to start you on the highway of discernment so you can apply the principles I have given you. I taught you previously there are times when just discernment and repentance, renouncing, taking responsibility and resisting do not work. My ministry began when this failed. So we are looking deeper into this picture, looking deeper into our hearts, our souls.

We are looking for the roots and blocks, for what is preventing you from receiving after repentance so renouncing and resisting can start to work in your life, thus allowing God to sanctify you in a particular area of your existence. There has to be a heart change on the inside.

I believe healing and deliverance come as a direct result of sanctification; I also believe disease prevention can be a direct result of sanctification. A lot of times, the people who believe in healing have done Christianity a disservice because they believe we can have our blessings and keep our sins. It is just not going to happen in the long-term.

I come from a different perspective. When people find out pastors are talking about disease and healing, they shudder and have visions of some of the excesses they have seen around healing. I hope I have not increased that image and I hope we have been able to talk about real life and real things from a very practical, biblical perspective while also doing something that is very scientifically and medically accurate. I hope we have achieved some of this in your lives.

I know many of you will never be the same after this study. God, through the Holy Spirit, will start to deal with you and many of you will not get the diseases that would have come upon you because you had not heard. I trust the Holy Spirit deals with you. God the Father loves you at this level as the Word of God dwells richly within your hearts and I hope that not only your lives, but the lives of your family, friends and enemies are enriched.

I teach in two dimensions. I believe in the traditional, fundamentalist position of God's grace being sufficient for us. I believe God when He told Paul that His grace was sufficient for him:

> **And he said unto me, My grace is sufficient for thee: for my strength is made perfect in weakness. Most gladly therefore will I rather glory in my infirmities, that the power of Christ may rest upon me. 2 Corinthians 12:9**

This is a scriptural, biblical principle and it includes us when we are in our problems as well as out of our problems.

If it were not for God's sustaining grace in our lives in disease, we would be most miserable in it. So I thank God for the principles of the **sustaining grace** of God. They are scriptural and are very Pauline. However, I have also come to **another understanding** in the Pauline teachings, as being a **greater grace**.

> **⁴And my speech and my preaching *was* not with enticing words of man's wisdom, but in demonstration of the Spirit and of power: ⁵That your faith should not stand in the wisdom of men, but in the power of God. 1 Corinthians 2:4–5**

> **¹¹And God wrought special miracles by the hands of Paul: ¹²So that from his body were brought unto the sick handkerchiefs or aprons, and the diseases departed from them, and the evil spirits went out of them. Acts 19:11–12**

> **⁸And it came to pass, that the father of Publius lay sick of a fever and of a bloody flux: to whom Paul entered in, and prayed, and laid his hands on him, and healed him. ⁹So when this was done, others also, which had diseases in the island, came, and were healed: Acts 28:8–9**

*The greater grace is **a more excellent way**™ with respect to sustaining grace.* The *greater grace* does not negate the *sustaining grace and* the *sustaining grace* does not negate the *greater grace*. The *greater grace* is the absence of the problem, where God alone receives all the glory. The *sustaining grace* is His provision of grace and mercy in our lives at all times, including the problem. To Him we give the glory in all things.

Now I have brought you a principle of my life. I teach both *sustaining grace* and *greater grace and* neither one are in opposition to the other. Both are scriptural. Both are positionally correct and in them God meets all of us, regardless of who we are and regardless of our circumstances in this journey as pilgrims. We are in a world that is going to be changed one day and is even now being changed through the Church.

> **…they [Paul and Barnabas] speaking boldly in the Lord, which gave testimony *unto the word of his grace,* and granted signs and wonders to be done by their hands. Acts 14:3**

You and I are pilgrims, called by God, called by His name and sealed by His Spirit. We are not as we shall be, but in a twinkling of an eye we shall be changed. In that is our hope—the redemption of our bodies and the establishment of the kingdom of God in righteousness. You and I, one day, regardless of the curse and the fall of Adam and Satan and sin, will partake of the glorious promise God, given to us through Jesus Christ.

Scripture has said eye hath not seen, ear hath not heard, nor has it entered into the heart of man, the things which God has prepared for those who love Him.

> **But as it is written, Eye hath not seen, nor ear heard, neither have entered into the heart of man, the things which God hath prepared for them that love him. 1 Corinthians 2:9**

I say to you, "Father, I love You." I think maybe I should say this so you understand I am not trying to negate *sustaining grace.*

What if we know the spiritual roots of our problem? What if the root of our disease biologically or psychologically does, in fact, have a spiritual component? We see it from the Word and from medical science. The confirmation is there. Is there any guarantee we will be healed of a malady or disease?

Even though you know the roots of the disease, there may be blocks to prevent God from moving in your life. You see, discernment is just the opening of the door to understanding.

In Isaiah 5:13, God said His people had gone into captivity because they had no knowledge.

> **Therefore my people are gone into captivity, because *they have* no knowledge: and their honourable men *are* famished, and their multitude dried up with thirst. Isaiah 5:13**

Again, Hosea 4:6 says God's people perish for lack of knowledge.

> **My people are destroyed for lack of knowledge: because thou hast rejected knowledge, I will also reject thee, that thou shalt be no priest to me: seeing thou hast forgotten the law of thy God, I will also forget thy children. Hosea 4:6**

So, discernment brings us to a place of observation of spiritual principles.

In Hebrews 5:14, Scripture says he who is able to handle strong meat (who is spiritually mature) is one who, by reason of exercise of his senses, is able to discern both good and evil.

> **But strong meat belongeth to them that are of full age, *even* those who by reason of use have their senses exercised to discern both good and evil. Hebrews 5:14**

We come to a place of maturity when we take a look at all things and judge them on the basis of discernment. Does discernment alone produce freedom? Not necessarily, because there may be blocks.

You know, I still find in the Bible these words: *if, then,* **and *but.*** I also am reminded in many Scriptures of the conditions for receiving God's promises. His promises are all yea and amen...

> For all the promises of God in him *are* yea, and in him Amen, unto the glory of God by us. 2 Corinthians 1:20

...but we have to *appropriate them through our obedience*, which is better than sacrifice:

> ²²And Samuel said, Hath the LORD *as great* delight in burnt offerings and sacrifices, as in obeying the voice of the LORD? Behold, to obey *is* better than sacrifice, *and* to hearken than the fat of rams. ²³For rebellion *is as* the sin of witchcraft, and stubbornness *is as* iniquity and idolatry. Because thou hast rejected the word of the LORD, he hath also rejected thee from *being* king. ²⁴And Saul said unto Samuel, I have sinned: for I have transgressed the commandment of the LORD, and thy words: because I feared the people, and obeyed their voice. 1 Samuel 15:22–24

We come to a place where we understand the words of Christ when He said, If you love Me, you will keep My commandments.

> If ye love me, keep my commandments. John 14:15

In the keeping of the commandments of the LORD, we find a provision in the Torah (the first five books of Moses) for when blessings will come (Deuteronomy 28). The blessings are automatic when we are obedient to God.

I also taught you about the principles of blessings and curses. Blessings come from God. Curses come as the blessings of the devil in our life. We choose what we shall have: blessings or curses, life or death.

I discussed Mt. Gerizim and Mt. Ebal. We found the mountain of curses was Mt. Ebal and Mt. Gerizim was the mountain of blessing. In this type and shadow, we saw the separation of God's people as God taught them a very graphic lesson. The Torah (Moses and the books of the law) bears witness to the truth that our obedience to God brings the blessing and they are very close and near by; however, our disobedience to God will eventually bring the curse. It is a long way off, but it will surely come (see Deuteronomy 28 and Deuteronomy 11:29). God has built the principles as well as the types and shadows to show that His grace overextends His judgments and He gives us a measure of time so we may apply our hearts to righteousness and to figure it out. Even under the law, grace and mercy was a factor of God's nature.

Here we are today under grace and mercy, but *the fact we are under grace and mercy does not negate our responsibility for obedience to the living God and His Word.* I have to obey His commandments, but I don't do it because the law requires it. I do it because I love God and I love the Lord Jesus. It is a small thing for me to be obedient to One I love.

The teaching of blocks to healing has allowed me to help more people get free, as well as knowing their spiritual roots.

The Spirit of the Lord is in the midst of us; where two or three are gathered together in His name, there He is in the midst of us.

> **For where two or three are gathered together in my name, there am I in the midst of them. Matthew 18:20**

The Holy Spirit within you bears witness with my spirit we are sons of God and the Spirit of God bears witness to truth.

> **The Spirit itself beareth witness with our spirit, that we are the children of God: Romans 8:16**

> **Howbeit when he, the Spirit of truth, is come, he will guide you into all truth: for he shall not speak of himself; but whatsoever he shall hear, *that* shall he speak: and he will shew you things to come. John 16:13**

I assume you are still reading this teaching because the things you read have borne witness. If they have not borne witness then you should be concerned. If they do not bear witness corporately, then I should not be teaching, for then we have come to a place of mere observation.

In beginning to understand the blocks to healing, let us remember Proverbs 26:2: As a bird by wandering and the swallow by flying, so the curse causeless does not come.

> **As the bird by wandering, as the swallow by flying, so the curse causeless shall not come. Proverbs 26:2**

*In other words, the enemy does not have the right to afflict your life just because he wants to. There must be open doors, historically, both in your family tree and in your personal life, in which you have wandered outside the parameters of God's knowledge, His provision and His covenant.*

We find ourselves opening the doors to many things. Some diseases have a right to be in our lives because somewhere along the line we or our ancestors opened the door. Satan does not have the right to arbitrarily afflict us. If it were the case, he could have eliminated the body of Christ worldwide within one year. Since that has not happened, it indicates to me the same parameters of protection are here today as were in the days of Job.

The open doors for Job to be sifted by the devil first involved fear. Job said in chapter 3 that the thing he feared most came upon him.

> **For the thing which I greatly feared is come upon me, and that which I was afraid of is come unto me. Job 3:25**

The areas of spiritual pride and arrogance in his life can be seen in the description of Behemoth and Leviathan in chapters 40 and 41 of Job and also in the great discourse in which God spoke to Job.

> **He *is* the chief of the ways of God... Job 40:19**
>
> **...he *is* a king over all the children of pride. Job 41:34**
>
> **¹Moreover the LORD answered Job, and said, ²Shall he that contendeth with the Almighty instruct *him?* he that reproveth God, let him answer it. Job 40:1–2**

The bitterness, fear, arrogance and spiritual pride were *open doors* in Job's life, but he got the message. God restored to him double what he had lost.

Today, I still believe there are parameters God has placed against the enemy. The way the enemy gets into our lives is that we have opened the door historically and genetically through familiar spirits of ancestry or we have wandered away from the path God has called us to.

You may or may not agree, but this is my position. Proverbs 26:2 amplifies my position by saying the curse without a cause does not come. Deuteronomy 28 says the curse involves all manner of disease and the blessing involves all absence of disease.

As we begin our teaching on blocks to healing, I have listed 33 blocks for the purpose of this teaching (and more can be found in Scripture). They must be considered because they reveal another dimension of separation from God. These blocks are very common to all men, including Christians. They hinder us from fully walking in the Spirit and receiving the blessings of God. Blocks need to be repented of with a heart change, just as repentance is needed in dealing with the roots.

## □ 1. Unforgiveness

The first block to healing is lack of forgiveness *(unforgiveness)* and this is the most important one. In fact, we go here first with every person to whom we minister. If we don't get this first block dealt with, *we are going no further in any dimension.* We are wasting our time with roots or the other possible blocks. We are wasting our time even talking to God on the subject. I want to take you to Mark 11:22–24: And Jesus, answering, saith unto them: Have faith in God. For verily I say unto you, whosoever shall say unto this mountain, Be thou removed, and be thou cast into the sea; and shall not doubt in his heart but shall believe those things which he saith shall come to pass; he shall have whatsoever he saith. Therefore I say unto you, what things soever ye desire, when ye pray, believe ye receive them, and ye shall have them.

> [22]And Jesus answering saith unto them, Have faith in God. [23]For verily I say unto you, That whosoever shall say unto this mountain, Be thou removed, and be thou cast into the sea; and shall not doubt in his heart, but shall believe that those things which he saith shall come to pass; he shall have whatsoever he saith. [24]Therefore I say unto you, What things soever ye desire, when ye pray, believe that ye receive *them,* and ye shall have *them.* Mark 11:22–24

> [14]For if ye forgive men their trespasses, your heavenly Father will also forgive you: [15]But if ye forgive not men their trespasses, neither will your Father forgive your trespasses. Matthew 6:14–15

It is clear from the Scriptures that we are to ask and expect to receive the object of our prayers.

There are now those in the body of Christ who build a doctrine around the first portion of this Scripture by saying you can have all the blessings of God just by asking or just by confessing in faith. This position may become a presumptuous faith, not taking responsibility and accountability for sin, especially the sin of unforgiveness found in context of this promise. In fact, this position totally negates the conditions of receiving found in Mark 11:25–26.

When you read Mark 11 and move into verses 25 and 26, there is a conditional Scripture attached that is never quoted when people are trying to make God a bubble gum machine (just putting a quarter in and getting something back). It says that when you stand praying (in order to receive something from God), forgive anyone who has wronged you so that your Father in heaven may forgive you your trespasses. But if you don't forgive, neither will your Father Who is in heaven forgive your trespasses.

> [25]And when ye stand praying, forgive, if ye have ought against any: that your Father also which is in heaven may forgive you your trespasses. [26]But if ye do not forgive, neither will your Father which is in heaven forgive your trespasses. Mark 11:25–26

*I say this to you, with the great authority of the Scriptures: God's forgiveness for you is in direct relationship to how you forgive your brother.* I know what it says in 1 John 1:9: if we confess our sins, He is faithful and just to forgive us our sins and to cleanse us from all unrighteousness.

> If we confess our sins, he is faithful and just to forgive us *our* sins, and to cleanse us from all unrighteousness. 1 John 1:9

I believe this. At the same time, I believe that forgiveness is in direct relationship to our own choice to be obedient in forgiving others following the example of Christ, being perfect as He is perfect in the area of forgiveness.

> Then said Jesus, Father, forgive them... Luke 23:34

Many people struggle with a Scripture quoted out of context because it accuses them and makes them feel unworthy. There is a Scripture found in Matthew 5:48 that tells us to be perfect even as our Father in heaven is perfect. However, this Scripture has nothing to do with your perfection in relationship to the totality of God's holiness; it is specific to having a nature like His in forgiveness. I could say it this way: be ye therefore perfect in forgiveness toward others even as your Father in heaven is perfect in His forgiveness toward you.

> **⁴⁴But I say unto you, Love your enemies, bless them that curse you, do good to them that hate you, and pray for them which despitefully use you, and persecute you; ⁴⁵That ye may be the children of your Father which is in heaven: for he maketh his sun to rise on the evil and on the good, and sendeth rain on the just and on the unjust. ⁴⁶For if ye love them which love you, what reward have ye? do not even the publicans the same? ⁴⁷And if ye salute your brethren only, what do ye more *than others?* do not even the publicans so? ⁴⁸Be ye therefore perfect, even as your Father which is in heaven is perfect. Matthew 5:44–48**

> **³⁶Be ye therefore merciful, as your Father also is merciful. ³⁷Judge not, and ye shall not be judged: condemn not, and ye shall not be condemned: forgive, and ye shall be forgiven: ³⁸Give, and it shall be given unto you; good measure, pressed down, and shaken together, and running over, shall men give into your bosom. For with the same measure that ye mete withal it shall be measured to you again. Luke 6:36–38**

Jesus is saying our forgiveness from God the Father is not a one-way street. Our forgiveness from God the Father begins vertically to the degree that we make it work horizontally. This Scripture in Mark 11:25–26 is one of the toughest Scriptures in the Bible because it says if you don't forgive your brother his trespass, your Father which is in heaven will not forgive you your trespasses.

> **²⁵And when ye stand praying, forgive, if ye have ought against any: that your Father also which is in heaven may forgive you your trespasses. ²⁶But if ye do not forgive, neither will your Father which is in heaven forgive your trespasses. Mark 11:25–26**

I have had many people come to me over the years in ministry who have gone to the altar every service, every week, every month, every year, yet still cannot get free of their bondage. I have talked to people who have fasted and prayed. They have begged God to be free of certain vices, certain bondages, certain things in their life and the harder they try, the more they pray, the more in bondage they find themselves. The skies of heaven seemed closed to their prayers.

When they came to me and indicated they had been begging God for something and it had not happened, the first thing I asked them was, "Who gives you this high octane ping in your spirit when you think about their name or when you face them? Who is it?"

I have found someone there without exception. The high octane ping goes off inside you when you think about someone in the past who has wronged you or hurt you and they may already be dead. You know how many people have unforgiveness against dead people? It is a tragedy!

How can you make it right with a dead person? How do you correct a wrong when the person is dead? You cannot. The same is true even about people who are alive when you do not know where they are. Sometimes this applies to people who refuse to interact with you about past wrongs.

I believe this is how God judges it: He judges it by your heart attitude toward it. If you have something from your past and it is not possible for you to personally make it right with the person, then sincerely make it right with God. It is taken care of; you do not have to carry the guilt about this issue any longer.

*The first block to receiving from God is you are going to have to make peace in your heart with every person you have ever known and get it resolved before God.* This does not mean you have to make peace with them personally if they are not available. It does mean you have to get it right with God concerning them.

The Word of God says those sins you retain are retained and those sins you remit are remitted.

> **Whose soever sins ye remit, they are remitted unto them; *and* whose soever *sins* ye retain, they are retained. John 20:23**

I would say to you very carefully and very strongly: make sure in your Christian experience that you are a *remitter* of sins. This will make you perfect like your Father Who is in heaven (Matthew 5:48).

*Forgiveness is an attitude of your heart toward others in love.* The biggest problem we have in the area of forgiveness is when someone has sinned against us, we also make the sin equal to them. We have a perfect hatred for the sin and we have a perfect hatred for them in the sin.

You see, what you have to do is separate the person from their sin as God separated you from your sin when He saved you. When God saved you, He separated you from your sin in His heart. He sees the sin, but He sees you without it. He is able to separate you from your sin. He has loved you from the foundation of the world.

> **[3]Blessed *be* the God and Father of our Lord Jesus Christ, who hath blessed us with all spiritual blessings in heavenly *places* in Christ:**
> **[4]According as he hath chosen us in him before the foundation of the**

world, that we should be holy and without blame before him in love:
⁵Having predestinated us unto the adoption of children by Jesus Christ to
himself, according to the good pleasure of his will, ⁶To the praise of the
glory of his grace, wherein he hath made us accepted in the beloved.
**Ephesians 1:3–6**

We need to have faith and expectation of who we are in the Father
because of Christ.

You don't forgive people who have wronged you because you feel like
it; you need to forgive them because you are obedient to Christ and His
commandments. You don't do it from an intellectual standpoint. You don't do
it because it is a law. You need to do it because it is just the way you are. If
you are just a lovebug who will forgive all manner of sin, then you are just
like your Daddy, your Father in heaven.

You can do this because you are all indwelled by the Spirit of God and
the Spirit of God gives you the ability to think like your Father, act like your
Father, talk like your Father and forgive like your Father, whether you feel
like it or not. I promise you: God forgives whether He feels like it or not. Are
you with me? *In the area of forgiveness, it is an attitude of the heart, not a
ritual of performance.*

Unforgiveness has to be dealt with. You are either a remitter of sin or a
retainer of sin. I made up my mind: in my life I am going to forgive all
manner of sin to all men.

## ☐ 2. Ignorance or Lack of Knowledge

Ignorance or *lack of knowledge*, the second block to healing, can be
found in Isaiah 5:13–14 and Hosea 4:6. In Isaiah, we read God's people had
gone into captivity because they had no knowledge.

> ¹³**Therefore my people are gone into captivity, because** *they have* **no
> knowledge: and their honourable men** *are* **famished, and their multitude
> dried up with thirst.** ¹⁴**Therefore hell hath enlarged herself, and opened
> her mouth without measure: and their glory, and their multitude, and
> their pomp, and he that rejoiceth, shall descend into it. Isaiah 5:13–14**

Hosea said,

> ⁶**My people are destroyed for lack of knowledge: because thou hast
> rejected knowledge, I will also reject thee, that thou shalt be no priest to
> me: seeing thou hast forgotten the law of thy God, I will also forget thy
> children.** ⁷**As they were increased, so they sinned against me:** *therefore* **will
> I change their glory into shame. Hosea 4:6–7**

One day, I was dead in my trespass and sin and it was ignorance, but in
*my* thinking, it was correct knowledge. **Ignorance is a form of knowledge.**
People who are ignorant don't know they are ignorant. The beginning of all

wisdom begins with knowledge. You cannot have wisdom unless you first have knowledge. You cannot have wisdom if you don't preface it with knowledge. Knowledge apart from wisdom is foolishness. It is vanity and it is humanistic in nature.

> The fear of the LORD *is* the beginning of knowledge: *but* fools despise wisdom and instruction. Proverbs 1:7

> The fear of the LORD *is* the beginning of wisdom: and the knowledge of the holy *is* understanding. Proverbs 9:10

How many of us have found ourselves ignorant in our lifetime and we still are in many areas? The Bible says very clearly that we still see through a glass darkly, but when that which is perfect has come, that which is in part shall be done away with, He shall be known and we shall be known. We shall see Him as He is.

> For now we see through a glass, darkly; but then face to face: now I know in part; but then shall I know even as also I am known. 1 Corinthians 13:12

Knowledge ties the past to the present and wisdom ties the present to the future. God wants you to understand your past, your present and your future. This is why teaching on spiritual roots of disease and blocks to healing is so important. It gives you knowledge, understanding and discernment so the wisdom of God for your future can include healing and prevention of disease. **This is *a more excellent way*™.**

## □ 3. No Relationship with God According to Knowledge

The third block to healing is *no relationship with God according to knowledge.* In Mark 7:24–30, we see a difference between lack of knowledge and no relationship with God according to knowledge. They seem to be similar, but they are different. Many times we come to a place in our relationship with God where we are not meeting Him according to Scripture.

> ²⁴And from thence he arose, and went into the borders of Tyre and Sidon, and entered into an house, and would have no man know *it:* but he could not be hid. ²⁵For a *certain* woman, whose young daughter had an unclean spirit, heard of him, and came and fell at his feet: ²⁶The woman was a Greek, a Syrophenician by nation; and she besought him that he would cast forth the devil out of her daughter. ²⁷But Jesus said unto her, Let the children first be filled: for it is not meet to take the children's bread, and to cast *it* unto the dogs. ²⁸And she answered and said unto him, Yes, Lord: yet the dogs under the table eat of the children's crumbs. ²⁹And he said unto her, For this saying go thy way; the devil is gone out of thy daughter. ³⁰And when she was come to her house, she found the devil gone out, and her daughter laid upon the bed. Mark 7:24–30

Do you remember when Jesus was ministering on the border of Tyre and Sidon and He came across a certain woman whose young daughter had an unclean spirit? She had heard of Him and came and fell at his feet. The woman was a Greek who had looked for Him so He would cast a devil out of her daughter. But Jesus said unto her, "Let the children first be filled: for it is not meet to take the children's bread, and to cast it unto the dogs" (Mark 7:27). What Jesus was saying to her was: you do not qualify, you are not in covenant, you are not with God according to knowledge, you are outside and you are separated from God. You are asking for something not belonging to you.

In Mark 7:28, she answered Him, "Yes, Lord: yet the dogs under the table eat of the children's crumbs." He said unto her, "For this saying go thy way; the devil is gone out of thy daughter." When she came to her house, she found the devil was gone and her daughter laid upon the bed.

I struggle sometimes with people who are unsaved, yet they want God to heal them. For many years, 40 percent of those we minister to nationally was unchurched and unsaved. People are coming from all over America; many of them are unchurched and unsaved or from New Age and false religions. They ask us, "Will God heal me if I don't accept Him? Do I have to accept Jesus in order to be healed?"

We tell them, "No, you can be healed without being in covenant," because we see this scripturally. You can be healed when you are not in covenant, but if you are healed outside of covenant, it would behoove you to get into covenant quickly because He who has healed you is He whom you should follow the rest of your days. This is our position. After they are healed, they are grateful and they do come to the saving knowledge of the Lord. This is wonderful! God has healed people in our ministry, even though they weren't born again.

I don't know where you are theologically, but I do know they are not going to die first and be born again last. We try to get them healed and born again first, before they die. If they die, we can never get them saved. There is no provision for getting saved after death. There is no stopping-off point or reincarnation facility. It is appointed unto men to die and then judgment.

> **And as it is appointed unto men once to die, but after this the judgment: Hebrews 9:27**

Sometimes people don't receive from God because they do not have a relationship with God according to knowledge. In Mark 7:6, Jesus answered and said unto them: Well hath Isaiah prophesied of you saying that you honor Him with your lips, but your heart is far from Him.

> **Wherefore the Lord said, Forasmuch as this people draw near *me* with their mouth, and with their lips do honour me, but have removed their heart far from me, and their fear toward me is taught by the precept of men: Isaiah 29:13**

> He answered and said unto them, Well hath Esaias prophesied of you hypocrites, as it is written, This people honoureth me with *their* lips, but their heart is far from me. Mark 7:6

It also says in Hebrews 11:6 you must believe God is and that He is a rewarder of them that diligently seek Him.

> But without faith *it is* impossible to please *him:* for he that cometh to God must believe that he is, and *that* he is a rewarder of them that diligently seek him. Hebrews 11:6

If you want to make God a slot machine, it is not going to work. Do you remember the Scripture where the Bible says that sometimes we pray and God doesn't hear?

> Ye ask, and receive not, because ye ask amiss, that ye may consume *it* upon your lusts. James 4:3

This really is referring to a prayer of vanity. So we learn when we are praying prayers of vanity that God is not interested in honoring them. God is not interested in answering fraudulent prayers.

The way I see it, according to knowledge, is to seek after God and pursue relationships. The first phase of relationship is fellowship with our Creator. Fellowship involves talking to God. Going to church and reading the Bible does not guarantee fellowship and relationship. Relationship involves going to church and Bible reading, but it also involves conversation with God, conversation with God about the desires, plans and purposes of His heart, not just your heart. If I read the Bible correctly (I could be wrong—I don't have all the answers), the first thing to come is fellowship with our Creator. This is the way I see it.

Draw nigh to God and He will draw nigh to you.

> Draw nigh to God, and he will draw nigh to you. Cleanse *your* hands, *ye* sinners; and purify *your* hearts, *ye* double minded. James 4:8

Seek ye first the kingdom of God and His righteousness.

> But seek ye first the kingdom of God, and his righteousness; and all these things shall be added unto you. Matthew 6:33

The next thing coming after *fellowship* is *worship*, because when you are in fellowship, then you will be in worship. Then, finally and lastly, comes the *petition*. If you come to petition first and you have not already come to fellowship and to worship, then your petition is fraudulent. It is not according to knowledge. Are you with me? Many people begin with God, petitioning first; then they don't understand why their prayers are not answered.

You have to reverse the order. You have to go back to fellowship first and don't skip worship. Then petition is always last. What *you* want is last.

The first thing you have to do is approach God because of *Who* He is…and what He has done for you from the foundation of the world, whether He gives you anything or not.

> **But the hour cometh, and now is, when the true worshippers shall worship the Father in spirit and in truth: for the Father seeketh such to worship him. John 4:23**

The gift of salvation is enough. The rest of it is just icing on the cake, but the foundation is salvation. Rejoice not that the spirits are subject unto you, but rather rejoice because your names are written in heaven:

> **Notwithstanding in this rejoice not, that the spirits are subject unto you; but rather rejoice, because your names are written in heaven. Luke 10:20**

I find many people coming to this ministry from all over America wanting to get well from psychological and biological diseases, but they do not want my Boss (God). They do not want my Father. They do not want the Holy Spirit, who would seal them and do the work to begin with. They just want the "fix."

Well, they are really in for a rude awakening because what they get from me first is that I take them to fellowship. They want me to go to petition. I go to fellowship and they gnash their teeth. They're trying to get the fix without the fellowship. It will never happen. *A hindrance to our healing, sometimes, is the attitude of our heart.*

Sometimes, part of this *"no relationship with God according to knowledge"* is that we are approaching God, not with what the Word has said about it, but by what some religion or man has said we should do to get it. So if you are going to approach God, it is not from what some man teaches you; it has to be on the basis of what you can prove in Scripture.

I don't believe there is any canon available to us that cannot be found already written. I am not into advanced revelation that cannot be supported by Scripture already written. I have taken a firm stand on this as a believer.

I say it this way: when you have mastered the Bible from Genesis to Revelation, then bring me your new esoteric knowledge and maybe I'll listen. But I haven't found anyone yet who has mastered Scripture from Genesis to Revelation in its entirety. Maybe you have, but I haven't.

Every time I think I understand the Word, I go to read it some more and see something new in there I did not see before. Did you ever have this happen to you? I thought I had just mastered this thing; I went back, reread it again and it was fresh all over again. A whole new understanding opened up to me. Oh, it is a wonderful thing to read the Word!

Now we have dealt with the fact that sometimes people want something from God, but they are not in covenant. At the same time, we must always make provision for people who are not in covenant. They came to Jesus, not because they wanted to be in covenant, not because they wanted to repent and be baptized, but they came to Jesus because they were sick. Then, He taught the gospel. He never healed and He never delivered until He first preached the gospel. Read it in Matthew, Mark, Luke and John. He preached first and healed second.

So the first thing we do is teach the ways of God. In the meantime, if people come because they want to get healed and Jesus heals them, it is great.

In Scripture, after Jesus healed, they followed Him. He was always telling people, "Follow Me." Paul said, "Follow me as I follow Christ."

> **14I write not these things to shame you, but as my beloved sons I warn you. 15For though ye have ten thousand instructers in Christ, yet *have ye* not many fathers: for in Christ Jesus I have begotten you through the gospel. 16Wherefore I beseech you, be ye followers of me. 1 Corinthians 4:14–16**

> **Be ye followers of me, even as I also *am* of Christ. 1 Corinthians 11:1**

I say to you, follow Henry as he follows Christ.

## ☐ 4. Personal and Family Sins

The fourth block to healing relates to *personal and family sins*. Isaiah 59 tells us that the LORD's hand is not so short that it cannot save; neither is His ear so dull that it cannot hear. But your iniquities have made a separation between you and your God and your sins have hid His face from you that He will not hear.

> **1Behold, the LORD'S hand is not shortened, that it cannot save; neither his ear heavy, that it cannot hear: 2But your iniquities have separated between you and your God, and your sins have hid *his* face from you, that he will not hear. Isaiah 59:1–2**

Isaiah 59:1–2 says that our sins can separate us from our God. Not only can our sins separate us from our God, but also the consequence of our ancestors' sins can transfer into us. We have evidence of this through genetically inherited disease.

Not only do we have genetically inherited disease, but the psychiatric industry over the years has determined that certain non-genetic factors such as disposition, personality quirks and idiosyncrasies can also be passed down through family trees without a genetic component being seen or known. These are iniquities.

In Exodus 20:5, it says that the sins of the fathers shall be passed on to the children, on down to the third and fourth generations. We also read this in Deuteronomy, so we have a confirmation of this in two different verses of the Bible.

> **Thou shalt not bow down thyself to them, nor serve them: for I the LORD thy God *am* a jealous God, visiting the iniquity of the fathers upon the children unto the third and fourth *generation* of them that hate me; Exodus 20:5**

> **Thou shalt not bow down thyself unto them, nor serve them: for I the LORD thy God *am* a jealous God, visiting the iniquity of the fathers upon the children unto the third and fourth *generation* of them that hate me, Deuteronomy 5:9**

In Nehemiah chapters 8 and 9, Ezra the scribe/priest called all the people together—the mommies and the daddies and their children. It was one of the longest church services in the history of the Bible—it was twelve hours. For six hours, they stood and heard the Word of God. The next six hours they worshipped and confessed their sins and the sins of their fathers before God.

> **²And Ezra the priest brought the law before the congregation both of men and women, and all that could hear with understanding, upon the first day of the seventh month. ³And he read therein before the street that *was* before the water gate from the morning until midday, before the men and the women, and those that could understand; and the ears of all the people *were attentive* unto the book of the law…⁶And Ezra blessed the LORD, the great God. And all the people answered, Amen, Amen, with lifting up their hands: and they bowed their heads, and worshipped the LORD with *their* faces to the ground…⁸So they read in the book in the law of God distinctly, and gave the sense, and caused *them* to understand the reading. Nehemiah 8:2–3, 6, 8**

> **⁹:¹Now in the twenty and fourth day of this month the children of Israel were assembled with fasting, and with sackclothes, and earth upon them. ²And the seed of Israel separated themselves from all strangers, and stood and confessed their sins, and the iniquities of their fathers. Nehemiah 9:1–2**

In Nehemiah 9:2, it says they stood there and confessed their sins and the sins of their fathers. Why? So they could be freed from the curse of sin generationally.

God holds the fathers responsible for the spirituality of the family. The sins of the fathers are passed on to the third and fourth generations of them that hate Me…

> **…for I the LORD thy God *am* a jealous God, visiting the iniquity of the fathers upon the children unto the third and fourth *generation* of them that hate me; Exodus 20:5**

...but blessings to thousands who love God and keep His commandments. Thousands of what? Thousands of generations.

> **And shewing mercy unto thousands of them that love me, and keep my commandments. Exodus 20:6**

Not only do we have this knowledge in Exodus and Deuteronomy, but we also have it in Nehemiah. We also see the evidence today that the curse of the fathers is still here. So we not only have to consider personal sins separating us from our God, we have to consider inherited family tree sins.

It is amazing to me to see the rollover and the similarity between generations and the bondages and the diseases following down family trees, including insanity, including personality characteristics and all the rest. In fact, when people come to me for the first time for ministry, I sit down and just listen to their personal case history for about ten minutes. I can usually tell them (I don't know the people's names, I don't know their lifestyle or where they work) their spiritual dynamics back four generations of the family. Often, I can tell them about their mother, their father, their grandmother, their grandfather and all the spiritual problems they've had. I am usually correct.

How do I know this? Is it some kind of esoteric knowledge? No, this is by pragmatic observation of the family tree and also by what the Word has to say about generational curses flowing from family to family.

## ☐ 5. Not Having Faith in God

The fifth block to healing can be found in Mark 11: *not having faith in God.* In Mark 11:22, Jesus told His disciples to have faith in God.

> **And Jesus answering saith unto them, Have faith in God. Mark 11:22**

The Bible also says without faith, it is impossible to please God.

> **But without faith *it is* impossible to please *him:* for he that cometh to God must believe that he is, and *that* he is a rewarder of them that diligently seek him. Hebrews 11:6**

Hebrews 11:1 says faith is the substance of things hoped for, the evidence of things not seen.

> **Now faith is the substance of things hoped for, the evidence of things not seen. Hebrews 11:1**

Matthew 21:21 says if you have faith and not doubt.

> **Jesus answered and said unto them, Verily I say unto you, If ye have faith, and doubt not.... Matthew 21:21**

Hebrews 4 says the children of Israel, coming out of Egypt under the leadership of Moses and Aaron, did not enter into promise, yet the same gospel preached to them was preached to us; preached to us and preached to them, but they did not enter into promise because of unbelief and doubt.

> **²For unto us was the gospel preached, as well as unto them: but the word preached did not profit them, not being mixed with faith in them that heard it...⁶Seeing therefore it remaineth that some must enter therein, and they to whom it was first preached entered not in because of unbelief: Hebrews 4:2, 6**

When Jesus went back to His hometown of Nazareth, preached and tried to help the poor folk He grew up with, Scripture says He did no great miracles in Nazareth because their unbelief and doubt was great.

> **⁵And he could there do no mighty work, save that he laid his hands upon a few sick folk, and healed *them*. ⁶And he marvelled because of their unbelief. And he went round about the villages, teaching. Mark 6:5–6**

In Mark 5:36–42, Jesus was about to raise a young lady from the dead and there were a lot of people around because she had died. They were ready to have a wake and He walked in and said, "But she's just sleeping." They laughed at Him and scorned Him. He put them out of the room, brought the family and His disciples into the room and He raised her from the dead.

> **³⁶As soon as Jesus heard the word that was spoken, he saith unto the ruler of the synagogue, Be not afraid, only believe. ³⁷And he suffered no man to follow him, save Peter, and James, and John the brother of James. ³⁸And he cometh to the house of the ruler of the synagogue, and seeth the tumult, and them that wept and wailed greatly. ³⁹And when he was come in, he saith unto them, Why make ye this ado, and weep? the damsel is not dead, but sleepeth. ⁴⁰And they laughed him to scorn. But when he had put them all out, he taketh the father and the mother of the damsel, and them that were with him, and entereth in where the damsel was lying. ⁴¹And he took the damsel by the hand, and said unto her, Talitha cumi; which is, being interpreted, Damsel, I say unto thee, arise. ⁴²And straightway the damsel arose, and walked; for she was *of the age* of twelve years. And they were astonished with a great astonishment. Mark 5:36–42**

Why did He put them out of the room? Because their unbelief and doubt would negate His power and ability to heal.

Do you have hearts of belief, or am I casting seed on the stony, rocky ground? If I am casting seed on good, fertile ground, then your faith is drawing my faith into a crescendo to move the hand of God.

If there is unbelief and doubt in your hearts coming at me, I would stagger under it and I could do only a few things for you. As we mix our faith together before God as we come here trusting Him to honor us, trusting Him to convict us and trusting Him to work with us, I am asking Him, in faith, to come to us.

> **I tell you that he will avenge them speedily. Nevertheless when the Son of man cometh, shall he find faith on the earth? Luke 18:8**

## ☐ 6. The Need to See a Miracle

The sixth block to healing is your *believing you need to see a miracle in order to receive from God.* Do you know how many people won't believe until they've seen a miracle? Well, what happened to the first person who saw a miracle? Who did they look back at?

There were two thieves on the cross in Matthew 27:38–44: those that passed by reviled Him, wagging their heads and saying, Thou that destroyest the temple and buildest it in three days, save Thyself. If Thou be the Son of God, come down from the cross.

> ³⁸**Then were there two thieves crucified with him, one on the right hand, and another on the left. ³⁹And they that passed by reviled him, wagging their heads, ⁴⁰And saying, Thou that destroyest the temple, and buildest *it* in three days, save thyself. If thou be the Son of God, come down from the cross. ⁴¹Likewise also the chief priests mocking *him,* with the scribes and elders, said, ⁴²He saved others; himself he cannot save. If he be the King of Israel, let him now come down from the cross, and we will believe him. ⁴³He trusted in God; let him deliver him now, if he will have him: for he said, I am the Son of God. ⁴⁴The thieves also, which were crucified with him, cast the same in his teeth. Matthew 27:38–44**

What did they want to see before they would believe? They wanted to see Jesus come off the cross, but it would have been the worst thing He ever did. You and I would not be here today if He had done that. You know what Jesus said to Peter when He was preparing the disciples for His crucifixion: He said He would be going to Jerusalem and He would be betrayed and be crucified. So Peter rebuked Him. Remember this? Peter rebuked Jesus and kind of told Him off. Jesus turned to him and told him what? Get behind Me, Satan. Thou savorest the things of men and not the things of God.

> **But when he had turned about and looked on his disciples, he rebuked Peter, saying, Get thee behind me, Satan: for thou savourest not the things that be of God, but the things that be of men. Mark 8:33**

Well, do we have to see a miracle in order to believe we can receive a miracle? The chief priest in verse 41 and 42 echoed the same thing (Matthew 27:41–42): "Likewise also the chief priests mocking Him, with the scribes and elders, said, He saved others; Himself He cannot save. If He be the King of Israel, let Him now come down from the cross and *we will believe Him.*"

> [41]Likewise also the chief priests mocking *him,* with the scribes and elders, said, [42]He saved others; himself he cannot save. If he be the King of Israel, let him now come down from the cross, and we will believe him. Matthew 27:41–42

Wow! "We will believe Him." Two classes of people would not believe until they could see some proof. Well, Jesus dealt with this issue with Thomas. Thomas said he would not believe until he what? Until he saw the scars. So Jesus showed him the scars in His hands and in His side. Then Thomas said, My Lord and My God, and Jesus said, Blessed are those who do not see and yet believe rather than those who believe because they see.

> [28]And Thomas answered and said unto him, My Lord and my God. [29]Jesus saith unto him, Thomas, because thou hast seen me, thou hast believed: blessed *are* they that have not seen, and *yet* have believed. John 20:28–29

Another great area of investigation is having to see a miracle to believe God. Let's go to Matthew 4. I believe God heals and delivers today. Do you know how many people ask me to prove it? Lots! I have had people come to me and say, "Do this, do that, do this, do that."

I cannot do anything. I don't have any powers. I could not heal a fly with a toothache. I don't have any abilities. Who do you think I am? What are they doing? They are tempting me to tempt God. They come to me because they are sick, but in their hearts they are saying, "Henry, if thou be the anointed son of God, do something," and in their hearts they are also saying, "If you cannot, then you're not."

Let's see how Satan tempted our Lord Jesus in this area. Matthew 4:1–3 says Jesus was led up of the Spirit into the wilderness to be tempted of the devil. When He had fasted forty days and forty nights, He was afterward an hungered. And when the tempter came to Him, he said, *If Thou be the Son of God* command that these stones be made bread.

> [4:1]Then was Jesus led up of the Spirit into the wilderness to be tempted of the devil. [2]And when he had fasted forty days and forty nights, he was afterward an hungered. [3]And when the tempter came to him, he said, If thou be the Son of God, command that these stones be made bread. Matthew 4:1–3

Do you know what people say to me? "If thou be anointed then do something." *This is a hindrance to healing because you are NOT to look to me.* You are to look to Him, to the sanctifying work of the Holy Spirit and to the Word of God. All I am is His slave, His servant.

If you are looking at me and do not see Him behind me, or the sanctifying work of the Word behind me, or the love and purpose of the

Father behind me, if I do not become invisible so all you see is Him, then you have a block.

So here we see the temptation of Jesus: *"Do something."* How many of us have asked God? How many of us have put up fleeces? God, if you will do this, then I'll believe You. Why don't we just believe Him to begin with? If He wanted to do it for us, He would anyway. He would come to us and deal with us.

## ☐ 7. Looking for Signs and Wonders

A seventh block to healing from God is *looking for signs and wonders*. People are chasing signs and wonders rather than seeking the Word of God. I believe in signs and wonders, but I don't go chasing signs and wonders. I hope you don't, either, but signs and wonders do follow those who believe. There is a difference between chasing signs and wonders and having signs and wonders follow you.

The issue is a matter of perspective. We must seek God and His Word, not the signs and wonders as the foundation of our faith. Disease is a fruit of the separation from God in some area of your life. The key is faith in God and His Word on the basis of relationship, not on the basis of signs and manifestations.

Romans 10:17 says that faith comes by hearing and hearing by the Word of God.

> **So then faith *cometh* by hearing, and hearing by the word of God. Romans 10:17**

Some people are looking for signs rather than the Word of God. John 4:46–48 says, So Jesus came again into Cana of Galilee where He made the water wine. And there was a certain nobleman whose son was sick at Capernaum. When he heard that Jesus was come out of Judea into Galilee, he went unto Him and besought Him that He would come down and heal his son, for he was at the point of death. Then said Jesus unto him, Except ye see signs and wonders, ye will not believe.

> [46]**So Jesus came again into Cana of Galilee, where he made the water wine. And there was a certain nobleman, whose son was sick at Capernaum.** [47]**When he heard that Jesus was come out of Judaea into Galilee, he went unto him, and besought him that he would come down, and heal his son: for he was at the point of death.** [48]**Then said Jesus unto him, Except ye see signs and wonders, ye will not believe. John 4:46–48**

Matthew 12:38–39 is another Scripture about an evil and an adulterous generation looking after a sign.

**38Then certain of the scribes and of the Pharisees answered, saying, Master, we would see a sign from thee. 39But he answered and said unto them, An evil and adulterous generation seeketh after a sign; and there shall no sign be given to it, but the sign of the prophet Jonas: Matthew 12:38–39**

The issue is that we are not seeking something like healing from God first—we are seeking God first. Disease is a fruit of the separation.

## ☐ 8. Expect God to Heal on One's Own Terms

The eighth block to healing can be found in 2 Kings 5:8–14. Some people *expect God to heal them on their own terms*. They tell God exactly what He is going to do, when He is going to do it and how He is going to do it. Then they expect Him to do it just this way on the terms they have set forth.

Second Kings 5:8–14 tells the story of Naaman, who had leprosy. I want to say something to you: this was a real important individual. Naaman was the captain of the host of the king of Syria. He was a great and honorable man, valued by his master. He had leprosy. He came a great distance to find this man of God who (he had heard) could heal him or fix him and get him right.

Now the real kicker of this story is when Elisha did not go meet him at all. He sent his servant. This takes care of idolatry, doesn't it? You know, you have to be careful that you don't make your spiritual leaders into icons. You have to be careful you don't make those who rule over you greater than they really are. I am not greater than you. I am a sheep just like you. I am not greater than you. God doesn't love me more than He loves you. I don't have more of an edge with God than you do; He is no respecter of persons.

**Then Peter opened *his* mouth, and said, Of a truth I perceive that God is no respecter of persons: Acts 10:34**

What He has done for one, He will do for another. In my experience as a pastor, I am one among equals. I am just like you. I am not greater than you—I am with you. My only problem is this: I will get judged with a double judgment one day and you won't. Scripture also says that I'll get double honor, but I'll wait and see about that.

**Let the elders that rule well be counted worthy of double honour, especially they who labour in the word and doctrine. 1 Timothy 5:17**

It is the double judgment that bothers me.

**My brethren, be not many masters, knowing that we shall receive the greater condemnation. James 3:1**

You know I have to stand before God one day in an area you don't even have to. I have to give an account to God of how I conducted myself with the souls of men. I take this very seriously. I might have a little fun once in a while just to kind of lighten it up a little, but I consider this very serious business. My Boss is listening and watching every move I make.

In 2 Kings 5:10–12, Elisha sent a messenger unto him saying, "Go and wash in the Jordan seven times and thy flesh shall come again to thee and thou shalt be clean." But Naaman was wroth and went away and said, "Behold, I thought, He will surely come out to me"—there you go: there is that pride—"and stand and call on the name of the LORD his God and strike his hand over the place and recover the leper" (Naaman).

> ¹⁰And Elisha sent a messenger unto him, saying, Go and wash in the Jordan seven times, and thy flesh shall come again to thee, and thou shalt be clean. ¹¹But Naaman was wroth, and went away, and said, Behold, I thought, He will surely come out to me, and stand, and call on the name of the LORD his God, and strike his hand over the place, and recover the leper. ¹²*Are* not Abana and Pharpar, rivers of Damascus, better than all the waters of Israel? may I not wash in them, and be clean? So he turned and went away in a rage. 2 Kings 5:10–12

Well, Naaman figured out how it was going to be. But what did Elisha tell the messenger to say? Go down to the river and wash seven times. What? You don't know who you are talking to. You don't know who I am. I want *you* to come out here, Elisha, call unto your God in heaven, strike your hand over the place and cause a miracle so I can go home and rejoice!

So our subject is this: sometimes we expect God to heal us on our own terms in the way we think it should go. Well, do you think Naaman had a spiritual problem? Can you think of a spiritual root? Pride!

So he turned and went away in a rage. What was his next spiritual problem? Bitterness, resentment, unforgiveness, rage, anger. This is a good place to start receiving from God, isn't it? Verse 13 says his servants came near and asked him, "My father, if the prophet had bid thee to do a great thing, would thou not have done it?"

> And his servants came near, and spake unto him, and said, My father, *if* the prophet had bid thee *do some* great thing, wouldest thou not have done *it*? how much rather then, when he saith to thee, Wash, and be clean? 2 Kings 5:13

So who had the wisdom for the matter? His servants! He went down and dipped himself seven times in the Jordan, according to the saying of the man of God and his flesh came again like unto the flesh of a little child and he was clean.

> Then went he down, and dipped himself seven times in Jordan, according to the saying of the man of God: and his flesh came again like unto the flesh of a little child, and he was clean. 2 Kings 5:14

Well, this is God dealing with a Gentile again. Do you think God loves those unsaved Gentile sinners? You say, "Well, it looks like He loves the unsaved Gentile more than me. I've been a saint for 48 years and I'm still waiting for my healing!" Watch it now! Watch it now! *Sometimes we expect God to heal us on our own terms.*

## ☐ 9. Looking to Man Rather Than to God

The ninth block to healing is *looking to man.* We find this in Jeremiah 17:5. I want to say something to you very carefully. I am not against physicians. I am not against psychiatrists. However, we expect physicians to do something they are not qualified to do: heal us of spiritually rooted diseases. They are not qualified to heal you of spiritually rooted diseases because, first of all, you have to be born again to do it. Second, as far as I can tell from Scripture, you have to be a spiritual leader to set it in motion.

Once again, I am not against physicians. I am not against psychiatrists. Don't you think for a minute that because I am in the healing business I automatically do away with the doctors and physicians. What I do have to say to you is this: the Church has negated its role in the healing of disease. It has asked doctors to become spiritual healers and they are not qualified to do it. They are not listed in the fivefold ministry giftings of Ephesians 4. They are not qualified to heal you of spiritually rooted diseases. This has been ordained by God to be the role of the Church with the body healing the body as set forth in 1 Corinthians 12.

Doctors have their place, but in the area of spiritually rooted disease, they will not be able to bring forth the healing. The best they have to offer in these cases is disease management. I do not have a problem with your going and checking out your life. I am all for your getting a diagnosis. I don't play games with people's lives. I have to meet people in their faith and also in their faithlessness. What we need are doctors who understand there are spiritual components to disease and who will work with those who also understand the role of the Church in the healing of disease.

The point we are making is that looking to man—to doctors—for the healing *before* seeking God and *without giving consideration* to the spiritual dynamics behind the curse of disease is a block to healing.

Jeremiah 17 says, Thus saith the LORD; Cursed be the man that trusteth in man and maketh flesh his arm and whose heart departeth from the LORD. Blessed is the man that trusteth in the LORD and whose hope the LORD is. The heart is deceitful above all things and desperately wicked: Who can know it? I, the LORD, search the heart, I try the reins, even to give every man according to his ways and according to the fruit of his doings.

> ⁵Thus saith the LORD; Cursed be the man that trusteth in man, and maketh flesh his arm, and whose heart departeth from the LORD...⁷Blessed *is* the man that trusteth in the LORD, and whose hope the LORD is...⁹The heart *is* deceitful above all *things,* and desperately wicked: who can know it? ¹⁰I the LORD search the heart, *I* try the reins, even to give every man according to his ways, *and* according to the fruit of his doings. Jeremiah 17:5, 7, 9–10

One of the great blocks to healing from God is to look to man to be your source. I am not your source. I am a road sign along the highway, pointing out the way you should go.

I remember a joke I heard one time. I am from Northern Maine; I was born and raised there, way up in Aroostook County where they grow potatoes. Down south, they have the "downeasters," and "ya know they talk kinda funny." They're a strange crew, those downeasters, down around Cherryfield and Machias and places like that. They told me a story one time about one of those city slickers from Boston who came up riding through Maine and got to looking at stuff out there in the middle of nowhere, outside of Cherryfield. He came to a four-way crossroads, where there were no signs. There was a house with an old guy sitting there, kind of rocking in his chair, surveying the situation.

The city slicker got out and walked up and said, "How are you doing, sir?"

The old guy said, "Howdy."

Then he said, "I'm trying to get to Augusta. Can I take this road?"

The old man looked over and said, "Yeah, yeah, I suppose you would get there eventually."

And he said, "Well, how about that road over there?"

"Yeah, yeah, I've been that way a couple of times and that'll eventually get you there."

"Well, how about this road over here?"

"Well, I've never been down that road too far, but they tell me down that road you can get to Augusta, too."

Well, by this time the city slicker had enough and he said, "You don't know much, do ya?"

The old guy said, "Yeah, maybe so, but then again I'm not lost either!"

So sometimes I could be a road sign for you: this is the way you should go, but I am not your source. I am just your friend. A lover of your soul. A lover of your life. Do not look to me, because if you look to me, you need to understand that I am looking to somebody else: my Boss—Jesus Christ—and the Father who sent Him.

Second Chronicles 16:7–12 contains the story of Asa. Very clearly, it says that he died. One of the reasons he died was because he did not seek the LORD first, not only in war, but also in his personal life when God had already proven Himself to be on his side in previous wars. His heart had hardened in his apostasy and in his darkness and disease it was unto death, **Asa sought first not to the LORD but to physicians.**

> **⁷And at that time Hanani the seer came to Asa king of Judah, and said unto him, Because thou hast relied on the king of Syria, and not relied on the LORD thy God, therefore is the host of the king of Syria escaped out of thine hand. ⁸Were not the Ethiopians and the Lubims a huge host, with very many chariots and horsemen? yet, because thou didst rely on the LORD, he delivered them into thine hand. ⁹For the eyes of the LORD run to and fro throughout the whole earth, to shew himself strong in the behalf of *them* whose heart *is* perfect toward him. Herein thou hast done foolishly: therefore from henceforth thou shalt have wars. ¹⁰Then Asa was wroth with the seer, and put him in a prison house; for *he was* in a rage with him because of this *thing*. And Asa oppressed *some* of the people the same time. ¹¹And, behold, the acts of Asa, first and last, lo, they *are* written in the book of the kings of Judah and Israel. ¹²And Asa in the thirty and ninth year of his reign was diseased in his feet, until his disease *was* exceeding *great:* yet in his disease he sought not to the LORD, but to the physicians. 2 Chronicles 16:7–12**

Wow! Let me say this to you again: I am not against physicians. I do not have a problem with your getting a diagnosis. So I do not have a problem with your going and checking out your life. I do not play games with people's lives. I have to meet people in their faith, but I also have to meet them in their faithlessness. In other words, I am not sure where people are with God at any given moment in their life.

Why don't you take time out and seek the Lord first? Why don't we take time and go to the Lord? I want to say this to you: sometimes our diseases are unto death because we sought not the Lord first as His people. This is a hard word, isn't it? But it is a word I have to give you because Jeremiah 17:5 says, cursed be the man that trusteth in man.

> **Thus saith the LORD; Cursed be the man that trusteth in man, and maketh flesh his arm, and whose heart departeth from the LORD. Jeremiah 17:5**

Although this is a hard word, it is hard because the Church has failed in its mission at this level to represent God. The people have nowhere to turn except to man. Granted, many churches teach their people to believe in God, but they just do not understand disease and the cause for it, which is spiritually rooted in 80 percent of all cases.

## □ 10. Not Being Honest and Transparent

The tenth block to healing is *not being honest and transparent.*

Two big reasons for not being honest and transparent are fear and pride. You may ask, "What do you mean by fear?" The answer would be fear of rejection, fear of man, fear of failure, fear of abandonment and fear of not being loved. The pride issue is very dangerous because it makes you appear holy when you are not and you are stuck with a real problem. This is a fraudulent existence. In other words, you are living a lie. It is a high price to pay because pride produces a fall and much disease.

> **Pride *goeth* before destruction, and an haughty spirit before a fall.**
> **Proverbs 16:18**

Do you know how many people get nervous and jerky when I start probing into their personal life? What are they afraid of? God already knows. God knows everything. He knows you so well that the hairs of your head are numbered. He knows the secret thoughts of your heart. You ain't hiding nothing! Did you forget God sees you? He hears every word I am saying here. He knows my thoughts; He knows your thoughts.

James tells us to confess our faults one to another that we may be healed.

> **Confess *your* faults one to another, and pray one for another, that ye**
> **may be healed. The effectual fervent prayer of a righteous man availeth**
> **much. James 5:16**

Galatians 6:1 tells us if a brother is overtaken in a fault, those of you who *"consider yourself"* spiritual, restore such an one in a spirit of meekness and consider yourself also, lest you be tempted in like manner and fall away. Verse 2 says bear ye one another's burdens and so ye fulfil the law of Christ.

> **⁶:¹Brethren, if a man be overtaken in a fault, ye which are spiritual,**
> **restore such an one in the spirit of meekness; considering thyself, lest thou**
> **also be tempted. ²Bear ye one another's burdens, and so fulfil the law of**
> **Christ. Galatians 6:1–2**

It is a scary thing to be transparent these days. I don't know if I can trust my life with you. Can you trust your life with me? Some of you have and I thank you for your transparency. Why is it so important to be transparent and confess our sins to God and to each other? Proverbs 28:13 gives you a clue. If you cover your sins, you shall not prosper. But if you confess them and forsake them, you shall have mercy.

> **He that covereth his sins shall not prosper: but whoso confesseth and**
> **forsaketh *them* shall have mercy. Proverbs 28:13**

Isaiah said this about God: The high and lofty One, He that inhabits eternity dwelleth also with him that is of a humble and of a contrite heart.

> **For thus saith the high and lofty One that inhabiteth eternity, whose name *is* Holy; I dwell in the high and holy *place,* with him also *that is* of a contrite and humble spirit, to revive the spirit of the humble, and to revive the heart of the contrite ones. Isaiah 57:15**

### *Do you know where God is?*
### *Right there in your mess, transparent one!*

God can be found with a humble and a contrite heart. This made David a man after God's own heart, in spite of sin and in spite of inherited sin.

> **Behold, I was shapen in iniquity; and in sin did my mother conceive me. Psalm 51:5**

This is because he had a perfect hatred for evil in the end. When he was convicted, he repented and turned away from it (read Psalm 51:1–17—it is most beautiful). Sometimes I don't use the Romans Road to lead people to the Lord; I use Psalm 51. To me, this psalm is the best foundation for the sinner's prayer you can find. It just says it all. Then, in the end, David says, in essence, "And I will convert sinners." In other words, when he has finished repenting, he is out trying to get someone saved! I love this guy. When I get to heaven, I am going to find Paul and David and give them bear hugs and say, "I appreciate you guys." I am! They are fantastic!

> **51:1To the chief Musician, A Psalm of David, when Nathan the prophet came unto him, after he had gone in to Bathsheba. Have mercy upon me, O God, according to thy lovingkindness: according unto the multitude of thy tender mercies blot out my transgressions. 2Wash me throughly from mine iniquity, and cleanse me from my sin. 3For I acknowledge my transgressions: and my sin *is* ever before me. 4Against thee, thee only, have I sinned, and done *this* evil in thy sight: that thou mightest be justified when thou speakest, *and* be clear when thou judgest. 5Behold, I was shapen in iniquity; and in sin did my mother conceive me. 6Behold, thou desirest truth in the inward parts: and in the hidden *part* thou shalt make me to know wisdom. 7Purge me with hyssop, and I shall be clean: wash me, and I shall be whiter than snow. 8Make me to hear joy and gladness; *that* the bones *which* thou hast broken may rejoice. 9Hide thy face from my sins, and blot out all mine iniquities. 10Create in me a clean heart, O God; and renew a right spirit within me. 11Cast me not away from thy presence; and take not thy holy spirit from me. 12Restore unto me the joy of thy salvation; and uphold me *with thy* free spirit. 13Then will I teach transgressors thy ways; and sinners shall be converted unto thee. 14Deliver me from bloodguiltiness, O God, thou God of my salvation: *and* my tongue shall sing aloud of thy righteousness. 15O Lord, open thou my lips; and my mouth shall shew forth thy praise. 16For thou desirest not sacrifice; else would I give *it:* thou delightest not in burnt offering. 17The sacrifices of God *are* a broken spirit: a broken and a contrite heart, O God, thou wilt not despise. Psalm 51:1–17**

I want to give you a story to shock you a little bit. It has to do with being honest and transparent without regard to pride, which is what we are discussing in this block. I was doing a seminar in Houston, Texas, and teaching on these same matters. I had a mixed audience which included about 30 percent New Age persons. I was trying to "tiptoe through the tulips." I was trying to be "all things to all men" so I might win one or two to Christ in this seminar. About 30 minutes into it (and I am not being funny when I tell you this), a voice came thundering into my head saying, "Henry, cut the crap and shut up!" I staggered. I said out loud to the audience, "Excuse me! I think God's talking to me!" In my heart, God said, "Listen, I called you here to represent Me, not to appease the devil. Get off this thing and do what I told you to do!"

I asked, "What did You tell me to do?" In the audience, the people were watching me; I was going back and forth—What? What? Then God spoke to my heart and said, "I want you to take yoga on for size." I said, "God, leave me alone! You don't know what You're asking me. Half of these people are into yoga, Eastern mysticism and meditation." Then in my heart God said, "Do what I tell you!"

I said, "God has said, I must deal with yoga." So as I started to reveal the foundation of kundalini and the divination principles of the Eastern mysticism of yoga, one-third of the audience got up and walked out. As I watched them go, I thought, "Oh, I must have heard the devil. I'm trying to save them, Lord." Then in my heart God said, "We have work to do!" Things changed in the seminar and the first night we went until one o'clock in the morning; the second night until four o'clock in the morning; the third night, two o'clock in the morning; the next Sunday went from nine in the morning until three in the afternoon. We had revival!

In the middle of this, as I was talking about yoga and explaining the fallacies of yoga, a woman got up in the audience. She was a very regal-looking woman who was Pakistani. She interrupted me and said, "I go to a Seventh Day Adventist church, but I practice yoga and Eastern mysticism with my husband. I am convicted." Then she started to confess. Well, she also had five diseases! She had diabetes; she had diseases in her feet; I don't remember all the things that she had, but she had five major diseases. She stood there and confessed, with tears running down her face, the sin of worshipping Satan through yoga. She stood there, humbling herself, this regal woman looking so majestic in her nationality, her pride, the way she carried herself and her stature. I was listening to her confess openly before a huge congregation and God spoke to me and said, "Because she has humbled herself before Me and before you and this congregation, I am going to deliver her and heal her."

I waited until she finished and when she had finished, I said, "Sister, God has spoken to me; He wants to deliver you and heal you. Would you come here?" So she walked to the front and I said, "You foul, unclean spirit of kundalini, of divination, come out of this woman in the name of Jesus Christ of Nazareth." That spirit of divination manifested in her and she told me later that it "wanted to tear you apart." But all she could do was just make a throat clearing/grunting noise and weakly pound her hands on my chest—and then it was gone!

God not only delivered her—He healed her of five "incurable" diseases! She came back to the next year's Houston seminar and gave her testimony. She is doing very well. She is getting on with God. She is free! Because she humbled herself and was transparent, God met her. Could it be that God stopped a service just to get and free one person He loved?

So, sometimes you just have to be transparent, don't you? I love it when people are honest with me. You do not have to worry about me condemning you. Who am I to condemn you? My rap sheet is probably longer than yours!

God hates pride, hypocrisy and fraud. But we are so afraid of each other and have been so murdered by each other that we cannot even trust each other anymore. This is in the Christian Church.

Perfect love covers a multitude of sins.

> **And above all things have fervent charity among yourselves: for charity shall cover the multitude of sins. 1 Peter 4:8**

> **There is no fear in love; but perfect love casteth out fear: because fear hath torment. He that feareth is not made perfect in love. 1 John 4:18**

Aren't you glad He is our Father? Amen!

## ☐ 11. Flagrant Sin or Habitual Sin

The eleventh block to healing is *flagrant sin or habitual sin.* Now there is a difference between temptation, falling into sin, then repenting and getting out of sin and living habitually in it. *Temptation is not sin.* Jesus was tempted in all points such as we are, yet without sin.

> **For we have not an high priest which cannot be touched with the feeling of our infirmities; but was in all points tempted like as *we are, yet* without sin. Hebrews 4:15**

So I know temptation is not sin. But in Galatians 5:19–21, in the great book against legalism and the great statement of grace and mercy, we find a real problem. It is right at the end of this great chapter of the book of Galatians, which Paul uses to defeat legalism and to establish our freedom from legalism. It says: Now the works of the flesh are manifest, which are these; Adultery, fornication, uncleanness, lasciviousness, idolatry, witchcraft [The word *witchcraft*, by the way, is not the word used in the Hebrew. The word *witchcraft* is found only one time in the New Testament and it is the Greek word *pharmakeia, Strong's #5331*, which means medication (pharmacy, sorcery). It is taken from the Greek root word *#5332, pharmakeus,* which means a drug, a druggist (pharmacist or poisoner, that is, sorcerer).], hatred, variance, emulations, wrath, strife, seditions, heresies, envying, murders, drunkenness, reveling and such like: of the which I tell you before, *as I have also told you in time past, they which do such things shall not inherit the kingdom of God* (Galatians 5:19–21).

This is pretty emphatic, isn't it? The only way we can survive and still maintain our freedom from legalism is to understand the context of God's grace and mercy. I believe I can quote Paul accurately, in light of the word study done on the word "do," which translates as: *those who habitually practice those things against God with a hardened heart as a way of life, they shall not inherit the kingdom of God.*

It is interesting to note in Galatians, the English word *do* has three different Greek root words and three different meanings. It is important to understand grace and mercy do not absolve us from responsibility for holiness.

> ¹**What shall we say then? Shall we continue in sin, that grace may abound? ²God forbid... Romans 6:1–2**

In some quarters, there are teachings removing responsibility for sin because of grace and mercy, but I will tell you, Church, that the wages of sin are still death.

> **For the wages of sin *is* death... Romans 6:23**

If there is any doubt in your mind about there being no consequences for sin in the New Covenant, *just look around at the psychological and biological diseases that have engulfed the Christian Church*, especially in light of Deuteronomy 28, which clearly states that all disease is a result of separation from God, His Word and disobedience to His Word.

Habitual, unrepented, flagrant sin is a major block to God healing you and meeting you in your life.

I have taken the position as a pastor—it may not be your position, but I am not your pastor so you don't have to believe a thing I say—I have taken the position in dealing with people that I can have one person over here doing this sin while another person over here is doing the same sin. One person is accepted before God in that sin and the other one over here is not accepted by

God in that sin. I have observed it. Please understand that God does not condone sin in our lives, but my point is that grace and mercy seem to be extended to one person and not the other. How can this be?

The person over here, who is not accepted before God—his heart is hardened toward God and he is just not going to change.

But the person over here who, because of temptation, has fallen into the sin—he still has a perfect hatred for it; his heart is right before God against the sin even though he is still in bondage. God is dealing with this person and working him over. God does not condone sin, but He has made a provision for it and a way out of the penalty because of it.

Are you with me? It is not the sin. It is your attitude of the heart toward the sin God is looking at. But if you are into flagrant sin and your heart is hardened, then it keeps the hand of God from meeting you, healing you and delivering you.

## ☐ 12. Robbing God in Tithes and Offerings

The twelfth block to healing is in Malachi 3:8–11 and deals with *robbing God in our tithes and offerings.*

> **⁸Will a man rob God? Yet ye have robbed me. But ye say, Wherein have we robbed thee? In tithes and offerings. ⁹Ye *are* cursed with a curse: for ye have robbed me, *even* this whole nation. ¹⁰Bring ye all the tithes into the storehouse, that there may be meat in mine house, and prove me now herewith, saith the LORD of hosts, if I will not open you the windows of heaven, and pour you out a blessing, that *there shall* not *be room* enough *to receive it.* ¹¹And I will rebuke the devourer for your sakes, and he shall not destroy the fruits of your ground; neither shall your vine cast her fruit before the time in the field, saith the LORD of hosts. Malachi 3:8–11**

It says you are cursed with a curse. Why? Because you have not brought the tithes and the offerings into the storehouse. You have robbed God. How do you rob from God? Everything you have belongs to Him. You think your paycheck is yours? It is God's. He is just loaning it to you.

In fact, the Bible says when you work for an employer, you are not working for him; you are working for the Lord. If he is an unjust employer, you are still working for the Lord. Everything we do is "unto the Lord," just or unjust. You do it unto the Lord. Is this how you are taught in your church? Everything we do is unto the Lord! Everything we have is His. He just loans it back to us. So robbing God is not just in tithes and offerings, but in the firstfruits of our substance, including our time.

If 10 percent is the standard and if we have 168 hours a week that God has given us to exist, then 10 percent of this is 16.8 hours a week. That time belongs to God. We have 90 percent for the rest. We have 90 percent of the 168 hours for the rest, so in each day—there are 8 hours for work, 8 hours for family and 8 hours for sleep—God will get His share of our time.

Well, I don't become legalistic in this, but I just offer it as a point of challenge, to challenge your hearts. Who we are and what we are involve a lot of things. I know most of you give your time and more than a 10 percent tithe.

## ☐ 13. Some Are Just Not Saved

The thirteenth block to healing is *some are just not saved*. They do not know Jesus or the Father. They perish because they received not the truth so they might be saved.

In 2 Thessalonians 2:10, it says, And with all deceivableness of unrighteousness in them who perish; because they received not the love of the truth that they might be saved.

> **And with all deceivableness of unrighteousness in them that perish; because they received not the love of the truth, that they might be saved. 2 Thessalonians 2:10**

This is a tough Scripture—God will give you over to a greater delusion. If you want to believe error, He'll allow more to come into your life.

> **And for this cause God shall send them strong delusion, that they should believe a lie: 2 Thessalonians 2:11**

God says, "This is your party. Do what you want to do. You're a free will agent, so go for it." Some people go into greater delusion and greater separation from God and cannot be healed and delivered because they are not in covenant and they are not saved. They have a zeal, but not according to knowledge.

## ☐ 14. Sin of Our Parents

The fourteenth block to healing is *the sin of our parents*. In 2 Samuel 12:13–14, there was a curse of death on David and Bathsheba's child. The child died because of the sin of adultery and murder.

In 1 Kings 14:1–13, there is a tremendous statement about God taking a child in death. It is the only Scripture I can find where God has taken anyone through a disease just to preserve them for Himself. This is a tremendous chapter because this was a son of Jeroboam and Jeroboam the king was very evil. God looked down from heaven, saw this child and knew if he was allowed to live, his evil parents would pervert his heart; and then He would lose him from Himself forever. So God took him in disease to preserve him in the resurrection.

About the same time, Abijah son of Jeroboam got sick. Jeroboam told his wife, "Disguise yourself so no one will know you're my wife, then go to Shiloh where the prophet Ahijah lives. Take him ten loaves of bread, some small cakes and honey and ask him what will happen to our son. He can tell you because he is the one who told me I would become king." She got ready and left for Ahijah's house in Shiloh. Ahijah was now old and blind, but the LORD told him, "Jeroboam's wife is coming to ask about her son. I will tell you what to say to her." Jeroboam's wife came to Ahijah's house, pretending to be someone else. But when Ahijah heard her walking up to the door, he said, "Come in! I know you're Jeroboam's wife—why are you pretending to be someone else? I have some bad news for you. Give your husband this message from the LORD God of Israel: Jeroboam, you know I, the LORD, chose you over anyone else to be the leader of my people Israel. I even took David's kingdom away from his family and gave it to you. But you are not like my servant David. He always obeyed me and did what was right. You have made me very angry by rejecting me and making idols out of gold. Jeroboam, you have done more evil things than any king before you. Because of this, I will destroy your family by killing every man and boy in it, whether slave or free. I will wipe out your family just as fire burns up trash. Dogs will eat the bodies of your relatives who die in town and vultures will eat the bodies of those who die in the country. I the LORD have spoken and will not change my mind! This is the LORD's message to your husband. As for you, go back home and right after you get there, your son will die. Everyone in Israel will mourn at his funeral. But he will be the last one from Jeroboam's family to receive a proper burial because he is the only one the LORD God of Israel is pleased with."

14:1At that time Abijah the son of Jeroboam fell sick. 2And Jeroboam said to his wife, Arise, I pray thee, and disguise thyself, that thou be not known to be the wife of Jeroboam; and get thee to Shiloh: behold, there is Ahijah the prophet, which told me that I should be king over this people. 3And take with thee ten loaves, and cracknels, and a cruse of honey, and go to him: he shall tell thee what shall become of the child. 4And Jeroboam's wife did so, and arose, and went to Shiloh, and came to the house of Ahijah. But Ahijah could not see; for his eyes were set by reason of his age. 5And the LORD said unto Ahijah, Behold, the wife of Jeroboam cometh to ask a thing of thee for her son; for he is sick: thus and thus shalt thou say unto her: for it shall be, when she cometh in, that she shall feign herself to be another woman. 6And it was so, when Ahijah heard the sound of her feet as she came in at the door, that he said, Come in, thou wife of Jeroboam; why feignest thou thyself to be another? for I am sent to thee with heavy tidings. 7Go, tell Jeroboam, Thus saith the LORD God of Israel, Forasmuch as I exalted thee from among the people, and made thee prince over my people Israel, 8And rent the kingdom away from the house of David, and gave it thee: and yet thou hast not been as my servant David, who kept my commandments, and who followed me with all his heart, to do *that* only *which was* right in mine eyes; ⁹But hast done evil above all that were before thee: for thou hast gone and made thee other gods, and molten images, to provoke me to anger, and hast cast me behind thy back: ¹⁰Therefore, behold, I will bring evil upon the house of Jeroboam, and will cut off from Jeroboam him that pisseth against the wall, *and* him that is shut up and left in Israel, and will take away the remnant of the house of Jeroboam, as a man taketh away dung, till it be all gone. ¹¹Him that dieth of Jeroboam in the city shall the dogs eat; and him that dieth in the field shall the fowls of the air eat: for the LORD hath spoken it. ¹²Arise thou therefore, get thee to thine own house: *and* when thy feet enter into the city, the child shall die. ¹³And all Israel shall mourn for him, and bury him: for he only of Jeroboam shall come to the grave, because in him there is found *some* good thing toward the LORD God of Israel in the house of Jeroboam. 1 Kings 14:1–13

This is a tremendous, tremendous insight. You cannot make a big doctrine out of it, but it certainly helps you understand more about the people who die in disease. Sometimes you just have to let God be sovereign. God wanted that child. What a tremendous statement!

Reflecting on this, I do not believe, as a rule, that God uses or needs disease to get someone to heaven, but in observing human nature, there is always a possibility someone who God really wants for eternity could be lost to Him by falling away or things in life totally separating them from God.

## □ 15. Sometimes the Sickness is unto Death

The fifteenth block to healing is *sometimes the sickness is unto death*. In 2 Chronicles 21:4–20, we read the story of Jehoram. He once knew God, but he turned away from Him. He killed his brothers and because of murder, he became sick and died. The Bible says it was a sin unto death. There are certain sins in the Bible from which people will die.

⁴Now when Jehoram was risen up to the kingdom of his father, he strengthened himself, and slew all his brethren with the sword, and *divers* also of the princes of Israel...⁶And he walked in the way of the kings of Israel, like as did the house of Ahab: for he had the daughter of Ahab to wife: and he wrought *that which was* evil in the eyes of the LORD...¹²And there came a writing to him from Elijah the prophet, saying, Thus saith the LORD God of David thy father, Because thou hast not walked in the ways of Jehoshaphat thy father, nor in the ways of Asa king of Judah, ¹³But hast walked in the way of the kings of Israel, and hast made Judah and the inhabitants of Jerusalem to go a whoring, like to the whoredoms of the house of Ahab, and also hast slain thy brethren of thy father's house, *which were* better than thyself: ¹⁴Behold, with a great plague will the LORD smite thy people, and thy children, and thy wives, and all thy goods: ¹⁵And thou *shalt have* great sickness by disease of thy bowels, until thy bowels fall out by reason of the sickness day by day. ¹⁶Moreover the LORD stirred up against Jehoram the spirit of the Philistines, and of the Arabians, that *were*

near the Ethiopians: [17]And they came up into Judah, and brake into it, and carried away all the substance that was found in the king's house, and his sons also, and his wives; so that there was never a son left him, save Jehoahaz, the youngest of his sons. [18]And after all this the LORD smote him in his bowels with an incurable disease. [19]And it came to pass, that in process of time, after the end of two years, his bowels fell out by reason of his sickness: so he died of sore diseases. And his people made no burning for him, like the burning of his fathers. [20]Thirty and two years old was he when he began to reign, and he reigned in Jerusalem eight years, and departed without being desired. Howbeit they buried him in the city of David, but not in the sepulchres of the kings. 2 Chronicles 21:4, 6, 12–20

In 1 John 5:16, it also talks about a sin unto death. What did John say? I would not that you pray for it.

[16]If any man see his brother sin a sin *which is* not unto death, he shall ask, and he shall give him life for them that sin not unto death. There is a sin unto death: I do not say that he shall pray for it. [17]All unrighteousness is sin: and there is a sin not unto death. 1 John 5:16–17

I do not know what sin unto death is, but it is a sin producing a disease unto death. It is a death sentence and praying for it to be healed is a waste of time.

I do not know personally what sin unto death is. This is a difficult Scripture, but this is how I understand it. If I see you sin a sin, but it is a sin not producing a disease that will kill you, then I shall pray God for you and He may heal you. *But if I see you sin a sin that is a sin producing a disease unto death, I shall not pray for you, because it is a sin unto death. Of the many diseases we have talked about in this teaching, many of them are unto death. Each one of them has a sin behind it. Unless the sin is dealt with, the disease will be a disease unto death. If I try to pray for a person, without the sin being dealt with, I am wasting my time. So before I pray, I have to be involved to deal with the "sin" issue first. Then I pray and minister around the sin issues. Many people are not healed after prayer because they do not understand this.*

Diseases coming out of bitterness and unforgiveness are diseases unto death. Here is where we have missed it. Rather than praying healing for these diseases, we must meet the person according to knowledge, as we are instructed in 2 Timothy 2:24–26 and Galatians 6:1 and then go to the person in love.

We must go in love because we want to remove the curse of death from their life. We must say to this person: according to the Word of God, I cannot pray for you. But because I love you, I have come to you and I want to instruct you from the Word to bring repentance to you so you may recover yourself from the snare of this death penalty. Then when you have repented, I can come before God and ask His healing for you and He shall give it to you.

Sanctification for healing is the dimension not being taught today in the Church. The Church is not teaching why healing does not come. Cancer is a disease unto death coming out of bitterness. *Diabetes (Type 1)* is a death disease coming right out of self-hatred. There is disease after disease which carries a death sentence. But it does not have to be this way, does it?

Do you know how tough it is for me not to automatically pray for healing when I am asked to? I do not become presumptuous with the gift of healing. I promise you, I operate in all nine gifts as the Lord wills, not as I will. I am very responsible when it comes to serving God and I take it very seriously. I am not a god; I am a servant of God. I am not greater than my Master. If a person is not listening to God, why should they listen to me? If I bring you truth that is truth from God and you don't listen to me, then why should I pray for you? Am I greater than my Master? I can do no more for you as a teacher of the gospel than you are already allowing God to do in your life. All I do is come along beside you, help you and assist you in the victory. I cannot do it against your will. I cannot ask Him to dishonor His Word by doing it for you and condoning your sin. My success rate, if I did not teach you properly, would be less than 10 percent and the other 90 percent of you would be mad at me and mad at Him because you did not get healed. The 10 percent would be rejoicing and the 90 percent would be sad. I want 100 percent of you to be happy. I am willing to take the time and the risk of offending you to bring you truth at this level. I don't like losing because my Boss never lost a battle. Jesus healed every single person who came to Him. So you say, "Why isn't that happening today?" Maybe God just gave you a clue to this question.

One day someone said, "Well, it is the HIV virus." But, I do not know if this is what it is. I have no idea. No one knows what it is. The point is this: sometimes there are sins and sicknesses unto death. Second Kings 1:2–8 is the story of Ahaziah. He dabbled in sorcery and under the Law of Moses, sorcery, witchcraft and occultism brought a penalty of death. This individual died because his sin was unto death.

> ²And Ahaziah fell down through a lattice in his upper chamber that *was* in Samaria, and was sick: and he sent messengers, and said unto them, Go, enquire of Baal-zebub the god of Ekron whether I shall recover of this disease. ³But the angel of the LORD said to Elijah the Tishbite, Arise, go up to meet the messengers of the king of Samaria, and say unto them, *Is it* not because *there is* not a God in Israel, *that* ye go to enquire of Baal-zebub the god of Ekron? ⁴Now therefore thus saith the LORD, Thou shalt not come down from that bed on which thou art gone up, but shalt surely die. And Elijah departed. ⁵And when the messengers turned back unto him, he said unto them, Why are ye now turned back? ⁶And they said unto him, There came a man up to meet us, and said unto us, Go, turn again unto the king that sent you, and say unto him, Thus saith the LORD,

*Is it* not because *there is* not a God in Israel, *that* thou sendest to enquire of Baal-zebub the god of Ekron? therefore thou shalt not come down from that bed on which thou art gone up, but shalt surely die. ⁷And he said unto them, What manner of man *was he* which came up to meet you, and told you these words? ⁸And they answered him, *He was* an hairy man, and girt with a girdle of leather about his loins. And he said, It *is* Elijah the Tishbite. 2 Kings 1:2–8

King Saul died prematurely because of his sins. Saul, first of all, disobeyed God and secondly, he contacted the witch of Endor, who had a familiar spirit. In 1 Chronicles it says when Saul committed suicide, he was judged in death because he disobeyed God and because he consulted with a familiar spirit. There are certain things that we have to pay attention to. In 1 Chronicles 10:13–14, there is a story about King Saul dying:

¹³So Saul died for his transgression which he committed against the LORD, *even* against the word of the LORD, which he kept not, and also for asking *counsel* of *one that had* a familiar spirit, to enquire *of it;* ¹⁴And enquired not of the LORD: therefore he slew him, and turned the kingdom unto David the son of Jesse. 1 Chronicles 10:13–14

Many times, in dealing with certain diseases, in order to get a healing from God for people, I have to bring people to a place of repentance before God for their involvement in occultism: the contacting of mediums, contacting witches, dabbling in sorcery and things of this nature. In fact, when I minister to someone, I have a difficult time getting them healed if I do not get Ouija boards dealt with, because Ouija boards are a means of contacting an evil spirit. What do you think makes the board move and spell those words out? It is the first medium of contact with Satan in children. Levitation, table tipping and spoon bending are all part of the kingdom and the power of Satan.

Many times occultism, involvement in spiritualism, involvement in mediumships, involvement in séances, involvement in this and that, will open us up unto the spirit of death. Under the law, dabbling on that other side carries a death penalty.

In His first commandment, God said, "Thou shalt have no other gods before me" (Exodus 20:3), and you had better get this one straight. Involvement in occultism is forgivable, but it can open the door to a curse of many diseases. Looking into the future or trying to control aspects of the future through any medium or person or mechanism as a replacement for consulting God and His Word is idolatry and makes this item or person a god to you in your life.

Take therefore no thought for the morrow: for the morrow shall take thought for the things of itself. Sufficient unto the day *is* the evil thereof. Matthew 6:34

Sometimes insanity is due to dabbling in the occult. Oppression can be the result of dabbling in the occult. It occurs because someone sought the guidance of a witch doctor, a wizard, a warlock or some other occultic practitioner to try to be healed of their disease. As a matter of fact, they should have been seeking God and His Word from the very beginning and finding the spiritual roots.

In Psalm 90, Moses indicated man's longevity would be 70–80 years as a promise. However, Solomon died prematurely at age 60 because of disobedience to God and following the gods of his pagan wives. God appeared to him two times about this issue, but he would not listen. He died early, losing one-quarter of his promised life expectancy.

## ☐ 16. Our Allotted Time in Life is Fulfilled

The sixteenth block to healing is simply that *our allotted time in life is fulfilled*. You know, sometimes we just have to be like the flower which fades away; it is time to go. Well, how soon should you go? I'll say this to you. In Psalm 90, God, by His Spirit through Moses, established the longevity of man as threescore and ten (70) comfortable years or fourscore (80) with some trouble. Today, the average longevity of mankind in America is no more than 76 or so.

> **The days of our years *are* threescore years and ten; and if by reason of strength *they be* fourscore years, yet *is* their strength labour and sorrow; for it is soon cut off, and we fly away. Psalm 90:10**

As far as I am concerned, until the coming of the Lord and the first resurrection, you won't find much extension, as an average, of what was declared by God in Psalm 90. This age will be over with before it happens. Psalm 90:12 says, so teach *us* to number our days so we may apply *our* hearts unto wisdom.

> **So teach *us* to number our days, that we may apply *our* hearts unto wisdom. Psalm 90:12**

*Anything less than 70–80 years of longevity on this planet is a curse.* God's promise is we should have longevity in order to establish His righteousness in our generation and we may number our days in righteousness and be part of His plan in His kingdom.

> **The fear of the LORD prolongeth days: but the years of the wicked shall be shortened. Proverbs 10:27**

Eighty years of life, if the Lord tarries, should be the minimum you are looking for. This is how I see it in the Word.

When you find men whose lives were shortened, it was always a curse. Solomon died at age 60 and the reason he died at age 60 was because he was following the heathen gods of his thousand women. God appeared to him twice and basically said, "You had better get it straight, boy." I do not know if you will see Solomon in heaven or not. The man, who was supposed to have the greatest wisdom to share with God's people, was the dumbest concerning himself!

**4For it came to pass, when Solomon was old, *that* his wives turned away his heart after other gods: and his heart was not perfect with the LORD his God, as *was* the heart of David his father. 5For Solomon went after Ashtoreth the goddess of the Zidonians, and after Milcom the abomination of the Ammonites. 6And Solomon did evil in the sight of the LORD, and went not fully after the LORD, as *did* David his father. 7Then did Solomon build an high place for Chemosh, the abomination of Moab, in the hill that *is* before Jerusalem, and for Molech, the abomination of the children of Ammon. 8And likewise did he for all his strange wives, which burnt incense and sacrificed unto their gods. 9And the LORD was angry with Solomon, because his heart was turned from the LORD God of Israel, which had appeared unto him twice, 10And had commanded him concerning this thing, that he should not go after other gods: but he kept not that which the LORD commanded. 1 Kings 11:4–10**

Paul said it like this: what a tragedy I win many to Christ and I myself am a castaway.

**But I keep under my body, and bring *it* into subjection: lest that by any means, when I have preached to others, I myself should be a castaway. 1 Corinthians 9:27**

## ☐ 17. Looking to Symptoms and Not to the Healer

Block number seventeen is *looking to symptoms and not to the Healer.* You know, when Peter was walking on the water, as long as he kept his eyes on the Lord, he was fine. When he took his eyes off the Lord, he went into unbelief and started to sink. Before you throw stones at Peter, remember that at least he tried. At least he tried, which is more than the rest of us have ever done. So we look to our symptoms and not to the healing.

I want to say this to you: If you are waiting for the symptoms of your disease to go away before you believe, you are going to be waiting a long time. *If you are waiting for the healing before you look for the Healer, you are going to be waiting a long time!*

You see, the symptoms of your disease are the fruit of the problem— not the root. Get your eyes off your pain; get your eyes off your disease; get your eyes back on the Lord and His Word and keep them there. Do not look at the symptoms!

I said to someone the other day who was really struggling with physiological pain, really dipping into it (and I am not being insensitive—I really care—and even though I teach at this level, it does not mean I am insensitive), but I finally looked at them and said, "You and I need to cut through this, darling." I said, "Are you born again?"

"Oh, yes, I'm born again."

"Where does the Spirit of God live in you?"

"In my heart."

"Wonderful. Is your human spirit a physical dimension or a spiritual dimension?"

"Oh…spiritual."

"Can your human spirit ever get sick from disease or feel pain?"

"No, it cannot."

"Then what is your problem?"

The Bible says the spirit of man shall sustain him in his infirmity.

> **The spirit of a man will sustain his infirmity; but a wounded spirit who can bear? Proverbs 18:14**

You may have disease and you may have pain at this point, but I will tell you that your human spirit is immune to it. Stay in the Spirit, stay before God and let your heart be complete. Then, as you are before God, ask Him for His mercy about the roots and blocks of the disease.

The question is asked, "Then how can you stay in the Spirit?" The Scriptures teach we are seated with Christ Jesus in heavenly places, far above all principalities and powers. Remember who you are and where you are in the battle.

> [19]**And what *is* the exceeding greatness of his power to us-ward who believe, according to the working of his mighty power, [20]Which he wrought in Christ, when he raised him from the dead, and set *him* at his own right hand in the heavenly *places,* [21]Far above all principality, and power, and might, and dominion, and every name that is named, not only in this world, but also in that which is to come: [22]And hath put all *things* under his feet, and gave him *to be* the head over all *things* to the church, [23]Which is his body, the fulness of him that filleth all in all. Ephesians 1:19–23**

> **And hath raised *us* up together, and made *us* sit together in heavenly *places* in Christ Jesus: Ephesians 2:6**

Remember, you are more than a physical body. Remember, you are more than a tormented soul. You must be born again and be a new creature in Christ Jesus. Then your spirit comes alive unto God. When you are alive unto God, the Spirit of God lives within you. The Bible says, let the same Spirit that raised Christ from the dead, dwell in you; He shall quicken your mortal bodies.

But if the Spirit of him that raised up Jesus from the dead dwell in you, he that raised up Christ from the dead shall also quicken your mortal bodies by his Spirit that dwelleth in you. Romans 8:11

*So we have to keep our eyes off the symptoms*
*and keep our eyes on the Lord.*

## ☐ 18. Letting Fear Enter Your Heart

The eighteenth block to healing is *letting fear enter your heart*. Fear will quench your faith and faith will quench your fears. You can choose which will rule you. Faith and fear are equal in this dimension—both demand to be fulfilled and both project into the future. "Faith is the substance of things hoped for, the evidence of things not (yet) seen" (Hebrews 11:1). The flip side of this Scripture would be this: fear is the substance of things not hoped for, the evidence of things not yet seen.

Information concerning fear is found in the book of Job:

²⁴For my sighing cometh before I eat, and my roarings are poured out like the waters. ²⁵For the thing which I greatly feared is come upon me, and that which I was afraid of is come unto me. ²⁶I was not in safety, neither had I rest, neither was I quiet; yet trouble came...¹⁴Fear came upon me, and trembling, which made all my bones to shake. ¹⁵Then a spirit passed before my face; the hair of my flesh stood up: Job 3:24–26; 4:14–15

This is God's antidote to the spirit of fear:

For ye have not received the spirit of bondage again to fear; but ye have received the Spirit of adoption, whereby we cry, Abba, Father. Romans 8:15

Let not your heart be troubled: ye believe in God, believe also in me. John 14:1

Peace I leave with you, my peace I give unto you: not as the world giveth, give I unto you. Let not your heart be troubled, neither let it be afraid. John 14:27

...for whatsoever *is* not of faith is sin. Romans 14:23

## ☐ 19. Failure to Get Away in Prayer and Fasting

The nineteenth block to healing is *failure to get away in prayer and fasting*. This block has to do with a lack of closeness in personal relationship with Jesus and the Father. There is much confusion in the body of Christ regarding prayer and fasting and the reasons for it. I believe this confusion exists because there is a misunderstanding about there being more than one kind of fast unto the Lord and their purposes are different.

Now I want to say something to you: you do not pray and fast to receive from God—*you pray and fast to meet God.*

Now I know what you have been taught from Isaiah 58:6, where it says, it is the fast He has called you to that will break every yoke. But you had better read this chapter in its context, because it has nothing to do with fasting from food and water. It is quite the opposite.

The fast of Isaiah 58 has to do with your service unto God on behalf of others. In your service unto God, He will meet you and heal you of your diseases. For as you give unto others, God will give back to you. This is the "fast" He has called you to. Service unto others breaks the yoke. This is what Isaiah 58 teaches us.

The prayer and fasting issue the disciples had to undergo was because they could not cast out the spirit of epilepsy. They were so involved in making a "science" out of this new ministry of healing in Christ that they forgot they were supposed to be in a tightly knit relationship with the Father and Jesus.

> [18]And Jesus rebuked the devil; and he departed out of him: and the child was cured from that very hour. [19]Then came the disciples to Jesus apart, and said, Why could not we cast him out? [20]And Jesus said unto them, Because of your unbelief: for verily I say unto you, If ye have faith as a grain of mustard seed, ye shall say unto this mountain, Remove hence to yonder place; and it shall remove; and nothing shall be impossible unto you. [21]Howbeit this kind goeth not out but by prayer and fasting. Matthew 17:18–21

Let me say this to you about prayer and fasting: if you do not pray and fast in your lifetime, it will be a block to the hand of God because this means you are not setting yourself aside before God to let Him enrich you and bring you back into the place of fellowship where He is your priority.

A time of prayer and fasting is not for the purpose of getting something from God. You pray and fast to meet God in relationship. This kind of fasting is not just the giving up of food as a sacrifice for so many days. This fast is for you to set aside everything, including eating, so as to have a period of time where you are completely alone with God and His Word for relationship purposes. It is setting yourself aside before God to give Him the opportunity to enrich you and bring you into His place of fellowship where He is your priority.

I have come to this understanding about prayer and fasting from these Scriptures. One day some of the Pharisees came to Jesus and asked, Why don't Your disciples fast and pray like John's disciples do? Jesus said unto them, Why should they? The reason for their prayer and fasting is here in the midst of them, but when I am gone, then they shall pray and fast. (That's my paraphrase; He was saying the relationship is right there in their midst). But when I am gone back to heaven, they will enter into that relationship, by faith, again in prayer and fasting.

> **And Jesus said unto them, Can the children of the bridechamber fast, while the bridegroom is with them? as long as they have the bridegroom with them, they cannot fast. Mark 2:19**

*Do not confuse petition with fellowship when it comes to prayer and fasting.* Prayer and fasting is primarily for fellowship out of which God blesses us, but many people only go into petition and have made prayer and fasting some type of spiritual mantra to automatically require God to do something.

## ☐ 20. Improper Care of the Body

The twentieth block to healing is *improper care of the body.* You know, if you are asking me to help you get well (and you are not, but if you were) and the disease is a result of your not taking care of the temple of the Holy Spirit, do you think God is going to answer my prayer for you? God's not going to answer my prayer for you if you are not getting good nutrition, if you are not drinking enough water and getting enough rest and sleep. If you are not taking reasonable care of yourself, you are going to pay a high price. This is the consequence of negligence.

So now there is another area in this improper care of the body. In Philippians 2, there is a story about someone serving the Lord who was sick unto death because he did not use wisdom in how much time he spent in ministry serving the Lord. Philippians 2:25–30 says, Yet I supposed it necessary to send to you Epaphroditus, my brother and companion in labor and fellow soldier, but your messenger and he who ministered to my wants. For he longed after you all and was full of heaviness because ye had heard he had been sick. For indeed he was sick nigh unto death: but God had mercy on him; and not on him only, but on me also, lest I should have sorrow upon sorrow.

> [25]**Yet I supposed it necessary to send to you Epaphroditus, my brother, and companion in labour, and fellow soldier, but your messenger, and he that ministered to my wants.** [26]**For he longed after you all, and was full of heaviness, because that ye had heard that he had been sick.** [27]**For indeed he was sick nigh unto death: but God had mercy on him; and not on him only, but on me also, lest I should have sorrow upon sorrow.** [28]**I sent him therefore the more carefully, that, when ye see him again, ye may rejoice, and that I may be the less sorrowful.** [29]**Receive him therefore in the Lord with all gladness; and hold such in reputation:** [30]**Because for the work of Christ he was nigh unto death, not regarding his life, to supply your lack of service toward me. Philippians 2:25–30**

Do you understand what was just said? This guy was sick unto death because he was burnt out serving Paul and serving the Lord.

I work long hours. Our ministry is going seven days a week, nearly 18 hours a day, 365 days a year. But I have to take it easy; I have to take time out. I have to measure my time and I have to allow my staff to measure their time because, if we do not, we will die prematurely trying to save people's lives. It is a high price to pay. So we are going to live and you are going to live, but we are going to take time out to make sure we do not end up in sin and become a block to our own healing and, even better, we will prevent a disease from getting a foothold.

## ☐ 21. Not Discerning the Lord's Body

The twenty-first block to healing is *not discerning the Lord's body.* First Corinthians 11:27–31 describes a situation where Paul was talking about a physical disease problem in God's people: Many are weak. Many are sickly. Many sleep (this means they died prematurely) because they did not discern the Lord's body. The term *sleep* refers to the death of believers.

> **For this cause many *are* weak and sickly among you, and many sleep. 1 Corinthians 11:30**

It is the "Lord's body" we must discern. It is by His stripes we were and are healed.

> **⁴Surely he hath borne our griefs, and carried our sorrows: yet we did esteem him stricken, smitten of God, and afflicted. ⁵But he *was* wounded for our transgressions, *he was* bruised for our iniquities: the chastisement of our peace *was* upon him; and with his stripes we are healed. Isaiah 53:4–5**

> **That it might be fulfilled which was spoken by Esaias the prophet, saying, Himself took our infirmities, and bare *our* sicknesses. Matthew 8:17**

> **Who his own self bare our sins in his own body on the tree, that we, being dead to sins, should live unto righteousness: by whose stripes ye were healed. 1 Peter 2:24**

If we don't want to be sickly and die prematurely, then we must have faith in the healing provided by Christ, as well as forgiveness.

> **Jesus Christ the same yesterday, and to day, and for ever. Hebrews 13:8**

Nothing will be impossible with such faith.

> **And all things, whatsoever ye shall ask in prayer, believing, ye shall receive. Matthew 21:22**

> **Jesus said unto him, If thou canst believe, all things *are* possible to him that believeth. Mark 9:23**

> **²²And Jesus answering saith unto them, Have faith in God. ²³For verily I say unto you, That whosoever shall say unto this mountain, Be thou removed, and be thou cast into the sea; and shall not doubt in his heart, but shall believe that those things which he saith shall come to pass; he shall have whatsoever he saith. ²⁴Therefore I say unto you, What things soever ye desire, when ye pray, believe that ye receive *them,* and ye shall have *them.* Mark 11:22–24**

[12]Verily, verily, I say unto you, He that believeth on me, the works that I do shall he do also; and greater *works* than these shall he do; because I go unto my Father. [13]And whatsoever ye shall ask in my name, that will I do, that the Father may be glorified in the Son. [14]If ye shall ask any thing in my name, I will do *it.* [15]If ye love me, keep my commandments. John 14:12–15

Hitherto have ye asked nothing in my name: ask, and ye shall receive, that your joy may be full. John 16:24

This Scripture in 1 Corinthians 11 is talking about taking communion in unbelief, not realizing its true significance and not discerning the Lord's body and blood in order to receive the benefits by faith. It also refers to the saved or unsaved man who takes communion with sin in his life, without making confession unto salvation and acknowledging personal needs and without judging himself so as to escape the chastening of God.

There are three facets of this block to healing. I really want you to pay attention because this is very, very important.

Many do not discern the Lord's body correctly in communion. I say again, there are three aspects. You will find them in 1 Corinthians 11:27–31:

[27]Wherefore whosoever shall eat this bread, and drink this cup of the Lord, unworthily, shall be guilty of the body and blood of the Lord. [28]But let a man examine himself, and so let him eat of *that* bread, and drink of *that* cup. [29]For he that eateth and drinketh unworthily, eateth and drinketh damnation to himself, not discerning the Lord's body. [30]For this cause many *are* weak and sickly among you, and many sleep. [31]For if we would judge ourselves, we should not be judged. 1 Corinthians 11:27–31

Let me give you the three aspects of why communion represents a block. These are the blocks in it:

Aspect 1: When you take communion, it is one of the sacraments of the Church. There are only three of them: water baptism, communion and foot washing. Only three sacraments are found in Scripture as commandments. In communion, you are celebrating the remembrance of Christ in two dimensions: His shed blood and His broken body. The cup for the blood and the wafer, bread or cracker for His broken body.

When you unworthily partake of what forgiveness by God represents in communion and do not repent unto Him, then you are guilty of fraud and you have cursed yourself with a curse. This is partaking unworthily. You have cursed yourself with a curse because you make what Jesus did at the cross of no effect for you. It is not the sacrament that saves you—it is the *obedience.*

Part of this aspect is not judging ourselves with regard to sin as the spiritual roots of disease. We bring forth the repentance so the forgiveness, deliverance and healing can be appropriated and bring forth the full benefits provided in the Lord's Supper. Judging ourselves involves having the discernment to know specifically what is being repented for. Otherwise, we do not know what to stand against, what to change in our lives and what to renounce out of our lives. Generic repentance and asking in a generic way for forgiveness of our sins, without knowing what those sins are, accomplishes very little. Many people say, "Father God, forgive me of all my sins," and He does forgive, but there can be no repentance without knowing specifically the sin area needing to be sanctified out of our life.

Aspect 2: This aspect has to do with us "eating each other alive." This is "not discerning the Lord's body." In fact, it creates what we might call an "autoimmune disease" in the Church body. This is the body of believers attacking one another in relationships, in like manner as an autoimmune disease attacks the physical body. The Church is called the body of Christ. We must learn to discern one another as part of our body.

> **Now ye are the body of Christ, and members in particular.**
> **1 Corinthians 12:27**

> **Bear ye one another's burdens, and so fulfil the law of Christ.**
> **Galatians 6:2**

This aspect has to do with fellowship and relationship with one another in the Church—if you say you love the Lord, yet you hate your brother, the love of God is not with you.

> **We know that we have passed from death unto life, because we love the brethren. He that loveth not *his* brother abideth in death.**
> **1 John 3:14**

When we partake of the Lord's Supper (communion) in remembrance of Him, we are saying to Him that because of what He did for us, we are ready to do this for each other: not dying for each other's sins, but laying our lives down in service one to another. When we partake of communion and ignore our brother in his need and his disease, then we have negated the fellowship with him which communion represents and we are cursed with a curse. Communion is *koinonia (#2842, Greek, Strong's Concordance)*, or *fellowship*. We must focus on the horizontal relationship in the body of Christ, which is our relationship with each other, as well as on the vertical relationship with each of the three persons of the Godhead.

> [16]**The cup of blessing which we bless, is it not the communion of the blood of Christ? The bread which we break, is it not the communion of the body of Christ?** [17]**For we *being* many are one bread, *and* one body: for we are all partakers of that one bread. 1 Corinthians 10:16–17**

> **But if we walk in the light, as he is in the light, we have fellowship one with another, and the blood of Jesus Christ his Son cleanseth us from all sin. 1 John 1:7**

The cup (the blood) is for forgiveness of sins on the vertical level from God and on the horizontal level with each other. The bread is the bread of life for healing of our bodies through helping one another deal with the spiritual roots of disease and blocks to healing. It is the Church being the Church and ministering the life of God to each other. Then we can truly say:

> **For the kingdom of God is not meat and drink; but righteousness, and peace, and joy in the Holy Ghost. Romans 14:17**

Aspect 3: The third aspect of the block to healing taught in 1 Corinthians 11 is even more serious. It is addressed to churches who do not believe healing is for today. It is why, in many denominational churches, people are dying with insanity and disease because the very thing they need—healing—was provided for them at the cross and what the communion service represents is negated by half; that is, one-half is rejected in unbelief and doctrinal positioning while still being celebrated in the actual communion service.

Here's how it works. The shed blood of Jesus was not for the healing of disease. His shed blood was for the forgiveness of sins. Scripture is clear: without the shedding of blood, there is no remission of sins.

> **For this is my blood of the new testament, which is shed for many for the remission of sins. Matthew 26:28**

> **And almost all things are by the law purged with blood; and without shedding of blood is no remission. Hebrews 9:22**

So when we come into communion and take the cup, we acknowledge that what He did for us allows us to be able to repent, have cleansing and forgiveness of all sin.

> **⁷But if we walk in the light, as he is in the light, we have fellowship one with another, and the blood of Jesus Christ his Son cleanseth us from all sin. ⁸If we say that we have no sin, we deceive ourselves, and the truth is not in us. ⁹If we confess our sins, he is faithful and just to forgive us *our* sins, and to cleanse us from all unrighteousness. ¹⁰If we say that we have not sinned, we make him a liar, and his word is not in us. 1 John 1:7–10**

However, the broken bread represents the stripes that were laid on Jesus. The bread represents freedom from the curse and the curse is all manner of disease (Deuteronomy 28).

> **Who his own self bare our sins in his own body on the tree, that we, being dead to sins, should live unto righteousness: by whose stripes ye were healed. 1 Peter 2:24**

When we do not *believe* healing is for today and *teach* that it is not, and then take the bread of communion, which represents the freedom from the curse, but deny freedom is for today, we have brought a curse into our lives. We are cursed with a curse, which is the disease and we now say we cannot be healed from it; yet we celebrate the sacrament providing for that healing. There is something theologically wrong with this picture.

*This happens because we negate one-half of what Christ did at the cross.* In partaking of the bread, we curse ourselves in our ignorance and our apostasy—for these three reasons, many of us are weak, are sick and die premature deaths—because we are cursed with a curse we have brought upon ourselves because of unbelief.

This, too, is a tough teaching, isn't it? But this is what I see. Those who are not correctly discerning the body of Christ personally and what all the work He did at the cross represents, open the door for sickness and disease and premature death. It is a spiritual block to healing.

## ☐ 22. Touching God's Anointed Leaders

The twenty-second block to healing involves *touching God's anointed leaders.* If you have a leader who is in sin, or you have a pastor who is in error, the elders should be able to straighten him out. No one is an island unto himself. So, when you do not agree with what I teach, then come—we will have a Bible study. *I cannot afford to be wrong and neither can you.*

Do not touch God's anointed.

> *Saying,* **Touch not mine anointed, and do my prophets no harm.**
> **1 Chronicles 16:22**

> *Saying,* **Touch not mine anointed, and do my prophets no harm.**
> **Psalm 105:15**

A major curse comes with touching God's anointed. Many people are upset about one of our former presidents, but he just represented the mores and morality of this nation. So what you have in a president reflects what you have in the people and you know it is true. *God has just given us what we are to convict us of what we are not.*

Touching God's anointed carries more significance than most Christians understand. God's anointed are those set in place for leadership in a ministry and this includes their families. I don't care what you think about this man, Henry, who is writing this book. But I do care, for your sakes, how you handle it. If you have anything negative to say, you should say it to me directly. If you don't say it to my face, you are cursed with a curse if you say it to anyone else.

You can read for yourself in the Bible about Korah and the 250 elders of Israel who went into sedition against Moses. You will find this in Numbers 16. Also read about Miriam, Moses' sister, being struck with leprosy because of her murmuring against the wife of Moses (Numbers 12).

I use myself as an example, but I am not the only anointed one of God in your life. What you say about your leaders is very important to your health and well-being. People do not understand the seriousness of the sins of the tongue and the sin of division against God's leaders and those who minister under them.

I want to make a bold statement to you: never be a part of a church split. You will not prosper and every church born out of a church split will not prosper. It will split and resplit and split and resplit until the coming of the Lord, because there is a spirit ruling in the church that is a curse. If you want to leave the church, don't burn bridges. Love the leader, even if you do not agree with him for whatever reason and communicate and let him send you out in peace. Then, when you leave, do not be a division-maker and take others out with you. If you do, you will be cursed with a curse. Leave in peace and burn no bridges. Let God be God and stay out of it. Keep your mouth shut. Do not gather to yourself those who agree with you against God's anointed. If a church is not ministering to you and your needs, then find someplace where you can agree, but don't murmur against that leader. He is God's servant and God is the One who will deal with him.

## ☐ 23. Immoderate Eating

This twenty-third block involves *not taking care of the body in nutrition.* This ministry believes in temple maintenance. We believe in good nutrition and we believe this in moderation (temperance). You cannot expect to walk in health if you don't drink enough water and eat the proper mix of food.

> [19]**What? know ye not that your body is the temple of the Holy Ghost** *which is* **in you, which ye have of God, and ye are not your own?** [20]**For ye are bought with a price: therefore glorify God in your body, and in your spirit, which are God's. 1 Corinthians 6:19–20**

Our body belongs to the Lord and we have a responsibility to give them proper rest, exercise and good nutrition. You cannot expect to walk in health if you don't drink enough water and eat foods to nourish the body. These foods include whole grain cereals and breads, dairy products, protein and generous amounts of fruits and vegetables, especially the green leafy ones. The day should begin with a good breakfast. Many people have the idea that if they eat by faith and trust in God, then they can eat anything they want with no regard to nutrition. Foolish, presumptuous faith negates the wisdom of God in good eating and will not promote health of the body.

If you are concerned about excessive weight gain, you should know first of all this is a spiritual problem rooted in self-hatred. Not eating breakfast is not the way to deal with the fear of gaining weight. It is the morning meal that sets metabolism for the rest of the day and burns the calories. If you eat lunch and you haven't had breakfast, then lunch becomes fat because the metabolism is overloaded when it should have been set in motion at breakfast. If a person does not eat sufficient calories, then the metabolic fire goes on low so as to conserve everything eaten. The body will actually hoard fat because of the slowdown in metabolism.

With regard to vitamin supplements, we say that if you are concerned about it, then a one-a-day is all you need. Megadoses of vitamin and mineral supplements can unbalance body chemistry and even cause the body to go into levels of toxic poisoning. Mega-nutrition is only another of man's efforts to bypass the curse and maintain health artificially and unnaturally rather than the way God created it to be. Those who are caught up in mega amounts of vitamin, mineral and herb supplements are motivated by fear and are trying to jump-start themselves in health. Just because "a little" is essential and beneficial does not mean that "a whole bunch" will help more. The chemical imbalance coming out of this can be a major block to God's health and wholeness. If you are doing megadoses of supplements, it is not wise to go "cold turkey"; the body will not be able to handle the withdrawal shock. You need to take yourself off in a slow, gradual manner so as to give your body time to adjust back to normal. Good nutrition is absolutely important to our health, but nutrition cannot heal the defects coming from separation from God and His Word or deal with sanctification and sin issues and become roots to disease.

Another concern is the growing use of sugar substitutes now used in the foods we buy. We are finding these are contributing to depression, muscle spasms, headaches and chronic tiredness. Sugar in moderation is the better way to go. Get off these sugar substitutes and you will see the difference. It is not bondage to do a little label reading on the products you buy. It is wisdom to stay on top of the subtle effects of the marketplace that, in well-meaning efforts, through ignorance, become man's attempt to bypass the curse. I find that God likes a little sugar Himself.

> [23]**Thou hast not brought me the small cattle of thy burnt offerings; neither hast thou honoured me with thy sacrifices. I have not caused thee to serve with an offering, nor wearied thee with incense.** [24]**Thou hast bought me no sweet cane with money, neither hast thou filled me with the fat of thy sacrifices: but thou hast made me to serve with thy sins, thou hast wearied me with thine iniquities. Isaiah 43:23–24**

> [16]**Know ye not that ye are the temple of God, and** *that* **the Spirit of God dwelleth in you?** [17]**If any man defile the temple of God, him shall God destroy; for the temple of God is holy, which** *temple* **ye are. 1 Corinthians 3:16–17**

Our bodies are God's mobile homes. We must not take them for granted. We need to keep our spirits nourished with the Word of God and keep our lives free of devastating sin and occultism. We need to exercise wisdom in the care of our bodies so that we will enjoy greater and greater measures of divine health.

Moderation is the key, whether it be with regard to exercise, rest or what you eat. Moderation is one of the fruits of the Holy Spirit listed in Galatians 5:23 as "temperance."

There is a movement, even within the Church, to selectively remove many foods from our diet. I consider this to be evil because what God has created to be taken with thanksgiving is now being eaten or not eaten out of fear. You can call what God created evil, but I am not going to. In Genesis, in the creation, He did not say it was good—He said it was very good. In fact, the Scriptures indicate this in the Word.

> ⁴:¹**Now the Spirit speaketh expressly, that in the latter times some shall depart from the faith, giving heed to seducing spirits, and doctrines of devils; ²Speaking lies in hypocrisy; having their conscience seared with a hot iron; ³Forbidding to marry,** *and commanding* **to abstain from meats, which God hath created to be received with thanksgiving of them which believe and know the truth. ⁴For every creature of God** *is* **good, and nothing to be refused, if it be received with thanksgiving: ⁵For it is sanctified by the word of God and prayer. 1 Timothy 4:1–5**

## ☐ 24. Pure Unbelief

The twenty-fourth block to healing is *pure unbelief.* Mark 6:4–6 refers to the unbelief in Nazareth. This is the story of Jesus being unable to do great works in His own hometown because of unbelief.

> ⁴**But Jesus said unto them, A prophet is not without honour, but in his own country, and among his own kin, and in his own house. ⁵And he could there do no mighty work, save that he laid his hands upon a few sick folk, and healed** *them.* **⁶And he marvelled because of their unbelief. And he went round about the villages, teaching. Mark 6:4–6**

Paul, in Hebrews 4, addresses the issue of pure unbelief in those who came out of Egypt under the leadership of Moses and also the unbelief in those whom he was addressing in these Scriptures. Paul indicated that unbelief and doubt would keep us from our rest. When we find ourselves in unrest, rather than believing and accepting what God has said, we would then try to create that rest by our own labors. In fact, disease management is a form of this type of work intended to create a rest apart from God.

> ⁴:¹**Let us therefore fear, lest, a promise being left** *us* **of entering into his rest, any of you should seem to come short of it. ²For unto us was the gospel preached, as well as unto them: but the word preached did not profit them, not being mixed with faith in them that heard** *it.* **³For we which have believed do enter into rest, as he said, As I have sworn in my wrath, if they shall enter into my rest: although the works were finished**

from the foundation of the world. ⁴For he spake in a certain place of the seventh *day* on this wise, And God did rest the seventh day from all his works. ⁵And in this *place* again, If they shall enter into my rest. ⁶Seeing therefore it remaineth that some must enter therein, and they to whom it was first preached entered not in because of unbelief: ⁷Again, he limiteth a certain day, saying in David, To day, after so long a time; as it is said, To day if ye will hear his voice, harden not your hearts. ⁸For if Jesus had given them rest, then would he not afterward have spoken of another day. ⁹There remaineth therefore a rest to the people of God. ¹⁰For he that is entered into his rest, he also hath ceased from his own works, as God *did* from his. ¹¹Let us labour therefore to enter into that rest, lest any man fall after the same example of unbelief. Hebrews 4:1–11

## ☐ 25. Failing to Keep Your Life Filled Up with God

The twenty-fifth block to healing is *failing to keep your life filled up with God.* Jesus said in John 5:14, after He had just healed someone, Go your way, sin no more, lest a worse thing come upon you. What was He saying? Keep yourself *filled;* do not sin.

> Afterward Jesus findeth him in the temple, and said unto him, Behold, thou art made whole: sin no more, lest a worse thing come unto thee. John 5:14

There is a Scripture in Matthew 12:43–45 that says when the unclean spirit has gone out of a man, he walks through dry places, seeking rest and finds none. Then he says, I will return into my house from whence I came out; and when he is come, he finds it empty, swept and garnished. Then he goes and takes with himself seven other spirits more wicked than himself and they enter in and dwell there: and the last state of that man is worse than the first. Even so shall it be also unto this wicked generation.

> ⁴³When the unclean spirit is gone out of a man, he walketh through dry places, seeking rest, and findeth none. ⁴⁴Then he saith, I will return into my house from whence I came out; and when he is come, he findeth *it* empty, swept, and garnished. ⁴⁵Then goeth he, and taketh with himself seven other spirits more wicked than himself, and they enter in and dwell there: and the last *state* of that man is worse than the first. Even so shall it be also unto this wicked generation. Matthew 12:43–45

What is this saying? The bottom line: when God delivers you, you have an obligation to stay "filled up."

If I give you knowledge about how to get free, that same knowledge will keep you free. But if you fall back into the same roots of sin, then your chances of keeping your healing are not very good. However, if you keep yourself filled up spiritually, your chances of keeping your healing are excellent.

Many people say, "Well, they didn't keep their healing." Did you ever ask God why? They probably fell back into their old sins all over again. So keeping ourselves filled up is essential and if we don't, it is a block to keeping our healing and our well-being.

It is important to note that when the enemy is removed, he will come back to see if you are for real and if you are "filled up" with the knowledge of God and obedience to Him. The enemy is somewhat lazy and he takes the path of least resistance. He needs you in order to be fulfilled. In fact, when the enemy is within you, he is at peace and you are in torment. Then when the enemy is gone out of you, he is in torment and you are in peace. The enemy knows what it took to gain access to your life and he will try it again, but you have the knowledge and the tools that will keep you free.

## ☐ 26. Not Resisting the Enemy

The twenty-sixth block to healing is *not resisting the enemy.* Isaiah 38:1–5 tells the story of Hezekiah the king. Remember, Hezekiah was sick unto death. The prophet came and said, "Boy, you're going to die." What did Hezekiah do? He had a disease unto death. Did he roll over against the wall and curse God? Did he roll over against the wall and go into abject bitterness? Did he roll over against the wall and have a pity party? Did he call the undertaker?

What did he do? *He prayed and asked God for extended life.* Did God give it to him? Yes! Fifteen years! If you have a disease unto death, talk to God. Ask Him for fifteen more years. You have a Scripture to stand on.

> ³⁸:¹In those days was Hezekiah sick unto death. And Isaiah the prophet the son of Amoz came unto him, and said unto him, Thus saith the LORD, Set thine house in order: for thou shalt die, and not live. ²Then Hezekiah turned his face toward the wall, and prayed unto the LORD, ³And said, Remember now, O LORD, I beseech thee, how I have walked before thee in truth and with a perfect heart, and have done *that which is good* in thy sight. And Hezekiah wept sore. ⁴Then came the word of the LORD to Isaiah, saying, ⁵Go, and say to Hezekiah, Thus saith the LORD, the God of David thy father, I have heard thy prayer, I have seen thy tears: behold, I will add unto thy days fifteen years. Isaiah 38:1–5

This is one aspect of not resisting the enemy: not asking.

The enemy is always trying to devour mankind through temptation, but the Scriptures indicate you can defeat him and he will flee.

> ⁸Be sober, be vigilant; because your adversary the devil, as a roaring lion, walketh about, seeking whom he may devour: ⁹Whom resist stedfast in the faith, knowing that the same afflictions are accomplished in your brethren that are in the world. 1 Peter 5:8–9

> ⁷Submit yourselves therefore to God. Resist the devil, and he will flee from you. ⁸Draw nigh to God, and he will draw nigh to you. Cleanse *your* hands, *ye* sinners; and purify *your* hearts, *ye* double minded. James 4:7–8

> I call heaven and earth to record this day against you, *that* I have set before you life and death, blessing and cursing: therefore choose life, that both thou and thy seed may live: Deuteronomy 30:19

## ☐ 27. Just Giving Up

The twenty-seventh block to healing is *just giving up.* You look at your symptoms; you look at the prognosis; you look at the word *incurable*; and you agree and accept *this* as the truth, rather than pursuing healing in the face of what everything in the physical realm would indicate.

There are dozens of people walking around on this planet today who have come to this ministry and would have been dead if God and our ministry team had not been involved. The doctors had given up on them. They are alive today, staying "filled up" with God and His Word. Which is *a more excellent way*™—premature death or a longer life in which to fulfill the will of God in your life? **The Lord is more magnified in our healing than in a premature death.**

> ⁹Mine eye mourneth by reason of affliction: LORD, I have called daily upon thee, I have stretched out my hands unto thee. ¹⁰Wilt thou shew wonders to the dead? shall the dead arise *and* praise thee? Selah. Psalm 88:9–10

> What profit *is there* in my blood, when I go down to the pit? Shall the dust praise thee? shall it declare thy truth? Psalm 30:9

What kind of mentality do we have when we are not prepared to live our 70–80 years in blessing? *God does not need a disease to bring you to heaven.* Moses prophesied in Psalm 90—have you noticed David did not write all the Psalms? the heading of this Psalm is "A Prayer of Moses"—that the longevity of man would be threescore and ten (70) and if by reason of strength they be fourscore years (80), yet is their strength labor and sorrow, for it is soon cut off and we fly away.

> The days of our years *are* threescore years and ten; and if by reason of strength *they be* fourscore years, yet *is* their strength labour and sorrow; for it is soon cut off, and we fly away. Psalm 90:10

It doesn't say age 60 with some trouble. It doesn't say age 40 with some trouble. It doesn't say age 30 with some trouble. It says trouble doesn't start happening till you are age 80, then you have some trouble. So I just really, really, inside as a human being, get irritated when somebody gives the devil credit for getting someone to heaven. Are you with me? I just have to believe in *a more excellent way*™. Sickness and a disease are a curse and they don't have to be a way of life. We ought not to be dying prematurely. We are of no earthly good in heaven and God does not need us there before our allotted years on earth are fulfilled. God prophesied through Moses that He purposes for one's lifetime to be 70–80 years, so anything less than this would be a curse. Where did this term "retirement" come from? Moses was 80 years of age before he even started his ministry. We should give consideration to the possibility that, when we retire from our livelihood jobs at age 60–65, we would then spend the next twenty years devoted to the ministry of helping people get free of their diseases and preaching the gospel—the Good News!

## ☐ 28. Looking for Repeated Healings Instead of Divine Health

The twenty-eighth block to healing is *looking for repeated healings instead of divine health.* God's perfect will is not to heal you—*His perfect will is that you don't get sick.* Deuteronomy 28 says that if we disobey the LORD our God, the curse will come upon us. If we obey the LORD our God, get all this stuff straightened out and keep working on it, He'll put none of the diseases of Egypt upon us. *God's perfect will is for you not to get sick.*

> **And said, If thou wilt diligently hearken to the voice of the LORD thy God, and wilt do that which is right in his sight, and wilt give ear to his commandments, and keep all his statutes, I will put none of these diseases upon thee, which I have brought upon the Egyptians: for I *am* the LORD that healeth thee. Exodus 15:26**

> **And the very God of peace sanctify you wholly; and *I pray God* your whole spirit and soul and body be preserved blameless unto the coming of our Lord Jesus Christ. 1 Thessalonians 5:23**

*The same principles I am giving you will move the hand of God to heal you and, if you apply them to your life, will prevent the diseases from coming in the first place.* Which is easier? Working this stuff out to get well or working this stuff out not to get sick? The same amount of work and the same amount of sanctification are involved. It requires the same amount of fellowship and the same amount of coming before God.

> ### *Why don't we start getting right with God now, not when we "have to"? It is a more excellent way*™.

God is not interested in repeated healings for you. He is interested in you not getting sick to begin with. If you are looking for repeated healings, you have missed the mark. Third John 2 says, Dearly beloved, I wish above all things that you prosper and be in good health, even as your soul prospereth.

> **Beloved, I wish above all things that thou mayest prosper and be in health, even as thy soul prospereth. 3 John 1:2**

There it is; it is His will.

Do you think it is God's will to heal today? There it is. Do you think it is God's will for to you be in good health today? There it is. Do you think it is God's will for your poor head to be straightened out today? There it is.

Oh, by the way, this is a New Testament Scripture not found in Matthew, Mark, Luke, John or the book of Acts.

## ☐ 29. Rejecting Healing as Part of the Covenant for Today

The twenty-ninth block to healing is *rejecting healing in the atonement as part of the covenant for today.* First Peter 2:24 tells us by His stripes we are healed; Isaiah 53:5 says by His stripes we were healed; Psalm 103:3 says, I am the LORD thy God, the LORD who forgiveth thee of all thy iniquities and healeth thee of all thy diseases.

> **Who his own self bare our sins in his own body on the tree, that we, being dead to sins, should live unto righteousness: by whose stripes ye were healed. 1 Peter 2:24**

> **But he *was* wounded for our transgressions, *he was* bruised for our iniquities: the chastisement of our peace *was* upon him; and with his stripes we are healed. Isaiah 53:5**

> **Who forgiveth all thine iniquities; who healeth all thy diseases; Psalm 103:3**

I was at a meeting in my community sometime back and there was a person there who suggested that we pray for some who were sick. So we all prayed for them. We prayed, they would get well. Later, outside, we were talking about a specific disease and I said I believed God could heal. A pastor said, "I do not believe this is in the atonement today. I believe it passed away 2,000 years ago."

I said, "Just a minute. Weren't you just in the meeting praying for someone to get well?"

"Well," he said, "if He wants to…but it is not there…."

I do not know where you are in your theology—whether you believe healing is for today or not—but I am here to tell you: if healing is not for today in *your* theology, then healing will never happen!

## □ 30. Trying to Bypass the Penalty of the Curse

The thirtieth block to healing is *trying to bypass the penalty of the curse* without taking responsibility for the sin causing it.

For example, if you have malabsorption because of anxiety, then taking a medication to block it is an attempt to bypass the penalty of the curse, because the root is *fear and anxiety*, which is sin. The fruit of it is the malabsorption and the drug is an attempt to manage it apart from dealing with it. We are always looking around for ways to get out of disease without dealing with the root cause of the disease.

It is like this: reincarnation is an attempt by mankind to bypass judgment—to get around it. Sometimes we are trying to get well without going back to what God said; we are trying to get around what He has said.

Another example is cancer resulting from bitterness against a mother, mother-in-law or sister(s), which is sometimes what causes breast cancer. You do everything under the sun to try to get well, but what you should have done was go back and make peace with your mother, mother-in-law or sister(s). Do you understand what I am saying?

When we do not come before God to deal with the sin in the situation, when we do not deal with the root cause, then modalities of healings we come up with to try to get well are an attempt to bypass the penalty of the curse. We try to get well without doing it God's way (in obedience to Him).

This does not mean a person is never supposed to go to a doctor to find out what is wrong. What we are saying is that if your disease is spiritually rooted, the only way healing/wholeness will come is by dealing with the spiritual root through repentance and sanctification. If you do otherwise, you are wasting your time and money seeking modality after modality for healing. If a disease is spiritually rooted, then no modality is going to do anything more than be an attempt to manage the disease. The modalities often further complicate the disease with drug side effects and oftentimes bring in occultism, which becomes a block to healing. Many holistic practices are rooted in occultism.

This block is saying that you want your healing but you don't want to go through the right doorway to get it. You don't want to go the route of repentance and sanctification. You would rather put your trust in doctors and medicine as an attempt to bypass responsibility before God for the disease, which is a curse in your life.

**As the bird by wandering, as the swallow by flying, so the curse causeless shall not come. Proverbs 26:2**

Be in Health™ takes the position that proper medical care, including diagnosis, is highly recommended for everyone agreeing with this teaching. It should not be construed that I am against doctors and proper medical attention. This information is being offered as a spiritual insight to psychological and biological disease with regard to the etiology of various diseases and must be recognized in conjunction with the healing and/or prevention of these diseases.

## ☐ 31. Murmuring and Complaining

The thirty-first block to healing is *murmuring and complaining*. Look at Numbers 12:1–15 and read about Miriam's leprosy.

> 12:1**And Miriam and Aaron spake against Moses because of the Ethiopian woman whom he had married: for he had married an Ethiopian woman.** 2**And they said, Hath the LORD indeed spoken only by Moses? hath he not spoken also by us? And the LORD heard** *it.* 3**(Now the man Moses** *was* **very meek, above all the men which** *were* **upon the face of the earth.)...**10**And the cloud departed from off the tabernacle; and, behold, Miriam** *became* **leprous,** *white* **as snow: and Aaron looked upon Miriam, and, behold,** *she was* **leprous.** 11**And Aaron said unto Moses, Alas, my lord, I beseech thee, lay not the sin upon us, wherein we have done foolishly, and wherein we have sinned.** 12**Let her not be as one dead, of whom the flesh is half consumed when he cometh out of his mother's womb.** 13**And Moses cried unto the LORD, saying, Heal her now, O God, I beseech thee.** 14**And the LORD said unto Moses, If her father had but spit in her face, should she not be ashamed seven days? let her be shut out from the camp seven days, and after that let her be received in** *again.* 15**And Miriam was shut out from the camp seven days: and the people journeyed not till Miriam was brought in** *again.* **Numbers 12:1–3, 10–15**

First Corinthians10:10–11 warns us not to murmur as did those who murmured and were destroyed by serpents in the wilderness.

> 10**Neither murmur ye, as some of them also murmured, and were destroyed of the destroyer.** 11**Now all these things happened unto them for ensamples: and they are written for our admonition, upon whom the ends of the world are come. 1 Corinthians 10:10–11**

This was about the time of Aaron. Murmuring and complaining are signs of ungratefulness and will block God's movement in our lives.

In Philippians, Paul said:

> 14**Do all things without murmurings and disputings:** 15**That ye may be blameless and harmless, the sons of God, without rebuke, in the midst of a crooked and perverse nation, among whom ye shine as lights in the world; Philippians 2:14–15**

## ☐ 32. Hating and Not Obeying Instruction

The thirty-second block to healing is *hating and not obeying instruction.* Proverbs 5:11–14 says, And thou mourn at the last when thy flesh and thy body are consumed; and say how have I hated instruction and my heart despised reproof; I have not obeyed the voice of my teachers nor inclined mine ear to them that instructed me. I was almost in utter ruin in the midst of the congregation and assembly.

> ¹¹And thou mourn at the last, when thy flesh and thy body are consumed, ¹²And say, How have I hated instruction, and my heart despised reproof; ¹³And have not obeyed the voice of my teachers, nor inclined mine ear to them that instructed me! ¹⁴I was almost in all evil in the midst of the congregation and assembly. Proverbs 5:11–14

For example, this teaching has come to instruct you in righteousness so you may experience *a more excellent way*™.

In concluding this block to healing called *hating and not obeying instruction*, I would like to quote from Isaiah 28:8–19 and let the plumb line of God's conviction find its place in your heart. I suppose these verses sum up the entire problem of disease in the world and in the Church today.

> ⁸For all tables are full of vomit *and* filthiness, *so that there is* no place *clean.* ⁹Whom shall he teach knowledge? and whom shall he make to understand doctrine? *them that are* weaned from the milk, *and* drawn from the breasts. ¹⁰For precept *must be* upon precept, precept upon precept; line upon line, line upon line; here a little, *and* there a little: ¹¹For with stammering lips and another tongue will he speak to this people. ¹²To whom he said, This *is* the rest *wherewith* ye may cause the weary to rest; and this *is* the refreshing: yet they would not hear. ¹³But the word of the LORD was unto them precept upon precept, precept upon precept; line upon line, line upon line; here a little, *and* there a little; that they might go, and fall backward, and be broken, and snared, and taken. ¹⁴Wherefore hear the word of the LORD, ye scornful men, that rule this people which *is* in Jerusalem. ¹⁵Because ye have said, We have made a covenant with death, and with hell are we at agreement; when the overflowing scourge shall pass through, it shall not come unto us: for we have made lies our refuge, and under falsehood have we hid ourselves: ¹⁶Therefore thus saith the Lord GOD, Behold, I lay in Zion for a foundation a stone, a tried stone, a precious corner *stone*, a sure foundation: he that believeth shall not make haste. ¹⁷Judgment also will I lay to the line, and righteousness to the plummet: and the hail shall sweep away the refuge of lies, and the waters shall overflow the hiding place. ¹⁸And your covenant with death shall be disannulled, and your agreement with hell shall not stand; when the overflowing scourge shall pass through, then ye shall be trodden down by it. ¹⁹From the time that it goeth forth it shall take you: for morning by morning shall it pass over, by day and by night: and it shall be a vexation only to understand the report. Isaiah 28:8–19

## ☐ 33. Past and Continued Involvement with Occultism

*Past involvement and continued involvement in occultic practices*, thinking about modalities of healing and disease prevention not of God, may prevent healing.

Often, in following the various attempts by to help ourselves or heal ourselves, we may have opened ourselves up to occultic intrusion. It may be following a mind-set or action that is an abomination to God because these ways of thinking and actions do not even include Him and do not match His Word.

In fact, many times these philosophies, mind-sets and various activities are merely an attempt to bypass the penalty of the curse (which is the disease itself) without taking responsibility for the sin or spiritual defect causing the disease. It would be God's will for you to be sanctified in these areas and not managed or manipulated in your spirit, soul or body.

Psalm 90:12 says: So teach us to number our days that we may apply our hearts unto wisdom.

> **So teach us to number our days, that we may apply our hearts unto wisdom. Psalm 90:12**

Our knowledge and wisdom come from teaching that is based on the Word of God, not the study of creation such as the sun, moon and stars. God has given us the hours, days, months and years of time so in time (sometimes just in time) we may understand what He has said concerning our thoughts and actions and not what a diviner, astrologer, soothsayer, false prophet or prophetess has said about the past, present and future.

Even in the Church we have to be discerning in the application of the prophetic. Obedience is still better than sacrifice (1 Samuel 15:22). Sanctification and righteousness, including repentance from dead works (Hebrews 6:1), are still the foundation, not what the future holds.

Today is the day of salvation (2 Corinthians 6:2). Take no thought for tomorrow, for the evil of today is sufficient unto itself (Matthew 6:34). Future revelation does not replace obedience to past revelation. Yet in certain sectors, I see an attempt to produce a better future through declaration and prophetic revelation. Yet the problems these declarations and revelations are aimed at are the result of disobedience to past declarations and revelations of the Word. Recognition of this and repentance are in order, not more occultic motion to be gods unto ourselves in order to fix ourselves apart from repentance for sin.

When we exalt the wisdom of the gods (gods with a little "g" meaning the wisdom of this world or the doctrine of devils as referred to in the New Testament), insanity and mental confusion often come. Refer to Daniel 5:17–21 in regard to King Nebuchadnezzar and his insanity when he suggested he was a god. When King Saul obeyed the voice of men and not God, he consulted with a woman who had a familiar spirit and insanity came. When the Spirit of God departs, all man has left is his own tormented mind, or a spirit of insanity from the devil. The first evidence of this is fear and torment. First John 4:18 says fear has torment.

Occultism always projects a fear issue and the enemy's thoughts and mechanisms to seemingly solve the problem when, in fact, there is no real solution—just thoughts and actions and the accompanying torment going with it. You might say it is like a blind dog chasing his tail: always in motion, but no ending.

The first line of defense against occultism is knowing the Word of God. Perfect peace belongs to them whose minds are fixed on the LORD (Isaiah 26:3) and the LORD is the Word of God. Many of the occultic modalities out there may offer various forms of spirituality, but they are often missing the Word of God as a foundation. Then, when Scripture is used, it is used out of context; or worse, is used to manipulate or create future promises of blessing without any regard to righteousness, holiness and sanctification.

We are either establishing the kingdom of God in the earth, or we are establishing the kingdom of Satan through men.

Some observable characteristics of occult bondage and influence are:

Deep confusion
Hatred of God
Distrust of God
Inability to sleep, night torment, night terror
Hostility, aggression and conflict
Fear of authority
Fear of relationships
Impatience
Control of others
Suspicion
Frustration
Insanity
Depression
Oppression

Tormenting thoughts

Certain types of pain, especially in relationship to the central nervous system

Feelings of isolation

Out-of-body experiences

Feelings of accusation against others and one's self

Division makers and trouble makers

Fear

Obsessions

Inability to hear God's voice

Falling asleep in church

Falling asleep while reading the Bible

Rebellion

Stubbornness

Disobedience to God's Word (chronic activities)

Losing interest in attending church and reading God's Word

Inability to develop a prayer relationship with God

In conclusion, occultism always offers itself as the real thing from God when, in fact, the real thing is obscured and hidden.

Satan always wanted to be like the Most High God and will disguise himself in order to accommodate himself to men. The Scriptures say that Satan is the god of the world.

> **In whom the god of this world hath blinded the minds of them which believe not, lest the light of the glorious gospel of Christ, who is the image of God, should shine unto them. 2 Corinthians 4:4**

What I have given you are some ideas from the Word and some examples that should challenge you, because sometimes knowing the root is not always the only solution. Sometimes there is a block hindering your healing.

> *It is just as important to know the blocks to healing*
> *as it is to know the spiritual roots.*

## Chapter Ten
# Closing Remarks

Hopefully, your hearts are challenged by the insight of roots of disease and blocks to healing so in your lives you can come before God according to knowledge and not according to ignorance. Then the Holy Spirit can convict you and work with you, so your lives can be better lives because God is working in your midst according to knowledge and His good will may be performed in your lives. Amen.

As I finish my teaching, we are going to come together and come before the Lord. I am going to lead you in prayer and we are going to ask the Lord to do some things in your life.

I will read from Nehemiah 8 to prepare your hearts.

**8:1And all the people gathered themselves together as one man into the street that *was* before the water gate; and they spake unto Ezra the scribe to bring the book of the law of Moses, which the LORD had commanded to Israel. 2And Ezra the priest brought the law before the congregation both of men and women, and all that could hear with understanding, upon the first day of the seventh month. 3And he read therein before the street that *was* before the water gate from the morning until midday, before the men and the women, and those that could understand; and the ears of all the people *were attentive* unto the book of the law.**

**4And Ezra the scribe stood upon a pulpit of wood, which they had made for the purpose; and beside him stood Mattithiah, and Shema, and Anaiah, and Urijah, and Hilkiah, and Maaseiah, on his right hand; and on his left hand, Pedaiah, and Mishael, and Malchiah, and Hashum, and Hashbadana, Zechariah, *and* Meshullam. 5And Ezra opened the book in the sight of all the people; (for he was above all the people;) and when he opened it, all the people stood up: 6And Ezra blessed the LORD, the great God. And all the people answered, Amen, Amen, with lifting up their hands: and they bowed their heads, and worshipped the LORD with *their* faces to the ground. 7Also Jeshua, and Bani, and Sherebiah, Jamin, Akkub, Shabbethai, Hodijah, Maaseiah, Kelita, Azariah, Jozabad, Hanan, Pelaiah, and the Levites, caused the people to understand the law: and the people *stood* in their place.**

**8So they read in the book in the law of God distinctly, and gave the sense, and caused *them* to understand the reading. 9And Nehemiah, which *is* the Tirshatha, and Ezra the priest the scribe, and the Levites that taught the people, said unto all the people, This day *is* holy unto the LORD your God; mourn not, nor weep. For all the people wept, when they heard the words of the law.**

**10Then he said unto them, Go your way, eat the fat, and drink the sweet, and send portions unto them for whom nothing is prepared: for *this* day *is* holy unto our Lord: neither be ye sorry; for the joy of the LORD is**

**your strength. ¹¹So the Levites stilled all the people, saying, Hold your peace, for the day *is* holy; neither be ye grieved. ¹²And all the people went their way to eat, and to drink, and to send portions, and to make great mirth, because they had understood the words that were declared unto them. ¹³And on the second day were gathered together the chief of the fathers of all the people, the priests, and the Levites, unto Ezra the scribe, even to understand the words of the law. ¹⁴And they found written in the law which the LORD had commanded by Moses, that the children of Israel should dwell in booths in the feast of the seventh month: Nehemiah 8:1-14**

And it goes on…so now let's go to chapter 9, verse 2:

**²And the seed of Israel separated themselves from all strangers, and stood and confessed their sins, and the iniquities of their fathers. ³And they stood up in their place, and read in the book of the law of the LORD their God *one* fourth part of the day; and *another* fourth part they confessed, and worshipped the LORD their God. Nehemiah 9:2–3**

*This is what happens when conviction comes. We get the engrafted Word of God, we come before the Lord, we worship Him, our hearts are circumcised and we stand and take responsibility, not just for our sins, but for the failures of our ancestors.*

Why? So genetically inherited diseases can be canceled and the familiar spirits of our generations ruling us, in our soul, can also be defeated.

I want you to take whatever time you think is necessary for you personally. If you want to, get down on your knees or just sit quietly in your chair, if you want God to move in your life because of what we have been teaching. We have been giving you the Word and the understanding. If you want God to heal you and deliver you from something or to set something in motion so things will change in your life, if God is dealing with your heart, I want to take a little time here. I want you to come before the Lord. I want you to confess the areas you are dealing with. Then, if you see it in your family tree, I want you to bring it to the Lord and say, "Forgive my fathers also." When you have your little checklist done in your heart, then you will be done.

I want you to take this time now until you are finished. Then I will offer you a prayer…so I'll bring you into a prayer now. Then I am going to pray another prayer at the end of this discussion. I am going to ask God to honor you and to heal you right where you sit, corporately and individually.

This is what I see in 2 Chronicles 29 and 30—that after this was done, *the LORD heard the voice of Hezekiah and He honored the voice of Hezekiah and He healed the people.*

**⁵And said unto them, Hear me, ye Levites, sanctify now yourselves, and sanctify the house of the LORD God of your fathers, and carry forth the filthiness out of the holy *place.* ⁶For our fathers have trespassed, and**

done *that which was* evil in the eyes of the LORD our God, and have forsaken him, and have turned away their faces from the habitation of the LORD, and turned *their* backs....[10]Now *it is* in mine heart to make a covenant with the LORD God of Israel, that his fierce wrath may turn away from us....[15]And they gathered their brethren, and sanctified themselves, and came, according to the commandment of the king, by the words of the LORD, to cleanse the house of the LORD....[31]Then Hezekiah answered and said, Now ye have consecrated yourselves unto the LORD, come near and bring sacrifices and thank offerings into the house of the LORD. 2 Chronicles 29:5–6, 10, 15, 31

I am not Hezekiah; I am Henry. But I am going to ask the Lord to do this and match the integrity of your hearts. I am going to ask Him to heal you in the areas in which you are asking Him for healing and to set in motion those things that will bring the conviction necessary to get you out of the bondage and into a place of freedom.

Could we do that now, please? Let me pray…

*Father, I consider this a very sovereign time; I ask that You sanctify these people in the name of the Lord Jesus Christ, where they sit and as they come and where they're at.*

*I ask that You will meet them in the integrity of their hearts and as they come before You, having heard the Word of God, mixing it with their faith, I ask that You hear them and receive their petitions unto You and forgive them their trespasses and release them from the curse of their generations. I ask You this, Father, in the name of our precious Savior, our Lord Jesus Christ, as the work of the Holy Spirit, I release it, Amen. Thank You, Father.*

*Lord, hear our hearts; hear our prayers and receive us. Hide not Thy face from us. Forgive us; release us from the sins of our fathers; forgive us of our sins and our trespasses as we forgive those who trespass against us. Lord, heal us; heal our families. Save us, O God; save our families. We pray for our enemies and those who spitefully use us. Lord, regard not the iniquities of Your people. May Your mercy and Your grace overshadow us. Heal us personally. Heal our marriages; heal our children. Heal our churches. Heal our political leaders. Heal our nation. God, let Your salvation be spread to the islands of the sea from the rising of the sun to the setting of the sun. Let the earth be filled with the knowledge of the living God. God, we pray that this planet shall be inhabited in righteousness. Let Your Spirit move in our midst; convict us of sin; deliver us from all evil. Heal our land.*

*Father, I thank You for being in our midst. Lord, be Lord of our hearts. We are Your people, the sheep of Your pasture. Your mercy endureth forever. Blessed be the Name of the Lord. Thank You, Father. Hear our prayer, O*

*God. Send Your Spirit. Thank You, Father. We give You thanksgiving, Lord; we have not made ourselves, but You have made us. You are He that forgiveth us of all our iniquities and You are He that healeth us of all our diseases. You are He that daily loadeth us with benefits; yeah, even the Elohiym of our salvation. Lead us not into temptation, but deliver us from evil.*

*Thank You, Father. In Jesus' name, Amen.*

Did you make some peace with God in your private time? Good!

I'm going to bring this teaching to a close with a Scripture and then I'm going to pray. Then we'll be finished. Read this passage from 2 Chronicles 30:15–20:

> **¹⁵Then they killed the passover on the fourteenth *day* of the second month: and the priests and the Levites were ashamed, and sanctified themselves, and brought in the burnt offerings into the house of the LORD. ¹⁶And they stood in their place after their manner, according to the law of Moses the man of God: the priests sprinkled the blood, *which they received* of the hand of the Levites. ¹⁷For *there were* many in the congregation that were not sanctified: therefore the Levites had the charge of the killing of the passovers for every one *that was* not clean, to sanctify *them* unto the LORD. ¹⁸For a multitude of the people, *even* many of Ephraim, and Manasseh, Issachar, and Zebulun, had not cleansed themselves, yet did they eat the passover otherwise than it was written.**
>
> **But Hezekiah prayed for them, saying, The good LORD pardon every one ¹⁹*That* prepareth his heart to seek God, the LORD God of his fathers, though *he be* not *cleansed* according to the purification of the sanctuary.**
>
> **²⁰And the LORD hearkened to Hezekiah, and healed the people. 2 Chronicles 30:15–20**

This is a powerful Scripture about God's love, not just in the area of total sanctification, but in the area of partial sanctification. God pardoned them and healed them. These Scriptures really affect me. So now I am going to pray. I believe everyone is very sincere. I trust you have believing hearts and are expecting. So I am going to ask God to meet you at whatever and wherever it is possible for Him to do this in conjunction with Who He is.

I am going to ask God to meet you in your life (spirit, soul and body) and for the many things you are believing in for your life. He will then make them start coming to pass. Even now, many of the oppressions and depressions and many of the things you are dealing with will start to change.

I have to believe this, because it is in the Word.

*Father, I stand before You and I sanctify myself before You. God, I repent for my failures and my sins and for the sins of my ancestors. God, in my uncleansed state, I tell You that I love You and by faith I accept Your provision in my life and the work of the Holy Spirit of sanctification in my life. And, God, as I represent You to the best of my ability, I ask that as in the days of Hezekiah, that You will hear from heaven and You will heal.*

*Father, I come to You in the name of the Lord Jesus Christ and I ask that You be a Father to the people reading this book. These are Your children; these are the sheep of Your pasture; these are those who have been called by Your name, sanctified and set aside for You forever. God, I know that You are on the throne. I know that You sit high above all things, that You look down to see that we do understand. God, we understand and we seek Your face and Your mercy and Your person in our lives, our families and in every area of our lives. So, God, right now I pray that as these people have come before You, that You will come before them and that You will meet them, every one, according to Your good pleasure through the work of the Holy Spirit.*

*I pray this in the name of the Lord Jesus Christ. Amen.*

# Bibliography

Anderson, Dr. Neil T. and Dr. Michael Jacobson. *The Biblical Guide to Alternative Medicine*. Ventura, CA: Regal Books, 2003.

"Danger in the Diet Pills?" *Time*, July 21, 1997.

"Deadly Rx: Why are drugs killing so many patients?" *USA Today*, April 24, 1998.

"Greater Expectations," *Newsweek*, September 24, 1990.

"Hormonal Reaction to Stress Tied to Disease, Researchers Say." *Dallas Morning News*, November 16, 1996.

Jones, E. Stanley. *The Unshakeable Kingdom and the Unchanging Person*. 1972, reprinted 1995.

McCance, Kathryn L. and Sue E. Huether. *Pathophysiology: The Biologic Basis for Disease in Adults and Children*. Mosby, 2nd edition, 1994.

*Merck Manual*. Rahway, NJ: Merck & Co., 16th edition, 1992.

Miller, Claudia S. and Nicholas A. Ashford. *Possible Mechanisms for Multiple Chemical Sensitivity*. http://www.ul.cs.cmu.edu/books/multiple_chem/mult143.htm

"Mysteries of Stress Probed." *Houston Chronicle*, May 28, 1998.

*Physician's Desk Reference*. Medical Economics Company, 55th edition, 2001.

Strong, James. *The Exhaustive Concordance of the Bible*. Hendrickson Publishers.

"The Power to Heal." *Newsweek*, September 24, 1990.

Tortora, Gerard J. and Nicholas P. Anagnostakos. *Principles of Anatomy & Physiology*. Harper & Row, 2nd edition, 1978.

"When Drugs Do Harm." *Newsweek*, April 27, 1998.

# Glossary of Medical Terms

This is not intended to be a comprehensive glossary. Rather, it is a supplement to the definitions that are already included in *A More Excellent Way*™.

Adrenal Cortex: The outer portion of the adrenal gland located on top of each kidney. The adrenal cortex produces steroid hormones that regulate carbohydrate and fat metabolism and mineralocorticoid hormones that regulate salt and water balance in the body.

Adrenal Gland: One of a pair of small glands, each of which sits on top of one of the kidneys. The adrenal gland is made up of an outer wall (the cortex) and an inner portion (the medulla). The adrenal glands produce hormones that help control the heart rate, blood pressure, the way the body uses food and other vital functions.

Adrenal Medulla: The adrenal medulla makes adrenaline and noradrenaline.

Adrenaline: A hormone secreted by the adrenal gland in response to low blood levels of glucose and to exercise and stress; it causes the breakdown of the storage product glycogen to glucose in the liver.

Alveoli: Tiny air sacs located at the very ends of the bronchioles within the lungs. The exchange of gases (oxygen and carbon dioxide) takes place in the alveoli.

Amygdala: A gland located in the brain's medial temporal lobe. It is believed to have strong connections to the mental and emotional reactions of the person. It is linked to fear responses and nervous reactions. Conditions such as autism, depression and OCD are also suspected of being linked to the amygdala.

Amenorrhea: Absence or cessation of menstruation.

Anaphylactic Toxic Reaction: A response to an allergen that the immune system has become sensitized to over a period of time. A person may experience flushing (warmth and redness of the skin), itching (often in the groin or armpits) and hives, which are common initial findings. Throat and tongue swelling resulting in hoarseness, difficulty swallowing and difficulty breathing frequently follow. Vomiting, diarrhea and stomach cramps may develop.

Aneurysm: An aneurysm is a localized widening of an artery, vein or the heart. At the area of an aneurysm, there is typically a bulge and the wall is weakened and may rupture.

Anterior Pituitary: The front portion of the pituitary, a small gland in the head, called the master gland. Hormones secreted by the anterior pituitary influence growth, sexual development, skin pigmentation, thyroid function and adrenocortical function.

Autoimmune Disease: An illness that occurs when the body tissues are attacked by the body's immune system. The immune system is a complex organization within the body that is designed normally to "seek and destroy" invaders of the body, including infectious agents. Patients with autoimmune diseases frequently have unusual antibodies circulating in their blood that target their own body tissues.

Catecholamine: These include epinephrine (adrenaline), norepinephrine (noradrenaline) and dopamine, which act as hormones or neurotransmitters.

Cortisol: A steroid hormone produced by adrenal cortex, the primary stress hormone.

Dopamine: An important neurotransmitter (messenger) in the brain; a precursor (forerunner) of adrenaline and noradrenaline.

Epinephrine: Adrenaline is a synonym of epinephrine.

Genitourinary (GU): Pertaining to the genital and urinary systems.

Glycogen: Considered to be the principal storage form of glucose (carbohydrates) and is stored mainly in liver and muscle.

Gluconeogenesis: The formation of glycogen in the liver from non-carbohydrate sources such as fats and proteins, amino acids and lactate.

Glycogenolysis: This is the process in which glycogen is broken down into glucose to form either pyruvic acid or lactic acid.

Hippocampus: An area buried deep in the forebrain that is associated with the regulation of emotions and the transfer of information from short-term memory to long-term memory. Helps regulate emotion and memory.

Limbic System: A group of brain structures, in particular the hippocampus and amygdala, that govern emotions and behavior involved in several emotions such as aggression, fear, pleasure and the formation of long-term memory. It is closely associated with the sense of smell. It affects both the endocrine system and the autonomic nervous system.

Lymph: A clear-to-white fluid that bathes the tissues and is transported through a network of lymph nodes and lymph ducts. It contains some proteins and fats, some red blood cells and many white blood cells, especially lymphocytes.

Lymphatic system: A complex circulatory system composed of a network of organs, lymph nodes, lymph ducts and lymph vessels that produce and transport lymph from tissues to the bloodstream. The lymphatic system is a major part of the body's immune system.

Macrophage: A type of white blood cell that ingests (takes in) foreign material. Macrophages are key players in the immune response to foreign invaders such as infectious microorganisms.

Neurotransmitter: A substance such as epinephrine or acetylcholine that transmits nerve impulses across a synapse to another nerve, muscle or gland. A neurotransmitter is a messenger of neurological information from one cell to another.

Noradrenaline: A hormone secreted by the adrenal medulla; it also serves as a neurotransmitter. It is a precursor of epinephrine in the body.

Serotonin: A hormone produced in the pineal gland and found in blood platelets, the digestive tract and the brain. It is both a neurotransmitter and a powerful vasoconstrictor.

Vasoconstriction: Narrowing of the diameter of blood vessels, especially as a result of vasomotor action.

Vasodilation: Widening of the diameter of blood vessels.

## Appendix A
# Walking Out to Wholeness

Now that you've finished reading *A More Excellent Way™*, it is time to apply it to your life. We call this application process Walk Out. There won't be time for a dress rehearsal or a test drive. This is real life. Issues will come up. Challenges will knock on your door. Choices will have to be made. But now you have tools.

In *A More Excellent Way™*, you were introduced to the 8 Rs to Freedom. The first step, the first R, is to **Recognize**. Once you have recognized the "issues" in your life, then you can do one of two things:

1.  Fall back into a comfort zone of denial, or

2.  Step out and deal with them.

Yes, thoughts and behaviors can be changed. Psychologists say that it takes weeks or even months to break a habit. So give God a little time to work on you. As you renew your mind, He will renew you! When issues come up and check you out, your renewed mind will be tested. Will you react the way you have always reacted in the past or will the mind of Christ be revealed in your actions?

Walk Out is simply the process of renewing your mind. It is making God's mindset your own. You must walk away from those old, instilled habits. You must walk out of old, ungodly ways of thinking—and into new, godly ones.

**And be renewed in the spirit of your mind; Ephesians 4:23**

## You Are Not Alone

It is true that not all of us live in a perfect, Norman Rockwell family. The more stressed and harried your life may be, the more you will need to employ these simple steps. Your world may not seem quite as safe and supportive as you would want it to be. This is okay! You may now find yourself on your own in your beliefs and have no one who understands the new things you have just learned. This is normal. You may even ask yourself, "How am I ever going to do this alone?"

Well, you are never alone. The living God is with you. This is as "un-alone" as you can get. God's Word is always true; He will guide you in your thinking and behavior.

## Give Yourself Time

This is not a quick fix; it is for the long haul! As you walk out, you will replace wrong thoughts, behaviors and habits with godly ones. It may take weeks or even months to firmly establish new habits. As you appropriate your freedom day by day, your obedience will create new long-term memory patterns of righteous behavior.

Remember to get your self-worth from God and His Word—not from other people and their evaluations.

## Take Every Thought Captive

How does one handle ungodly thoughts such as doubt, unbelief, self-hatred, addictions or behaviors? By holding every thought captive!

✓ Recognize the thought for what it is—**temptation**.

✓ Temptation is not sin; it is only Satan's kingdom checking you out.

✓ Take that thought captive and cast it out of your mind before it becomes your sin.

For example, someone throws fiery darts at you because of your child-rearing skills. You are tempted right away to get angry and throw some fiery darts back at them. You could be tempted to take offense and feel rejected. You could feel guilty and ashamed. You could get into strife with the other person. So you now have a decision to make.

You can say to yourself, "I know this is the enemy tempting me. God's Word says I should not sin in my anger. I won't go there anymore! I know the Bible says I should cast down any imagination that does not agree with God's Word."

> **Casting down imaginations, and every high thing that exalteth itself against the knowledge of God, and bringing into captivity every thought to the obedience of Christ; 2 Corinthians 10:5**

> **For the word of God is quick, and powerful, and sharper than any twoedged sword, piercing even to the dividing asunder of soul and spirit, and of the joints and marrow, and *is* a discerner of the thoughts and intents of the heart. ¹³ Neither is there any creature that is not manifest in his sight: but all things *are* naked and opened unto the eyes of him with whom we have to do. Hebrews 4:12–13**

## Know the Tricks of the Enemy

Remember separation. Those thoughts may not be coming from you! Something may be trying to gain access to your spirit, coaxing you to accept its lies. It would try anything to convince you these thoughts are just your own innocent ideas! Beware! Recognize the source.

## What Do I Do If I Fail?

Remember, the Holy Spirit brings conviction. Guilt and condemnation come from the enemy.

Confess your sins to God and to one another so the sin may be exposed and forgiven. Thus, it will no longer have a hold over you. Then, hold your head high and walk in the light of God.

### Apply the "8 Rs to Freedom"

1. **Recognize** an issue in your life that is not from God.

2. Take **Responsibility** for what you have recognized. Don't blame God or anyone else.

3. **Repent** for your participation with the enemy and the problem you have recognized.

4. **Renounce.** Fall completely out of agreement with your sin.

5. **Remove** the sin from your life. Cast it out.

6. **Resist.** Draw nigh to God and resist it coming back. Absolutely refuse to get involved with the sin. Flee from and resist evil temptation.

7. **Rejoice.** Give thanks to God for your freedom.

8. **Restore.** Help to restore others held captive.

## What Do I Do if I Do Not Receive the Healing I Expected?

Prayerfully consider:

1. Consider whether your confession was just mental assent or whether you really have turned your heart away from those things you confessed as sin.

2. Consider the "**Spiritual Blocks to Healing**" in *A More Excellent Way*™.

3. It just may not be God's timing for you. He knows what healing would be appropriate for you and at what pace.

4. Seek help from a trusted godly friend, pastor or family member from whom you will accept the truth. Keep in mind it may be difficult to discern things in yourself.

## How Do I Continue to Walk in Victory in the Light of Christ?

1. **Keep your house filled** with the Word of God and praise and worship. Strengthen your relationship with the Godhead.

   **That he might sanctify and cleanse it with the washing of water by the word. Ephesians 5:26**

2. **Fellowship with other Christians.** You may have to reevaluate some of your old relationships. Establish fellowship with positive, likeminded people in your area.

   **And they continued steadfastly in the apostles' doctrine and fellowship, and in breaking of bread, and in prayers. Acts 2:42**

3. **Hold every thought captive.** Discern good from evil. Separate lies (even from a loved one) from God's truth. Replace the lies of the enemy with the Word of God. The battle starts in your mind.

   **⁴For though we walk in the flesh, we do not war after the flesh: ⁴(For the weapons of our warfare _are_ not carnal, but mighty through God to the pulling down of strong holds;) ⁵Casting down imaginations, and every high thing that exalteth itself against the knowledge of God, and bringing into captivity every thought to the obedience of Christ; ⁶And having in a readiness to revenge all disobedience, when your obedience is fulfilled. 2 Corinthians 10:4–6**

4. **Dwell on godly thoughts and promises.** Reflect on things with virtue and praise and thanksgiving. Think about positive things.

   **Finally, brethren, whatsoever things are true, whatsoever things _are_ honest, whatsoever things _are_ just, whatsoever things _are_ pure, whatsoever things _are_ lovely, whatsoever things _are_ of good report; if _there be_ any virtue, and if _there be_ any praise, think on these things. Philippians 4:8**

5. **Quit thinking about the past.** Let go of past failures and traumas. Self-pity is the superglue of hell that ties you to the past. Keep your mind on God.

   **..._this_ one thing _I do,_ forgetting those things which are behind, and reaching forth unto those things which are before, Philippians 3:13**

6. **Guard your heart.** Guard against doubt, unbelief, discouragement and despair. Have patience. God's timing and ways are perfect.

   **Keep your heart with all diligence; for out of it are the issues of life. Proverbs 4:23**

7. **Have faith in God.** Without faith it is impossible to please Him. Believe God's Word, no matter what we see in natural circumstances.

   **For we walk by faith, not by sight. 2 Corinthians 5:7**

8. **Watch your mouth!** Your words today will create your life tomorrow. If it is not godly, don't say it. The tongue determines life or death.

> **6**And the tongue *is* a fire, a world of iniquity: so is the tongue among our members, that it defileth the whole body, and setteth on fire the course of nature; and it is set on fire of hell....**8**But the tongue can no man tame; *it is* an unruly evil, full of deadly poison. James 3:6, 8

9.  **Guard your eyes and ears.** Your eyes are the windows to your soul. Be careful of what you see and hear. Be selective of movies, television programs and books. Be very discerning about what kind of music and radio programs you listen to.

> **15**He that walketh righteously and speaketh uprightly; he that despiseth the gain of oppressions, that shaketh his hands from holding of bribes, that stoppeth his ears from hearing of blood and shuteth his eyes from seeing evil; he shall dwell on high... Isaiah 33:15–16

10. **Separate people from their sin.** Observe their actions without judging them.

> Judge not, that ye be not judged. Matthew 7:1

11. **Indecision leads to ungodliness.** Choose God in everything. Decide to be in peace.

> A double-minded man is unstable in all his ways. James 1:8

12. **Be willing to go into the fire** (see Daniel 3). The battle is in the fire. Stop making an idol of illness or programmed behavior. Face your fears and stressors in order to overcome them.

> Stand fast therefore in the liberty wherewith Christ hath made us free, and be not entangled again with the yoke of bondage. Galatians 5:1

13. **Remember, all good things come from God.**

> Every good gift and every perfect gift is from above, and cometh down from the Father of lights, with whom is no variableness, neither shadow of turning. James 1:17

## MY WALK OUT

This section is a handy reference to reclaiming your life and lands. Use it as often as you need.

## Ministry Prayer Model

Here is a sample prayer that you can use to converse with God the Father when you recognize a need for His cleansing and healing from sin in your life.

1.  **RECOGNIZE**—Recognize the sin issue participated with or connected to the disease.

**Note:** It is important to determine if the sin issue has been connected to the disease and, in fact, a spiritual dimension the person actually struggles with. If you are ministering, check with leaders you trust and consult the insights of Be in Health™.

*Person being ministered to says:*

Father God, I come to You in the name of Jesus. I recognize I have participated with this sin of (_____) in my life. [If you recognize your family line has served the same sin,] I recognize my generations have served this sin of (_____) also.

2. **RESPONSIBILITY**—Take responsibility with God the Father.

*Person being ministered to says:*

Father, I take responsibility for participating with and serving this sin of (_____) in my life.

3. **REPENT**—Repent to the Father in the name of Jesus and ask for forgiveness.

**Note:** Block to healing (Mark 11:26)—take time to remember, forgive and release those who have sinned against you, so you may be forgiven and released by God the Father.

*Person being ministered to says:*

Father, I confess my sin and the iniquities of my fathers. In the name of Jesus, I repent to You and ask You to forgive me for allowing this sin of (_____) to manifest through me. I also forgive all persons, living or dead, who have injured me or spoken evil toward me. I forgive them, so I also may be forgiven. By faith and in the name of Jesus, I now receive Your forgiveness, Father and ask to be released from the power of this sin over my life.

4. **RENOUNCE**—Take a stand against the sin you have recognized.

*Person being ministered to says:*

Sin of (_____), I renounce everything you stand for in my life. I will no longer serve you. I take a stand against you and everything you represent. I will discern you and help others discern you all of my days.

5. **REMOVE**—Remove the sin having been recognized, repented for and renounced.

*Person being ministered to says:*

Sin (spirit of_____), I have repented to my Father in heaven for serving you and allowing you to manifest through me. You must leave me and go into a dry place now in the name of Jesus. Now go.

*Person doing the ministry now says:*

Sin (spirit of_____), you heard their confession and declaration. You have to obey them in the name of Jesus. Spirit of (_____), go from this person in the name of Jesus.

## Specific Ministry Applications

**Note:**   Ministry to others differs in three locations:

1. Spirit

2. Soul

3. Body

Involving three different gifts of the Holy Spirit:

1. Discerning of spirits/casting them out

2. Gift of healing

3. Gift of miracles

### 1.  DISCERNING OF SPIRITS/CASTING OUT

*Person doing the ministry says:*

Spirit of (_____), I take authority over you in the name of Jesus and command you to leave this person now. You no longer have permission to stay and must leave.

**Note:** You don't lay on hands to cast out evil spirits. You calmly speak to them with authority to leave. Shouting is not necessary. They hear you very well.

### 2.  MINISTERING WITH GIFT OF HEALING

*Person doing the ministry says:*

In the name of Jesus, I speak healing to this body part (_____) that is diseased and command it to be restored.

**Note:** The ministry of healing is by the laying on of hands.

3.  **MINISTERING WITH THE GIFT OF MIRACLES**

*Person doing the ministry says:*

God has placed workers of miracles in the Church so, in accordance with Scripture, calling those things that are not as if they were and in the name of Jesus, I speak this body part (_____) into existence. Body part (_____) be formed as you were in Christ Jesus from the foundation of the world.

**Note:** Ministry of miracles is by speaking the body parts into existence, not by laying on of hands, although there is evidence Jesus and the apostles did it either way.

**Note:** Some body parts do not heal; that is why they have organ transplants. In these cases, the person ministering must minister in the gift of miracles. Examples include the following:

1.  Organs
2.  Brain tissue
3.  Nerve tissue
4.  Accident and injury malformations
5.  Birth defects

# MY PERSONAL STORY OF FREEDOM

The major issues of bondage in my life that I have identified were:
(check ✓ appropriate boxes)

- ❏ Bitterness
- ❏ Occultism
- ❏ Unloving Spirits
- ❏ Accusation
- ❏ Envy/Jealousy
- ❏ Addictions
- ❏ Rejection
- ❏ Doorpoints & Traumas
- ❏ Fear
- ❏ Blocks to Healing

I gained the most freedom from:

_____

_____

_____

The following issues still require attention:

_____

_____

_____

_____

## Walk Out Diary

A daily diary is a useful tool in your ministry of Walk Out. The following are elements that you might address each day when you face temptation.

## My Sin Issues

Here are some sin issues that have been identified in my life. I have to defeat the following issues: (check ✓ appropriate boxes)

| | | |
|---|---|---|
| ❏ Bitterness | ❏ Occultism | ❏ Unloving Spirits |
| ❏ Accusation | ❏ Envy/Jealousy | ❏ Addictions |
| ❏ Rejection | ❏ Doorpoints & Traumas | ❏ Fear |
| ❏ Blocks to Healing | | |

## Separation

In order to conquer these issues, I have to train myself to recognize them for what they are. In order to do this, I need to separate myself from anything that may establish the kingdom of evil through me (doorpoints), so my true identity in Christ is established.

## How Will I Recognize These Issues?

It may come to me as thoughts like these: (Remember, these are *lies*!)

- ❏ I hate you!
- ❏ You will never hurt me again.
- ❏ I wish you were dead.
- ❏ I will remember this forever!
- ❏ I am anxious about…
- ❏ If only I could be more like…
- ❏ I can do this better than you.
- ❏ What if…
- ❏ I am not worthy.
- ❏ I do not belong here.
- ❏ Do it my way or the highway.
- ❏ She does not like me…
- ❏ I must be perfect.

❑   I must have everyone's love and approval.

❑   My happiness comes from what I own and who loves me.

❑   Life is so unfair.

❑   If only other people would behave differently, I could be happy.

❑   My emotions and feelings are always right.

❑   My past will predict my future.

❑   I cannot admit that I was wrong.

❑   If those people would like me, I would be happy.

❑   My financial wealth and my material belongings define my self-worth.

And many other examples.

## Additional Help on Changing Habits and Thoughts

What is the habit or thought I want to change?

_____

_____

_____

Why do I entertain this habit or thought?

_____

_____

_____

When does it happen?

_____

_____

When did it start?

_____

_____

What is the godly alternative?

_____

_____

What is the lie I believed?

_____

_____

When you allow yourself to believe lies, your reactions to the world will be inappropriate and unhealthy.

## Notes to Reflect On

What were some sinful thoughts that came to me today?

_____

_____

_____

What did I do when I recognized them?

_____

_____

_____

What else do I need to do in order to renew my mind?

_____

_____

_____

What can I do to line up with God's Word about myself?

*Let God define who I am—not other people's opinions or my performance.*

_____

_____

What can I do to be in fellowship with others today?

*Avoid speaking criticism.*

_____

_____

What can I do to be in fellowship with the Godhead today?

Scripture:

_____

Action:

_____

*Papa, I love you!*

What am I grateful and thankful to the Lord for today?

*Reviewing your "praise list" builds up your faith.*

_____

_____

_____

_____

## I Yielded to the Temptation of Sin Today. What Do I Do Now?

☐ Apply the 8 Rs.

☐ Recognize guilt and condemnation wants to keep you from victory. A mistake is painful enough without creating further injury with emotional self-abuse and unforgiveness.

☐ Confess your faults one to another.

## Do I Need To Speak with a Trusted Friend Today?

☐ Yes, I desperately need help.

☐ I think I can make it another day.

☐ No, I am doing okay and I can speak to God, today and every day.

## Appendix B
# Testimonies

*Please note that Pleasant Valley Church, referred to many times in the following testimonies, has since been renamed Hope of the Generations Church.*

One of the most exciting benefits of working in the ministry at Be in Health™ is witnessing the dramatic changes in people's lives as they encounter the living God and receive His healing. True freedom comes only when we choose to love God by obeying His commandments.

We receive a constant flow of testimonies as to how He has touched lives in wondrous ways. Be in Health™ ministers to people from all around the world. Over the past year alone, several thousand have come for ministry, representing over 500 different disease diagnoses. While here, they are instructed in godly principles of health and disease prevention and are given tools to walk in righteousness. Many are healed physically and emotionally. And after that, they cannot keep quiet about God's loving touch.

Many more, who have never been to our campus, have applied the principles of *A More Excellent Way*™ and/or our tape series and received God's healing. It has been the truth alone that has made them free! Here is a sampling of their stories. Just read along and marvel with us at the goodness of God!

### *Testimony from Children's FML Program*

We just returned from the For My Life™ for Children program. Someone ministered to our daughter who is 11. Our 4-year-old was back home. Both girls have anxiety and fear, and I have fear and obsessive compulsive *tendencies*. (We are choosing that word because we are breaking the roots and habits daily with our 8 Rs and don't want to claim them as *traits* any longer.) There *was* occult, matriarchal control and freemasonry in our families.

Our little one also experienced the same kind of responses to fear and stress as mentioned. She has always been like a piece of Velcro on me. She was very afraid around meal time because of all the family food allergies.

So, the minister encouraged me to allow my husband to have his role as the spiritual head of our home. She encouraged him to take his place. She also encouraged him to read Psalm 91 over them while they are in bed during bedtime prayers. He has and, Praise God, she is able to walk through the house alone even if it means that she has to turn a light on in a place she is entering. She is eating again as we pray "Father God, we receive this food to bless our bodies in Jesus' name." No more night terrors or coming into our room in the middle of the night to sleep on our floor. No more Velcro.

We also began reading the Bible together as a family each day (mostly). I read Bible truths to her during the day, and when she talks about her fears, we try to stop, find a Scripture and counter the fear. We are home schooling much differently now.

We have *all* noticed that as he [my husband] has been in the word everyday by himself and taken over *most* of the burdens that I used to do… (He went to work and threw out the garbage and took care of the garage and outside… I did everything else and home schooled the girls) that he is happier and we are all a lot less stressed. I do think that once OUR home got into godly order, the girls could rest and not manifest with fear, stress and anxiety. He is also the go-to guy for them now, even if he is at work. It is an amazing transformation.

Secure, happy (not perfect) children; so much better than high strung, high maintenance, fearful children. Thank you, Father. Thank you everyone at Be in Health™. We would have never been able to do this without your help.

D.

## *Delivered of Seizures!*

7000 Project Journal Brings Healing and Relief. I wanted to share a success story regarding the Journal article on psychogenic seizures.

I was ministering to an individual who was walking out fear issues and the associated diseases that the enemy had put upon him. I received the Journal on seizures and was able to sit down with this individual and go through the article. The scientific and medical information lined up to what his doctors had been telling him. The doctors, however, had no hope for him or any answers as to whether his seizures were from electrical brain activity or not. They also told him that they could not offer any treatment options for him as they did not know the cause of his seizures.

He found victory and revelation in the journal article because he read that the type of seizures he was experiencing can be the result of past traumas. He recalled that before he had a seizure, he had thoughts of his past failures and unworthiness ruminating in his mind. These thoughts were lies coming from the enemy, and he believed these lies were true about himself.

Through this article, he was able to recognize that:

The thoughts were not true.
The thoughts were from the enemy.
He had the power to take every thought captive and not agree with it.
He could do the 8 Rs and take his life back with God.
His brain was fine and he could continue to think and function without fear.
There was hope for his future, as he had answers and a solution and a new found sense of love, power and a sound mind coming from the Godhead.

God has done a powerful work in this individual's life. This man has gained freedom from fear in the areas of: leaving his home, driving, going to public places in confidence, speaking to others without fear, and looking toward his future with hope and faith in his Father to take care of him. He calls God his best friend and has told me that he has never felt better physically, mentally, and emotionally in his life.

Praise God for patiently loving us, guiding us, and watching over us as we learn to recognize, renounce, repent, cast out, and take back our lives. We CAN grow and walk with Him out of our fears and insecurities and into His hope, truth and blessings.

Thank you to all who work so hard to put these resources together that help bring understanding of God's truth and healing. I am so appreciative to see people take back what the enemy has stolen from them and line up with what God says about them. Yea, Papa God!

B.

## Healed of MCS/EI and Chronic Fatigue Syndrome

I went to the Be in Health™ For My Life™ Program in January of 2005. I was healed by applying the principles they taught me and am writing this testimony almost four years later—still healed, still applying these principles in my life and thriving more and more with God.

When I went to FML, I had been severely ill for ten years. I had been bedridden for about 80% of the previous five years from Chronic Fatigue and had been almost totally housebound for several years due to MCS/EI. I also had Fibromyalgia, liver problems, insomnia, food allergies and 12 other conditions that were diagnosable but untreatable by the medical community.

I hadn't been in public in 1½ years without a carbon mask to protect me from chemicals. I had stopped going to friend's houses and church long before due to chemical exposures. On the rare occasion I did go somewhere, I needed to be pushed in a wheelchair to keep from exhausting myself. We had a big sign on our front door that said, "STOP! DO NOT ENTER!" We lived in our bedroom. We tore all the carpets up, we had an old bed. I spent the summer of 2004 lying on a bed outdoors in a pasture in the wilderness trying to prolong my life.

I had tried many different medical treatments—just about everything that was out there. I have a very generous mother who funded trips to Greece and Mexico and other places in this country to try to get me help. But I just got worse and worse and worse and worse. The doctors didn't know why I was failing, and they had nothing to offer.

At one time, from an exposure, I lost the use of the right side of my body for several days. I really went down physically, and we were pretty convinced that I was going to die. That was when I had the most peace because I thought I would finally get to go home and be with God and I would be done suffering. When I rallied physically a little and I really went into a depression; that was "it"; I gave up.

All during the decade of illness, I went through tremendous ups and downs: hope and no hope, faith and no faith. What it did to me emotionally and spiritually was devastating. I would read the Word, and the Word was so clear that God heals, but I was just getting sicker and sicker.

I tried all sorts of approaches to healing: medical, alternative and everything that you do when you really believe God and you have a heart for God. I went to all sorts of churches, I was prayed for and was anointed with oil, went to the healing rooms. I prayed and I stood, claimed and trusted. I pushed every button, pulled every lever. I tried every single thing that I could think of. I would read the Word and it was so clear, God's hope and His peace were right there in the Scriptures and I couldn't get a hold of it. I just kept thinking, "What is wrong with me?" I would talk with other people who had a lot of faith and I would think, "Well, I'm just a failure. I'm an absolute utter failure as a Christian, obviously, or I would have been healed by now." I knew that God wanted me perfectly healed, but I could not figure out how to grab a hold of it.

I tried everything that was out there.

And then eventually I just gave up and went into self-pity and stayed there a long time. I was not a happy camper and I was not a good friend. I was not a good wife. I was miserable and I was making everybody else miserable around me because I was really feeling sorry for myself. I was so confused in my faith about why I couldn't get through and find healing.

During all those years there was a driving need inside me to understand why I was sick—but we have an enemy. He misquotes Scriptures and he misuses the Word of God; especially when we're in places of pain. He did it to Jesus in the wilderness, and he's been doing it to human beings since the beginning. He did it to me, and he helped me try to rewrite my theology to match my experience.

I was really trying to understand how God could be responsible for my illness yet still be a loving God. I came up with some different theologies and tried these on for years on end, searching the Scriptures and reading other people's theologies and trying to find peace in them.

One that I tried on was that I was suffering for eternal purposes, to be more like Christ, and my suffering would make me more obedient and it would mold me and shape me, and His grace would be sufficient for me. But that led me into torment about trusting God.

Another one that I tried on was that this was just a trial. I would come to the end of it and I would be stronger as a Christian. But since this trial wasn't a trial from God at all and in many ways it made me a weaker Christian by destroying my faith in God, that one didn't hold water.

As a Christian, if you blame God (which I did), everyone gets all nervous and accuses you of not having faith! So I figured it must be my fault and that my problem was that I didn't have enough faith…and I was told by well meaning Christians that I just needed more faith and that's why I hadn't been healed.

Underneath all of this trying to find an answer, I was feeling condemned and worthless and wondering, "Why don't I qualify for God's healing? What is wrong with me?" I knew that His mercy was great but I couldn't figure out what I was doing wrong to be missing out on it. Eventually I pretty much gave up on God on the daily level of faith and love and trusting Him. And I certainly did not believe that He was a loving Father. I couldn't understand why He was doing this to me. Pastor Henry says, "To be prayed for and not healed is a staggering attack on our faith; it's a staggering attack on our trust in the living God." I found that to be so true.

Really I was trying to figure out if my illness was my fault or God's fault. These theologies were very insidious lies that the enemy was bringing to me to "help" me understand my life. Those lies were either blaming God or they were blaming me. The truth is that my illness was a curse being brought on me by the enemy. God was not the author of it, and I was not the author of it. Satan was the author of it! When I understood that, I was off the hook, God was off the hook, and Satan was on the hook where he should be.

I had read *A More Excellent Way*™ in 1999 but had no idea if it was the real thing or not. I don't know about you, but when I go into a Christian bookstore and I look at all of those books, I get pretty overwhelmed. How on earth do you know who is speaking the truth and who isn't, or what the blend of truth and deception is in all of those books, and who is who out there? I didn't know. So when I read *A More Excellent Way*™, I had no idea that his ministry was bearing the kind of fruit that it is.

Then in 2004 my mother told me she knew someone who had been healed there of what I had, so I called the woman, and I wanted so badly to be healed and got a glimmer of hope that it might be possible. Getting there was a challenge—I had to fly across the country and knew I could get very sick from it. I had already been taken off an airplane by an ambulance several years earlier and stopped flying. But as I reread AMEW, the hope grew that I could be healed, and I was willing to face the risk of traveling there. My husband pushed me through airports in my wheelchair and a mask, and God met me and I made it!

During the week, the first thing that I began to realize was that I was not a victim to the illness! It was a devastating thing to be a victim to this illness and not have any way out. They showed me that I wasn't a victim but that I was believing lies that were keeping me captive to it, and that I was in sin that I did not recognize was sin.

Nobody had taught me that the kind of stuff that I was doing that was keeping me under the curse was sin, things like "self-pity", "fear", or "self-hatred." Those are the kind of things that they teach about in the program. They're not talking about drinking and carousing; they're talking about the sins of the heart. And at the same time that they teach this, there's not one ounce of condemnation. I had been condemned by well meaning Christians for being ill but there was no condemnation at Be in Health™; there was just love and understanding and them saying, "Here, try this. We have some truth for you and God will set you free if you will just walk in this." It was so beautiful.

I was assured that I did have enough faith and I was so relieved.

I began to understand that God did want to heal me, and He could heal me and He would heal me and that He was going to heal me! Right now, NOW is the time. It wasn't going to happen twenty years from now when I had gotten qualified and I had gotten stronger and I had learned all my lessons; but it was whenever I could line up with God. He was eager to heal me.

And as the week progressed my life was completely transformed… permanently. God was able to give me the revelations that I needed to get to the point where, when I left on Sunday, I was pushing my wheelchair! I didn't have my mask on and I didn't have Chronic Fatigue. It was unbelievable; I had my life back.

I walked out of there a victorious Christian.

I found my Father there. Understanding that He wasn't making me sick for eternal purposes restored me to knowing that He is a loving Father.

I was restored to God and faith and trust again! I was able to walk the Christian life and it's been great; more than great—there's no word to describe what it is like to get God back after having given up like that.

During the week I had a mask and I kept trying to take it off and to fight the chemicals that were around. When you go there, they tell you not to wear fragrances because of people who go there with Chemical Sensitivity. What was really funny was that in the women's restroom there was this really fragrant hand lotion.

As I lay in my lounge chair, I would try to take off my mask to see if I would react. During breaks women would go lather up with this fragrant hand lotion and then come sit right near me. I was thinking, "You shouldn't be doing that! How dare you! I'm sick and I'm important." I would go into self-pity and victimization and anger and fear, but God was showing me my heart; that all that was sin. After several days He said to me, "Whenever you smell the fragrance, I want you to know that that is My love wafting over you." Boy did that transform that for me.

You know, there's a Scripture about an aroma that leads to death or leading to life, and that is what happened for me. Suddenly that cherry smell was God loving me, and I was thinking, "Bring it on in. I am going to have victory here." And I did; that was the end of that smell being a problem for me. It took a few months when I got home to take back every single thing that had been a trigger for me. I learned that when I had a reaction I needed to ask myself "What did I just think" not "What did I just smell?" That helped me take back everything very quickly and I'm completely free now. I remember standing in the detergent aisle in the grocery store smelling and saying, "I'm healed! I'm free! I can go anywhere!"

Now after 4 years I never even give chemicals or exposures a thought.

There were other physical and emotional issues that took much longer—like insomnia and healing of my heart from abuse. Everything that they teach that relates to physical healing relates to psychological healing, emotional healing, and spiritual healing as well. So all the tools that I learned there I have applied to every part of my being, and there are still things that I'm working on. But there's freedom, there's incredible change, incredible growth. It's WAY beyond health. It is about restoration at every level in everything in your life.

During For My Life™, I was shown the Gospel of love in a way that I had never seen modeled. I was transformed by the love of God.

Let me toss in my son's testimony. He was born with a very, very severe dairy allergy and, in fact, he had bloody diarrhea for the first year of his life. We had to take him to the Children's Hospital. He had other very severe symptoms. He didn't sleep for more than twenty minutes or an hour all night long when he was a really young child, waking up crying in pain. We took him off dairy and were managing the illness that way.

When we took him to Georgia, he was 9. He just sat by us and played. Nobody laid a hand on him, nobody prayed for him, and God healed him of his dairy allergy because his father and I were dealing with our issues, and those issues had transferred right down to him. It's called a *Generational Iniquity*. He is fine to this day—almost 4 years later.

H.M., Thomaston, GA

## Clean Bill of Health from Leukemia

Six months ago God set me free of leukemia!…I hold in my hand from Emory University Hospital (dated April, 2004) my "clean bill of health" from Acute Lymphoblastic Leukemia. You know, if you ask an oncologist what causes leukemia, they do not know. But then there's God. It turns out that God knows what the cause of leukemia is—which I'm going to show you in a minute, and He tells us in Psalm 103 that He heals ALL our diseases!

A close brother sometime last fall told me about a Bible study course in Thomaston, GA on the spiritual roots of disease (and therefore healing). As I completed that course, God made it extremely clear that almost all of our diseases, including leukemia, are a SPIRITUAL health condition. I'd like to show you what the actual cause of leukemia is.

Now, let me set this up a little bit.…Remember Ephesians 6:11–12: "Put on the whole armor of God, that you may be able to stand against the wiles of the devil. For we wrestle not against flesh and blood, BUT AGAINST THE INVISIBLE KINGDOM OF EVIL." And I want to remind you about Exodus 20: the sins of the father will be passed down on to the 3rd and 4th generations, right? "Deep-rooted [spirit of] bitterness coming out of unresolved rejection and abandonment by father, either literally or emotionally; [spirit of] death and destruction; [spirit of] fear, anxiety and stress; a broken spirit (heart)." "…for I the LORD thy God am a jealous God, visiting the iniquity of the fathers upon the children unto the third and fourth generation…"

Now, let me assure you that that was me. I was "text-book" leukemia. In the area of death and destruction: as a kid, youngest of four, I was what many people would describe as "very accident prone." My first memory is me falling out of the car going down the driveway to go to kindergarten!

I grew up in a Christian family—I'm a direct descendent of the founder of our denomination; my parents were deacons and all that stuff. As I grew up, I broke a finger, a toe, a collar bone; I swallowed a straight pin that got stuck in my throat (long story!), I needed stitches at least 3 separate times, 2 emergency eye doctor visits, and wrecked my brother's motorcycle [while he was out of town]. (There was more but we didn't always go for medical treatment!)

OK, the "Deep-rooted [spirit of] bitterness coming out of unresolved rejection and abandonment by father, either literally or emotionally..." When I was about 10 or 12 years old [and probably misbehaving...], my father told me that he and my mom wished they had not had me. Looking back, I now believe that my dad didn't know what he was REALLY doing at the time, by saying that to me. But, at the time, I bought it. I believed him. Rest assured that I've since completely forgiven him. In fact, God allowed me the privilege of leading my dad (and my mom) in verbally confessing Jesus as their Lord and Savior [Romans 10], as they had never done that!

Now, as I lived my life, I would compensate for my fear of further rejection by creating a facade. Anyone here ever create a facade? My facade would help me avoid rejection and made me SEEM like the nicest guy. But inside I was keeping a record of how you wronged me. Deep-rooted bitterness. Along with bitterness comes "retaliation." It became an art form—I had three insults to every one coming at me from my brother and sisters or classmates. Besides, gotta protect my broken heart! For some reason I had fear of man. Hmm...

Now, as an adult, I got BITTER with the Christian church. That's when I "accepted the call" into the so-called "new age" movement. That seemed perfect for me because it seemed like the other new-agers had some level of unforgiveness/bitterness with the Christian church, right?! PLUS there's no chance of REJECTION from God, because there's no consequence for sin and "all paths lead to the same God anyway," right?!

THAT belief just about cost me my life! 2½ years ago, I got so filled with self-bitterness that I tried to take my life—twice in one night. Hey, "ALL paths lead to the same God," right?! That was December 1, 2001. After getting out of the Psych Ward and 11 days later—on my birthday (December 12)—AT LAST, I accepted Jesus Christ as my Savior...AND LORD! Three weeks later, God connects me with the perfect Home Group. A few months later, I fire my therapist and begin Christian counseling. A year later, I'm completing a course for prayer ministry. Six months after that, I'm in a men's group. I'll tell ya, the psych ward is motivating!...And God is so faithful...He's showed me that I do not need to look anywhere else for my identity or approval, that He's mending my heart and...that bitterness is of the enemy! Thank God...He's so good!

Being set free of leukemia: Well, during that course that I mentioned in Thomaston, out of His loving-kindness, God allowed me to see Deuteronomy 28 and Exodus 15—that dis-ease is a result of disobedience—and Ephesians 6:12, that we do not wrestle against flesh and blood, but against the invisible kingdom of evil. And that I had to make a choice to clean up my act and (get this—this is crucial) that I needed to REPENT [Acts 3 and Revelation 2 and 3] for being in agreement with those things in MY generation as well as my generations before me, and appropriate what Jesus Christ did on the cross for me ["by His stripes, we're healed!"]. And I had to get those spiritual parasites [Ephesians 6:12], specifically, bitterness [Hebrews 12:15], fear [2 Timothy 1:7], and death and destruction **CAST** out of my spirit dimension! THANK GOD!

By the way, "the sins of the father will be passed down on to the 3$^{rd}$ and 4$^{th}$ generations," right? [Exodus 20]. Well, I went into the hospital because of leukemia on the very same DATE as my great-grandfather went into the hospital because of leukemia, 48 years earlier. Unfortunately, he died within 5 months. His son was diagnosed with leukemia, and great-great-great-granddaughter died of it.

Thank you for listening and I THANK OUR INVISIBLE GOD! AMEN!!

D.F., Atlanta, GA

## Free of Torment

I was a "recovering" alcoholic, drug addict, anorexic, bulimic, through a million 12-step groups. I also had fibromyalgia, chronic fatigue and endometriosis, by which Satan healed me through natural medicine and occultic practices. The problem, however, was I got so spiritually tormented, depressed, etc., that I was either going to a trauma hospital, a retreat run by nuns for "recovering" people or here (someone gave me a book). I ended up at Pleasant Valley, which is a testimony of itself (map quest directions to Molena address in old book). I got healed and totally set free of all torment and "recovering" illnesses which was total bondage (over 1600 12–step meetings I attended) by a couple of teachings and a million PVC tapes, notes left at my trailer and ministry in a trailer on the "anointed" campground. I've been back 3 times since then and the campground is part of my healings—the last 2 times in a <u>tent</u>. PRAISE GOD for your love for me!!!

M.P.J., Naples, FL

## Out of Occultism!

My allergies started with mononucleosis when I was 19 years old. I developed hepatitis when I was 26, and a few years later I became sensitive to synthetic fabrics and my chemical sensitivities expanded from there.

I worked as a medical social worker, and I had to cut back my hours to 3 days per week. Somewhere in the early 80s I began wearing a charcoal mask every time I went out. If I didn't, I would come down with respiratory flu-like symptoms that could put me to bed for weeks. Later I graduated from a charcoal mask to an industrial respirator. I could not be in a room with the windows open without becoming ill.

In 1986, I left work on a medical leave believing that if I got away from the stress of my job I would recover. Only I got worse. By then I was a universal reactor to all conventional allergens, multiple chemicals, foods, clothes, and the air I breathed.

I had an extremely difficult time finding clothes I could tolerate. Once I washed my clothes in anything, I could no longer tolerate them. At one point I was down to one pair of old worn-out-jeans and a checkered flannel shirt. I wore this every day for 10 months and I could not wash them as that was how I became sensitized to my clothes in the first place.

I had been diagnosed with:

Multiple Chemical Sensitivities aka MCS/EI

Hypothyroidism

Candida colonization hypersensitivity syndrome

Chronic viral myalgic encephalomyelitis secondary to EBV or CMV

Chronic intestinal protozoan parasitosis

Chronic fatigue immune deficiency-dysregulation syndrome

Tendonitis

Multiple allergies/universal reactor

Hypersensitivity urethritis

Autoimmune endocrinopathy

Electromagnetic frequency sensitivity

Asthma

Chronic back pain/degenerative disc disease

Depression

Diffuse fibromyalgia syndrome

Some time after a natural disaster, I hit an all-time low physically, emotionally, and spiritually. That is when I first heard about Henry Wright's ministry from a former roommate of a good friend of mine. This was a Jewish woman who had converted to Christianity and had been healed of similar medical problems by God. My friend and I contacted the church and began talking to them by phone on a regular basis. I got saved over the telephone when I was 50 years old.

I had not been raised in the church although my parents taught me Christian morality. I briefly explored Christianity in college but quickly became disillusioned. In my early 30s I became a disciple of a well-known Indian guru because I was in need of inner peace and he had promised this to those who followed him. I practiced his meditation and lifestyle for 18 years. This made me vulnerable to all kinds of new age and occultic activities. I became a student of astrology, Buddhism, E.S.T., radionics and the pendulum, etc., not to mention all the alternative medical practices that I tried. I mention these because becoming a born-again Christian was to the far right of my position both politically and spiritually.

In 1992 I got into an airplane using an oxygen tank and a respirator and I flew across the country to come to Henry Wright's church. The plane was sold out and someone wearing designer perfume was in close proximity to me. A miracle happened there on the plane when, after an hour of listening to some lively gospel music on my tape player, the overwhelming smell of the perfume dissipated. And when I changed planes in St. Louis, I did not react to the cigarette smoke although I could smell it. This alone was a miracle. Although I was experiencing massive fear, I had stepped out in faith and God met me.

Henry Wright put me into an apartment that had been prepared for someone who was very allergic. The second night I was served pork chops. This was a challenge because I had not eaten red meat in 18 years because of the vegetarian practice I had picked up from the guru. The people ministering to me read I Timothy

4:4–5, "For every creature of God is good and nothing to be refused, if it be received with thanksgiving, for it is sanctified by the Word of God and prayer."

I had a revelation that God wanted me to be able to eat anything. And He certainly didn't want me to follow strange diets any more. I ate pork chops and had no adverse reaction to it. I quickly took my foods back and then my clothes and afterward fresh air and chemicals. The church taught me the Word of God and helped me walk out my fears and occultism.

I am grateful to God for delivering me from disabling illness. I can truly say He has given me life more abundantly. Every occultic practice I did robbed me of my life and my health, but Jesus restored it.

Today I have freedom to move about in the world unhindered by environmental limitations. My energy has returned, and I can be productive. I can eat and drink anything I want. I can buy clothes and wear them off the rack. I can enjoy nature out of doors. Thank You, Father God, Jesus and the Holy Spirit, and the ministry of Henry Wright for giving my life back to me.

M.F., GA

## Uterine Cancer Disappeared!

I was diagnosed with Stage III uterine cancer in April of 2003. An emergency hysterectomy operation was performed, but the malignant tumor was still present. My doctor advised chemotherapy treatments, so I agreed to the first two in June of 2003.

I lost my hair and almost 25 pounds and felt awful. I was scared to go on with six more treatments and didn't know how I could keep on working as a real estate broker. Then things began to happen.

A $449,000 real estate listing came my way. The second day it was offered, I got a call from another broker whose customer gave full price. I arranged to meet the broker to complete the contract papers, and then came a surprise. After our meeting I asked him if he could stay for a while and chat with my husband and me. I had never met this man before, and I rarely discuss personal matters with strangers, but felt close to him and told him my story.

He listened patiently and then revealed that he had considerable experience in ministering at the VA hospital and hospice, and that he understood my concern. When I asked him what to do, he said, "I cannot really help you, but I have a booklet that tells you how to help yourself." The booklet was provided by Pleasant Valley, entitled "New Insights into Cancer." I read it that same evening, twice.

I began to realize the importance of forgiving others and that I had to get rid of the bitterness I had toward my ex-son-in-law. It was like a light bulb went off in my head. I had to forgive him, and I did. It happened in the driveway of my home just before he left my 11-year-old grandson to visit me. They were both in shock when I told him I was sorry and that I loved him. We both cried as we hugged each other. Wow!

This was on a Thursday, the day after I read the cancer booklet. The next day I went to my appointment for chemotherapy treatment, and to the surprise of both my oncologist and my radiologist, the cancer had completely disappeared! A miracle!

I know now that bitterness and unforgiveness were the cause of my cancer, but most important to me is that God heard my heart asking Him to forgive me for judging someone else. I call it a matter of DIVINE INTERVENTION of a God who loves me. I praise Him and worship Him. He has changed my life forever.

J.B.

### *Relationship Healed!*

My husband and I just got back from a life-changing spiritual journey. We feel it has saved our marriage, our sanity, and probably our lives. I felt writing this was the best way to express this so I won't bore those that aren't interested, and those that are interested can read on.

Whenever I looked at the fruits of the Spirit, I would think, why don't I have these? Patience and self-control was not in me. Serving others was not done with love. My husband's and my relationship was getting so bad that I didn't want to have anyone over; I felt so tired and stressed all the time. We tried so many diets trying to feel better, but things just got worse. I was so sick of repenting to God and my children daily for the same thing, my angry outbursts, etc. I had developed a bad case of reflux, foot pain and woke up frequently with horrible feelings about myself and fear about my relationship with my husband.

Thank God, we were introduced to a group of Christians who had been healed and delivered from many different things: allergies, pain, fears, and all kinds of diseases at the Pleasant Valley Retreat. It was a weeklong study of healing through God's Word. Some major things we learned were: God wants us healthy, and Satan wants us sick. Behind most diseases and sickness there is a spiritual root. Many diseases and sicknesses come from a generational curse and they can be removed. (Just think, our children can be freed from these curses.) The spiritual root to reflux and many diseases is fear, anxiety and stress. Fear is the opposite of faith. We can believe Satan's lies or God's promises. Negative thoughts are from Satan. Good thoughts are from God. We must take each thought captive. If we start believing Satan's lies about ourselves and others, they start snowballing in us and they start manifesting in us, and by the power of the Holy Spirit, they can be broken and cast out in Jesus' name. These are evil spirits we're dealing with. Certain buttons that were pressed would set my anger and fear in motion, and now I finally have control. I can say no to those thoughts, whereas before I couldn't and did not understand why.

They not only taught us all about the spiritual warfare going on within ourselves, but how to keep it out and away from our hearts. Satan continues to tempt us, but we recognize it and refuse it. I haven't had the foot pain since I've been there; I've only had reflux once since I've been back, and I knew where it was coming from and to deal with that fear immediately. If any of you would like any more details about this, my husband and I would love to tell you.

I urge any of you who are having marital or family problems, allergies, sickness or depression, etc., to check the web site www.pleasantvalleychurch.net. His book is a best seller and is titled *A More Excellent Way*™ by Henry W. Wright. It includes most of the information they teach: 60 Diseases and their Spiritual Roots, 30 Blocks to Healing (for example, unforgiveness and fear are big blocks to healing) and Scriptures to back these up. Pleasant Valley Church is only two hours away in Thomaston, Georgia.

God bless you, and please let me know if you've registered. I'd love to hear!!!

**Beloved, I wish above all things that thou mayest prosper and be in health, even as thy soul prospereth. 3 John 2**

GA

## What My Heavenly Father Has Done for Me to His Glory!

He loves me unconditionally in spite of myself. I am fearfully and wonderfully made! He has protected me through a violent, tormenting, raging, alcoholic, abusive, and satanic home, from emotional, physical, spiritual and sexual abuse including incest, rape and molestation and near drowning.

From birth to age 58, there were 45 years of bondage to my progressive diseases and diagnoses, specifically:

Allergies, asthma, bronchitis, sinusitis, emphysema, COPD (chronic obstructive pulmonary disease) including 2 near deaths, viruses, immune system shot, pneumonias, blepharitis, eyes, yeast infections and skin fungus, osteopio, hypothyroidism, acute schizophrenia, many mental breakdowns, anxiety attacks, nose bleeds, 20 shock treatments, mental institutions, psychotherapy, many attempted suicides, depression, obesity, obsessive compulsive disorder, manic depressive, multiple addictions to sugar, prescription drugs, shopping, etc., poverty, so much counseling, and programs, doctors, occult new age, self-death, destruction and mutilation.

In the summer of 2001, I purchased a book called *A More Excellent Way*™ by Henry Wright. I used the Bible with it as I was desperate for TRUTH about my life and in September 2001, I attended the For My Life™ ministry week at Pleasant Valley Church with a committed team to minister TRUTH about biblical principles.

I heard truth about God's purpose for my life that I had never heard before. This truth is setting me free. Since I can remember, I've wanted to be a whole person, loved and accepted. I'm on the way! My Father God loves me, and I have a new identity in Jesus Christ! I've been baptized for the right reasons, God's way. There is victory! Walk-out, taking what the Bible says as truth, the living Word (Jesus) and the power of the Holy Spirit. God the Father does know best!

I was taking eleven plus medications. Now, since December 2001 (10 months), I am taking close to zero; I'm on the lowest dose for hypothyroidism, which is to be eliminated any day. My thyroid is better, my blood and oxygen good, my lungs are clear, my immune system is normal, osteopio-bone density is normal, my eyes—I hardly need glasses, and I weigh 80 pounds less. I'm healed of so much and in God's mercy I'm forgiven, delivered and healed. My marriage is restored, my broken heart is mended concerning the death of my 10-year-old son, past Masonic and generational curses are broken, and so much more. I am better equipped to serve my Lord and Savior Jesus Christ. I've been empowered by the Holy Spirit, to the glory of God the Father, to minister in the prisons, etc., *FOR THEIR LIFE™!*

Thank you, Father God, for restoring my life from the pit, for restoring my health and for using Pleasant Valley Church staff and volunteers to help me to see the TRUTH OF THE WORD and for showing scriptural truth about sin and disease through ministry to myself and to others.

May God continue to bless you all!

C.H.

### Testimony of Healing of Sleep Apnea and Use of "Renouncing"

I had been diagnosed with Sleep Apnea in August 2003 and had been under a sleep mask with 14 pounds of pressure since that time. When I spent the night at the sleep clinic, I was told I stopped breathing 139 times during the course of 6 hours of sleep. Five times it was very severe, almost up to 2 minutes! I might add that I have two other sisters that have this problem. One sleeps with a mask and the other had major throat surgery about a year ago. The mask is much like a pacifier to a baby. Habit forming! Feels like security.

I was set free of Sleep Apnea during the Saturday morning prayer of *For My Life.* My freedom came when I specifically asked how "Freemasonry" came under the occult. I had felt a "bit of stirring" in my spirit during the teaching on occultism. My dad and granddad (mom's dad) were both in the Masons. My question prompted our group manager to inquire from the leader if this could be involved with sleep apnea.

As you know, the battle in "walk-out" began soon after I returned home. I had terrible nightmares. It did not wake me, but I had a very bad headache the following morning. In fact, it was the kind of headache I had when I did not get adequate oxygen to my brain. Medication never seemed to offer any relief. This was a strong "set back" for me. The doctor at the sleep clinic had told me it is possible to have a stroke or heart failure when one does not get adequate oxygen to the brain. I had suffered with this particular kind of headache off and on over the years, and very severely for at least a year prior to diagnosis of sleep apnea. I knew I could not allow this to happen to me.

A friend encouraged me to renounce and make my declaration out loud. THIS SAVED ME FROM GOING BACK UNDER THE MASK THAT VERY NIGHT! I looked at the mask and had a struggle but finally decided, "live or die," I was not going back under it. I believed God's Word to be truth, and I staked my claim to my deliverance and have remained free since April 30, 2004! Praise God! Hallelujah!! In fact, the mask has been packed away out of my sight.

I have continued to make my declaration every night that *"I am free of Sleep Apnea. I will have the sweet sleep promised to the beloved of God. I am free of Sleep*

*Apnea and whom the Son sets free is free indeed."* My sleep is sweet and I have not had any further symptoms. I AM FREE!! HALLELUJAH!

N.D., Anderson, SC

## Car Accident Testimony

It is my prayer that through this testimony I am about to share, God will bless those who are in pain from injuries received in accidents. I stand with those who read this to receive hope and be encouraged to trust God completely for their healing. Always remember that God is not a respecter of persons. God will work in cooperation with us. Based upon our choices, He will bring about His awesome faithfulness to complete in us what was already appropriated at the cross. May you apprehend Him because when you receive Him, everything else comes with it, including healing.

When someone is involved in an accident and there is loss of the ability to walk, provide for and take care of one's self, the enemy will always be standing by to bring tremendous fear, insecurity, doubt and unbelief into the picture. There is a torment that comes when we are gripped with pain and not sure if we are ever going to be able to do what we did before. But there also comes a time when we must really decide what we believe. I had settled in my heart what I really believed about God's faithfulness and promises before this accident happened. I had seen God's provision in my life so many times before. I knew that I would be in His constant care. By trusting and applying my faith in the past, and seeing Him always come through, I knew I could believe Him for an incredible healing now. That's when I realized that by believing Him, it was more of a statement about who God was and what He was willing to do than it was about me and what I was willing to accept. I simply refused to have a Plan B. I went with Plan A in which God enabled me to put my complete trust in Him. I encourage you to seek the type of relationship where you will allow Him be your all-in-all. Never question if it is God's will to completely restore you; know that it is.

After the accident I was unconscious for a period of time. I remember approaching the intersection at Sunnyside Grocery and a lady pulling out immediately in front of my car. I will never forget hearing the Holy Spirit pleading to me like a mother pleading for child—don't hit her. When I heard this voice, I saw the lady's face and her car door was directly in front of me. I had only a few seconds to turn the steering when in the opposite direction to avoid crushing her and most likely killing her from the impact. My choice to obey God meant I was choosing an undetermined course for my car to take because there wasn't any time to check for a clear path. Directly in front of her car and to my left was oncoming traffic and I remember seeing another car approaching the intersection. I had to go behind her car because to go in front of her would have placed me heading directly into the oncoming cars. This decision to avoid hitting her caused me to leave the road. My car hit a telephone pole head-on and the telephone pole broke in half. The bottom half of the pole, five feet high, was still in the ground and the top of the pole and power lines came down on my car. The car flipped and a portion of the corner of a house creased my driver's door. I was pinned between the house and crushed door, the steering wheel and the console in the jeep. The front windshield and the side glass were completely broken out. My head took the blow of the glass while my body received the impact of a head-on crash.

I will forever be grateful for every prayer because I know God spared my life. I can never thank Him enough for allowing me to live and walk again and without being in a wheel chair, without pain, and to be a part of all the wonderful things that He is doing. I praise God for His precious people and the hearts of everyone who blessed me so incredibly much through their prayers, love and support.

I vaguely remember the ride to the hospital in the helicopter. I remember thinking how bad this must be if I'm in a helicopter, not an ambulance. All I remembered was that I had to be cut out of my jeep and the terrific pain and trauma of realizing that my entire body was wrenched in pain. My left hip was dislocated; I had skull fractures from my left to right ear; the earring I was wearing was pressed into the side of my face and had to be cut out. My left ear required many stitches, which resulted in a plastic surgeon repairing the damage and in places reattaching my ear back to my head. My pelvic bone was cracked in two places and my lower backbone was fractured. I remember the pain I felt coming from the impact of my head and jaw against the side window of my car. The impact was enough that the glass was crushed. When I arrived at the hospital, the doctor first thought I was paralyzed, was sure that my jaw was beyond repair, and that my internal injuries could be so severe I would need immediate surgery. But amazingly God had already put me back together, and there was nothing that needed surgery or a cast.

The second miracle that God did after saving my life was saving my teeth. My jaw was swollen so much the doctor thought my jawbone was crushed. I will always believe God completely restored me while I was unconscious in my car before anyone arrived at the accident. I believe He put me back together because I was obedient to hear His voice and respond by not hitting the door of the car in front of me. I responded without questioning the outcome of that decision in regards to what would happen to my car. Amazingly, my jaw was not broken, and I did not have any crushed teeth; none of the teeth in my mouth were even loosened.

I was in the hospital five days and left without receiving physical therapy. Someone from the physical therapy department came by to evaluate me. At that point I really couldn't walk or do very much. Realizing I had no insurance in the natural (God is the most awesome insurance policy any one can ever have), they were eager to let me leave as soon as possible. Even the part about my hospital bills God took care of. After being home for 10 days, I had the stitches removed from my ear. That day in the emergency room, God graciously blessed me with a plastic surgeon to put the stitches in my ear, and there are almost no scars. Thank You, God, for providing a plastic surgeon at the hospital just when I needed one.

I did not go back to a doctor after I initially left the hospital. I did not have x-rays and follow up work done because I didn't need to. Praise the Lord. When I checked out of the hospital, I left in a wheel chair. And as I recovered, I moved from wheel chair to walker to two walking canes to one walking cane and then to no walking cane at all.

The first night I came home from leaving the hospital, I knew God was there. A friend spent the first night with me. I will never forget her ministering and caring for me. Later that night I sat on the side of my bed trying to get up on the walker. I heard the Holy Spirit say, "Walk, I am with you." And I also heard another voice say, "You will never be the same as before; you will never walk like you did before and you will always limp and be in pain." I knew I had to look at what God was capable of and not what I could do. I made a decision to be encouraged by and believe in the LORD.

That night and for the weeks that followed and from the time I was in the hospital, I had tremendous pain. I could not lie still and could not get comfortable any way I turned in bed. The decision to trust God enabled me to get off the bed that first night I came home from the hospital. It came from choosing to believe God's spoken word. I put action with what I believed about His faithfulness. I chose to believe His Word was true. It took persevering and many attempts to get up, but when I did get up with God's help, I began to move the left side of my body with the help of the walker. The amount of effort it took to move my body forward was incredible, but I began to praise God with my right arm and with my left hand renounce the devil. I remember the intensity of the warfare that I dealt with as I tried to walk. The further I got from the bed, the more I began to tire, then I turned to try and get back to the bed. But when I came to an end of all my own strength, when there was nothing left I could do and I realized I could not even stand any longer without collapsing, I called out to Jesus with all my heart, and I reached for His strength, knowing I had none left of my own to depend upon. Suddenly my legs became stronger, my arms became strengthened, and the presence of God that entered the room was incredible.

This was how I began to heal but it was also the beginning of more spiritual warfare. About a week after I was home from hospital, a pastor prayed for me for a spirit of infirmity. There was a heaviness and weakness that left me. Everyone in the room with me began to pray for the pain to leave and for the needed strength to overcome to be available. God answers prayer. I am living proof of that statement.

What was interesting was that the pain would leave in one area of my body and show up again somewhere else. The enemy lost the battle with pain in my back, but pain would then show up in my hip a few days later. But I began to notice that I was making the devil mad because I had figured out his game plan. The enemy was just testing me to see if he could gain access in another way. Would I believe the lie?

Another time I would try to get up out of a chair and there would be tingling, numbness, and loss of feeling in my hip, coupled with pain in the joint area. This happened after I started back to work after the initial pain had stopped. I remember saying, "You know, I must have pulled something in my hip because it wasn't hurting and it is now." This was after I made the connection and yielded to the temptation. I had a four week battle to fight out before I won. I had given place to the lie. Now I had to outlast the devil and renounce my own words, which lined up with Satan's kingdom, not God's! Perseverance and determination to stand and believe God's Word was true brought the victory. I got out of bed one morning pain free. Thank You, Jesus.

God also miraculously paid for all my hospital bills through the insurance company of the lady I was involved in the accident with. Her insurance also enabled me to replace my Jeep Cherokee with the same kind of vehicle I had before but one year newer. God has again and again provided for my needs, restored my strength to more than I had before the accident, and continues to bless and astound me with His provision and ability to provide for me in every way.

Trauma from an accident is a doorpoint for the enemy to keep you where God wants to see you set free. I encourage you to come to Pleasant Valley Church and go through the For My Life™ program. God will meet you in your understanding and help you overcome whatever the enemy has blocked you from receiving. There is hope, and God will never leave you and not show Himself strong in your life. Your part is to believe that and trust Him. As you allow Him, He will show you how to line up your thoughts, will, actions and words with the Word of God. Give Him your heart. When you hate what He hates and can love what He loves, you can begin to comprehend, apprehend and appropriate, and He will fulfill the desires of your heart.

S.D., Atlanta, GA

## Multiple Sclerosis

I am being healed of M.S.! The clock was turned back on my physical limitations by one year, and I am almost off all of my medications. You helped me get my life back.

Every day is like Christmas—I cannot wait to get up and see what has been restored today.

R.D.

## Allergy and Free From Arthritis Pain

Just reading the book and applying its principles has set me free from the horrendous allergies that I had been fighting for 30 years. My husband, who had been crippled with rheumatoid arthritis since he was 19, has also been set free from pain!

This book is real. The healing that you will find is real and not a bit of it is Hollywood. You can literally be free from disease by just applying the biblical principles that Henry Wright has outlined.

L.C.

## Fibromyalgia and Heart Problem Gone

Visiting Pleasant Valley Church changed my life around. After ministry, I was totally set free from the fibromyalgia that I had battled for 14 years. I am still free a year later and have eliminated other health issues as well, including a heart problem. I have a new life and can do so much more than I could ever do before. I've been hiking, and last week I did a four-mile trek up the side of the mountain that has a 1200–foot elevation.

I now purpose to "live and not die to declare the glory of the Lord."

D.W.

## Diabetes with Progressive Blindness

I had diabetes and progressive blindness with only 10 percent vision left. I went to the doctor for my laser treatment, and he said that the disease had reversed itself. At my next visit, he dismissed me because my eyesight had returned to normal.

M.B.

## No More Hypoglycemia Plus a Godly Husband

God has delivered me from numerous allergy problems and hypoglycemia. He has also blessed me with the truly wonderful love of a godly husband, which I never believed possible.

B.

## Crohn's Disease

The good news is that I am healed, not just in the faith but also in the body. Not only am I fully healed of Crohn's and ulcerative colitis, but I am also freed from the spiritual bondages and generational curses that I had carried for 50 years of my life.

S.W.

## Allergies

I had over 100 food allergies and was binging and using laxatives daily. I had no life except for thinking about my illness. I am now totally set free.

J.W.

## Irritable Bowel Syndrome

I just wanted you to know that God has healed the irritable bowel syndrome that has tormented me for over 8 years. I am no longer taking the probiotic supplement. Praise God!

J.C.

## Hypothyroidism

Much to my doctor's amazement, I have been healed of hypothyroidism and no longer need the two thyroid medications that were keeping me afloat.

R.R.

## I Can Walk!

I was healed of a condition in my hips (vascular necrosis) and am now able to walk!

V.B., San Mateo, CA USA

### Chronic Pain and Generational Curses Gone

The most amazing thing happened during the first week of the course. God took a physically and spiritually diseased Christian with occultic and pagan roots, and chose to heal me in spite of myself.

I was on the brink of filing for disability. My attorney said I would have no problem qualifying because fibromyalgia is a recognized disease. In fact, some of the patients "Dr. Death" Kevorkian treated were suffering from fibromyalgia and had finally lost all hope. Then someone gave me a copy of *A More Excellent Way*™.

Instead of filing for disability, I got on a plane to come to Thomaston, GA. I am now cured of an incurable disease and the chronic pain that went with it. I am no longer bed-ridden. Instead I now have God's peace and rest. Not only did He heal me, but also I learned that my perception of God was way too small. We are now expecting healing in every area of our lives.

R.H.

### Infertility

Through the use of *A More Excellent Way*™ and a dear sister, we have deepened our relationship with the Lord and broken many curses. The Lord has blessed us with our first child after 14 years of marriage!

K.J.

### Addictions Gone! And I Sleep Again!

I have been a Christian for many years yet continued to struggle in certain areas of my life both in my relationship with God and with myself.

The principles in this book have made such a difference! Not only is God healing me of addictions, back pain and insomnia, but my mom, who had a crippling fear of heights all of her life, has been healed and no longer has any fear!

D.G.

### PMS Gone!

I no longer have PMS. I can love and receive love from my husband. I have been healed of herpes simplex. I no longer have chronic pain in my hip, right gluteus and leg. I am no longer allergic to certain foods and this is just the beginning!

H.B.

### Creative Miracle in Ear

Just wanted to give you a praise report. I attended your seminar the week of May 25, 2003, and it changed my life. Your teachings on the Word seemed like revelation after revelation to me. On Friday morning during ministry, I was suddenly healed of 8 years of extremely painful chronic kidney stones by God's hot hand on my back, which nearly took my breath away. That night in your Friday night service, my knee (messed up after a bad fall) was healed, and then Saturday morning during ministry with each other, I got a creative miracle in my left ear. A doctor had surgically damaged my ear nerve and I had no ear drum, but I do now!

PRAISE GOD! The Lord had spoken to me a few days before I left to go to Georgia that He would "heal all my diseases" and He did!

I thank you for your faithfulness in seeking God and sharing the good news. He has overflowed my heart with your information and His love, and I am pouring out to as many as will listen and receive. Thank you again for your wonderful seminar.

P.B.

## Advanced Osteoporosis

While at Pleasant Valley, I had an incredible resolution spiritually to restore a breach I had with my brother and his family. Now, months later, I remain at peace about it. That alone was worth the trip, but God had more for me.

I had advanced osteoporosis. I was diagnosed years ago at age 47. Since leaving Pleasant Valley, I am noticeably straighter.

A.B.

## Lower Back Pain Gone

I have always believed in God's healing power, but now I have experienced it for myself. God has miraculously healed my lower back. I had been to a chiropractor, but it only got worse. I asked for prayer from one of the teachers here who uses your material, and to my complete amazement, I was able to stand up easily with NO PAIN! I believe this is just the beginning. I believe that God can and will restore me to perfect health. My faith has increased ten-fold.

J.D.

## Testimony Coming Out of the New Age

For as long as I can remember, I have been looking for peace. It brought me into some very weird places. After getting sick, when everything already seemed so surreal, the search continued into darker and darker places. There was no religion I had not tried. No method of invasive, alternative medicine I didn't subject myself to.

None of it worked. And I was still striving for peace. My MD at the time, a Jewish Buddhist, asked me point blank if I was a praying man, because medical science couldn't help me any longer. With a death sentence, I decided to find out who this God character was.

My main problem was an infection that moved into my brain and central nervous system. I had 24–hour nerve pain that nearly led me to suicide on many occasions. After a few weeks at Pleasant Valley, it left. Many may think it was from trading New York City-sized stress for a bucolic countryside. I know the healing came because I sought after God's peace and found it. Thus my nerves were healed. The power and peace of mind I searched for in the New Age came from getting to know God the Father—from the real truth, not the counterfeit.

M.S.

## Broken Heart Healed!

I have been a Christian for over 4 years. God drew me to Himself, and I surrendered my whole life to Him completely in 1999. I met and fell in love with my husband later that year. He is a strong, godly man who had loved the Lord for over 10 years at that point. We both determined we would live our lives to honor God and His commandments and waited to have sex until we were married. I was told I would have to take fertility drugs to get pregnant. The night of our honeymoon my husband prayed, believing that I would be healed. I got pregnant on our honeymoon. I say all of this to tell you that I was not a half-hearted Christian. God has been very present in my life, and I have desired nothing in my life but to please Him. I have been learning more and more about the Word of God and its instruction in truth of how to live my life. I was and have remained on fire for God.

I went to Pleasant Valley in my hunger to know more about God and to further deepen my relationship with Him. I went with a completely teachable spirit without spiritual pride. While I was down there, I was a witness to miracle healing in more than one person, each with various illnesses and life-threatening diseases. One person with acute leukemia was given one day to live by their doctor and hospital and was healed that week without any medicine!

I myself was not in need of such a miracle, I thought, since I had no diagnosed disease or illness. However, I highly underestimated the need for healing my heart from divorced parents, an angry and envious sister, sexual immorality and immorality in my adolescence, and many other common issues people deal with.

At Pleasant Valley, they explained the principalities we actually fight and how Satan works in this world. It is not flesh and blood we fight, but powers, principalities and wickedness in high places says the Bible. That baffled me before, because people tell you that, but they do not explain how principalities work. It doesn't do justice to tell you how awesome and life-changing this experience was. Next to my salvation, I place this experience as THE MOST IMPORTANT and the greatest experience in my life. When I say that, I mean even above my husband and child. Because of going to Pleasant Valley, I now can be the wife and mother God intends for me to be. Everyone has had something in their life hurt them, whether it be a person or an experience. Also, everyone has parents and grandparents and therefore generational issues. I didn't realize how much my past life experiences were still affecting me, my husband and my child and how some were related generationally. EVERY Christian and EVERY pastor no matter what denomination should go to Pleasant Valley's *For My Life*™ seminar.

H.K., GA USA

## Obsessive Compulsive Disorder Broken Off of Me

I saw Henry Wright on a Sid Roth television program and ordered the book. One Sunday I came up here for their service, where I spoke with Henry who suggested that I stay for the program that was beginning that evening. I did that and was set free of depression and Obsessive Compulsive Disorder. Man has no cure for OCD, but God does.

I am joyful and excited about life. I have gotten my hope back.

T.G.

## *Asthma*

I am completely 100 percent cured of very severe asthma. I no longer need the three inhalers and nebulizer I had to use every day. Here is the big one! I was able to go off of Zoloft, an anti-depressant, that I had been on for approximately five years.

T.R.

## *Scoliosis Gone!*

Last August (2001) you came to Abbotsford, Canada to minister and minister you did!

A friend of mine, who is in deliverance ministry, told me about your book *A More Excellent Way*™. After reading it, I was anxious to find where you would be teaching. I live in Oregon so Abbotsford seemed close enough. Being the last week in August, it was our week of setup for the new school year. I co-teach and my partner told me to go anyway—that it was too important. God is amazing!

The reason I wanted to attend was due to the fact that my brother-in-law is dying from a heart disease that is generational, and I believed he would be healed if he would attend. Bottom line was that he would not go (even though he is a believer) and instead I was healed! God is so very awesome!!

Try as I might, I could find no holes in your teaching. I had even asked my father-in-law (who is a Bible scholar) to come for one day to help me discern if you were right on. God tells us to test everything and so I do. However, your teaching is based solely on His Word, and you do not deviate from it. You have also seen how it is misused and abused in the realm of healing and expose those areas for what they are—the enemy's lies.

I could go on and on regarding my opinions (all positive) of what I saw happen at Abbotsford and how I feel about your ministry, but this letter would be endless. So I will get to the point of my healing.

The healing teams were wonderful. How awesome to use the body of Christ to minister to one another (like we are supposed to, as opposed to one person). Since I had only been there for half of the week, I could not minister, and though I would have loved to, your rules said I could not.

I asked for a couple of things. I had scoliosis since I was a teenager (I am 51 years old) and all the issues that go along with a curved back. I wanted to break all the generational fears and anxieties I inherited from my mother and my Italian/Catholic background. During our time of praying and seeking God, a captain helped us out by explaining the unloving spirit that I also had acquired in a past marriage that was abusive. Quite a package to be carrying all these years. However, I can truly brag on the Scripture that "Christ has come to set the captives free"! I am free! Gloriously free!!

It was so weird to be free of back pain. God gave me the best adjustment I ever received! I kept expecting it to be there around every turn. What joy in the freedom of physical movement. Truly miraculous!

As extraordinary as this is in and of itself, it was the other deliverance that has freed me in areas I would not have dreamed possible. Being set free from fear and anxiety is wonderful. When Philippians says, "be anxious for nothing," I can pretty much go there now. Before I used to think the Scripture was for others only. My overall health has improved so much I had to cut way back on the vitamin supplements I used to take (made my husband happy) because my body does not need them! Praise God!

Being released from the "unloving" spirit has also changed many things. I have been surprised at my reactions to things that happen. I seem to be able to handle most situations less emotionally and with a different attitude! I just love accepting God's love and my family's. I can see how I used to reject compliments from people and figured if I just did a good enough job as wife, mother, teacher, etc., that would prove I was a worthwhile person. What freedom there is in just being a child of God! How glorious!

I desire to pray with people and help them get well. Unfortunately, there are many people who do not wish to hear your teaching or about my healing. Our church teaches that you cannot be a Christian and have an evil spirit. I now know that is false teaching.

Thank you does not seem adequate for how my life has changed. May God continue to bless you, your family and the ministry.

R.T., Tualatin, OR USA

### *Healed of ADD*

Our daughter was there 5 weeks ago and has been doing fantastic! She had the beginnings of fibromyalgia, ADD, and some severe counseling challenges—all of which were healed at your classes! She is feeling terrific and is a changed person!

My wife has also been doing equally as well for the last 2 weeks. It is blowing me away!

I have been doing fine and have been released from feeling that I have let God down! I do not have any physical ailments that have been cured, but I am much more excited about life and what God is doing in our lives.

I hope this letter helps to encourage you and the staff in times of challenges. I consider it an honor to have met you all and to see the mighty work that God is doing through you all.

M.K., Cincinnati, OH USA

## *Look What the Lord Has Done!*

I grew up feeling insecure, confused and like I never fit in. Church didn't answer my questions that I couldn't even seem to voice, nor did anything else in my life break that insecurity. I do not know why much of it was. I had a loving family, a good home, but there was always something ever-present that was always with me, influencing everything I did. And now, after all these years, I know it was the spirit of fear. There were periods in my life where I was afraid of the dark, afraid of dying, afraid to leave home, afraid to stay there, afraid somebody would look at me… There was no peace. And I didn't know what was wrong as I had nothing that I had ever experienced to compare it with. I did not exactly understand how God was relevant to my life.

I did grow up going to church every Sunday and usually Wednesday nights. But I still felt out of place. I know now that an unloving spirit was affecting my life, making it hard for me to love people and very hard for me to accept love from others.

And finally a few weeks ago during CanaryCare's seminar in Houston, TX, which sponsored Pastor Henry Wright of Pleasant Valley Church and Ministries in Georgia, I learned about these things and why I had had all kinds of emotional upsets in my life. God had healed me suddenly of MCS/EI a year ago. At first I strongly smelled the chemical odors but did not react to them as I previously had. After a couple of months I no longer smelled many of them. And it took quite awhile to realize that I no longer had to do things the way I had done them for 6 years. I had CHOICES! I could even eat nearly everything. It has been quite an adventure to become reacquainted with food! And a growing experience!

As I prepared my generational chart in order to better understand myself and my problems, I could see lots of fear and anger coming down through my generations. There were generational curses—sins coming before allegiance to God in the lives of my ancestors (Exodus 20:5)—placed on my life that I was not even aware of. When I looked at myself and the things that were not me, the many things I was dealing with pointed to fear and anger, which go hand-in-hand. I was loaded. When I confessed the sins of my ancestors (Nehemiah 9:2) and repented of their sin (and my own) of giving that spirit of fear a place in my life, at the request of a special pastor, God broke the power of that spirit over me, and for the first time in my life I experienced the peace of God (Philippians 4:7). I realized that the many serious problems I was trying to deal with on my own all stemmed from the spirit of fear. Only God could help me with that, and I had not even known to ask Him.

At the Houston seminar this year, I learned that all disease with spiritual roots (as in MCS/EI) begins with a breakdown in relationships—first with God, then with self, then with man. I didn't have a relationship with God, certainly didn't even like myself, and definitely had a hard time getting along with other people. The way to healing is restoring the same situations in the same order—first, build a relationship with God; next, love yourself as God does; then love your neighbor as yourself (Matthew 22:36–39).

My life is changed now. God has called me to Him and given me a sense of belonging. I am growing more and more to understand who I am in Christ and separating out what is not me from how God sees me. And I'm growing to love others as they have suffered like trials as I have. I am a new creation! (2 Corinthians 5:17)

D.K., Clinton, LA USA

## Healing of Endometriosis

A friend's mom was at *For My Life*™ recently. When she returned home, she shared *A More Excellent Way*™ with her daughter, who has endometriosis. Since she didn't find much information about the disease in the book, she just began working on issues the book brought up, she prayed through rejection, bitterness, and everything that she felt pertained to her life. She already had her ovaries and uterus removed and was scheduled to soon have a 12–hour surgery to remove all endometriosis-related tissue from her neck down to her bladder. It had been affecting her lungs.

She went through the book getting her heart right with the Lord. She didn't think the issues she was praying through had to do with her physical health; she just wanted to be right with the Lord. After going through a series of repentance, that very night the Lord woke her up and told her to cancel the appointment for the 12–hour surgery. She did. She also cancelled her Medicaid so as not to have a back-up plan. As she hung up the phone with the Medicaid office, her physical pain ceased. She had been in extreme pain for 2.5 years and this was the first time it had ever stopped. She had been on extensive pain meds, but they never alleviated the pain, so she had already stopped taking them awhile back.

She has been free of pain and symptoms for six months. She does notice if her heart is not right with God, the pain returns, but she just repents and it goes away. She often repents to her children when she sins against them and then prays with them.

She read a book called the *Endometriosis Sourcebook*. She said the only good thing she got out of it was that one doctor said that endometriosis is the result of a woman hating herself and who she is. Many, many readers and doctors attacked the doctor's statement, but she took it and ran with it.

When I shared the current insight Henry had about endometriosis, of course, she totally agreed. The Lord had already led her through those issues. Amen!

L.H., Branson, MO USA

## No More Sciatica!

I feel so BLESSED! I've learned so much from you and pray that God is blessing you for helping so many!

After one week at your church, the Lord healed me of hives and allergies and tenderness in my body, which I associate with a broken heart! I am still on some high blood pressure medicine...though I do not feel that I now have fear of the future!

When I was sitting at my sister's house, I remember a strange sensation twice run down my back, and I have not had any Sciatica or back problems since...though two days later I was lifting some VERY HEAVY suitcases filled with old family mementos! PTL!!

C.O., GA USA

## My Son is Healed of Crohn's Disease! I am Healed of GERD!

My sister and I went to visit my son who was diagnosed with severe Crohn's disease. We were told later that even if he had the operation, that it would have done him NO GOOD because it was so far advanced.

We brought him the book *A More Excellent Way*™, and then we discussed his healing. He believed that God wanted him to have this disease as a cross to bear. A LIE….We told him that it was a lie that he was believing. I fasted for 5 days, and I had GERD or Acid Reflux for 11 years. I gave up my pills and put out a fleece and told the Lord, "When You heal me, then I know You have healed my son." I didn't know what to expect, but I began reading the book. I knew what I had to do.

So, on that Thursday my sister came in from Michigan and met me in Chicago, and we drove to Minnesota to speak to my son regarding the generational curses and the root of his disease. After talking to him for 6 hours, I got up and repented and asked his forgiveness for severely abandoning him when he was 4 years old, because his dad (a Pentecostal minister) left me and I had to go to work. I saw the change come into my son every time I left to go to work or go out with another man, he was so crushed.

I asked his forgiveness and I then broke the generational curses, which were many in my family with colon problems, Crohn's disease, throat cancers, Multiple Sclerosis, Manic Depression, double personalities, mental problems, Alzheimer's, heart diseases, cancers of lung, brain and kidney cancers, and ANGER…and on and on. I cursed the generational curses, and immediately he felt something release. He looked like death warmed over.

We convinced him to seek counseling at a church in Minneapolis. He went the next day (Saturday). On Tuesday, the next week, he went to visit his doctor who was going to do the surgery and told him that he was healed. The doctor didn't believe him and took a test and came back and told him to get rid of his pills because he was healed. He was plagued with this disease since he was 14 years old, and now he is 31 years old. He never testified, and now he is being asked to preach in his church because he was delivered.

I was also healed of GERD/Acid Reflux. Thank you, thank you, thank you….

N.W., Chicago, IL, USA

## Deafness Healed!

One cannot explain in simple layman's terms the blessings of the Holy Spirit and the Ministry of Pleasant Valley Church. I could not do it justice, but it would be even more of an injustice not to try. I started a book over three years ago. Pleasant Valley Church will be a wonderful chapter in this man's life.

Born in Honolulu, Hawaii. Living in a dysfunctional family with many occultic beliefs, I witnessed my mother's front teeth get knocked out by my dad and then my mother hitting my dad while he slept with an iron skillet. While our dad was in California looking for employment, my mother, my sister and I were kicked out of the house by our drunk uncle in a monsoonal rainfall in the dead of night with no place to go. Somehow, we managed to leave Hawaii for California.

My early years in California are a blur to me, but I was raised up from 6 years young to about 9 years old in an all black neighborhood. To say the least, of what I can remember, I was beat up, chased a lot, made fun of and always in fear. I didn't know it then, but I know it now…I met the evil spirits of hatred, anger, bitterness and prejudice.

We eventually moved to Gardenia; it was predominately Caucasian and Japanese. Strangely enough I even felt out of place there; everyone seemed to have parents with money (we were very poor), nice cars, nice houses, nice clothes, generally nice everything. Again, I was made fun of because my shoes were falling apart, clothes didn't quite fit, and I just wasn't like everyone else. So the pendulum of fear swung over to the other side, anger displayed in violence. I found every reason to get into fights; most fights were for the sake of defending underdogs, but they were still fights and still wrong. Especially since it caused me to meet up with more evil spirits, shame, jealousy, envy and prejudice toward my own nationality. I actually did very good in my studies, but my parents didn't care so my grades dropped, my attendance suffered severely, my attitude was terrible, and I got into trouble all the time; mostly because I was so afraid of fear I fought and got into trouble to hide it; also so that people would leave me alone. It worked in the opposite way I had hoped; suddenly I was surrounded by people who needed help or something.

Family life looked like it would never improve so I ended up in the Army at a very old age of 19. Four months later I found myself in Vietnam. Afraid out of my wits, I found I had to prove myself again. After two Bronze Star medals, a unit citation and a Presidential citation, I asked myself, "What are you doing? God, get me out of here, and I will attend church every Sunday for the rest of my life." He kept His promise; I went home. I didn't keep my promise.

I climbed to the top of the automobile manufacturing industry with American Honda Motor Company, Inc. I was the assistant national manager of the Acura Division. I went through three marriages. In the first marriage, I left three beautiful daughters. In the second marriage we had a beautiful son, a four-bedroom ranch style house in Phillips Ranch, two new cars in the garage and all the things we ever wanted. We were on top of the world. In my third marriage, I married into a world of hurt. She was possessed and had so much generational evil in her. Her recent past was a collection of more evil and sin and hatred. We divorced. Hello evil spirits of greed, lying, stealing, adultery and more.

After 24 years of having all the material things of the world, the world started taking its due fees…my life. Within two years my parents died, I left Honda, I lost my home and cars, my new son lived with his mother, and I became homeless. I've met the spirits of rejection many times before, but never have they been such a part of my everyday life. The spirit of depression tried to talk me into suicide, and the voice of the Lord stopped me.

The Lord led me to work for a church where I studied the Word, became the pastor's assistant and basically ran the church. I did this for four years, making $500.00 a month. Major spiritual attacks of the "unloving spirits" told me that I am worthless, that I'm hopeless and I'll never amount to anything. And then, the church didn't need me anymore; well, they said they couldn't afford me any longer. I had such a peace about that though. I knew that the Lord had something new and exciting planned for me.

I met with the vice president of broadcast engineering at Trinity Broadcasting Network. He told me he had 200 applicants. I told him that I did not have any experience in this field. I guess he didn't care; he hired me the next day. Serving the Lord here has been a wondering blessing to me. He, the Lord, gave me a great team of people. I lived the next few years in one room of a trailer. The roommate was a drug user, didn't work, acted like he had demons in him all the time; a very strange individual, with many strange habits. I remained faithful and thankful to the Lord that I had a roof over my head and a place to work and a life to give to the Lord.

One day, I found myself at work doubled over in severe pain. I was rushed to the hospital. The blockage was cancer of the colon. Two hours before going under the knife at the second hospital, my boss came in to tell me that the president of TBN wanted me moved to the best hospital in the area and to have his own doctor assigned to my case. They removed a third of my colon and ten lymph nodes, six of which had cancer. They wanted to treat me with chemotherapy and radiation. I told the doctors thank you but the Lord would take care of it. This was all in February of 2002.

My beloved wife persuaded me to read your book and listen to your tapes: Abbotsford, Cancer, Unloving Spirits. I loved what I read and heard. I flew to Pleasant Valley Church a day before the actual seminar, August 24th. I could feel the devil's attack, trying to keep me from going. A few days before departure, I knew without a doubt that the Holy Spirit was escorting me every step of the way. After staying in a hotel that evening, I went to PVC on August 25th. The studies were awesome, the prayers and deliverance were incredible, and the healings were miraculous.

During the prayers against the spirits of deafness, my ear popped. I haven't heard out of my left ear since Vietnam, 32 years ago. Suddenly I'm hearing in stereo. All during the week, I kept wondering if the Lord was working on the cancer. Well, it being something internal, I couldn't see if anything was happening. I truly believe that the Lord corrected my hearing so that I could have something tangible to reassure me that He was at work. It was like He was telling me, "Be still, know that I am at work." Anytime we discussed something related to cancer, I could feel something happening inside of me, right below and behind the incision from the operation. Each time that happened, I simply raised my hands and told the Lord, "Thank You for what You're doing in there. Thank You, Lord."

There was so much love, compassion, understanding and patience at PVC. Out at the retreat, I was so at peace....Well, the frog in my toilet did make me jump but besides that I was so at peace. I have a friend that will be at PVC next month. I had lunch with him on Sunday, showed him the pictures and reassured his wife. I told her that when he leaves for PVC say good-bye to the old man because the man that's coming back won't be the same one who left her two weeks ago.

God bless you all. What the Lord has done for me, through you, words cannot explain. By the way, I no longer need to use my distance glasses...my eyesight seems to have improved....Praise the Lord.

D.K., Tustin, CA USA

## I Can Eat and Run and Play and Laugh!

We've been very busy since we came home. We are all doing wonderful! I can see a big change in all of our lives since we came home from Georgia. I've been able to eat things that I can't remember being able to eat ever, and I can run and play and laugh and do all sorts of things that I could never do before.

I've always had terrible headaches all the time since I was six, and it has always been very hard for me to think and remember and to concentrate. I still have a headache all of the time but they are nothing compared to what they were before.

I'm still working hard to get rid of the last of my sickness. I've also been able to understand and learn things that have always been hard for me to learn because of the headaches and because I couldn't remember what I had already learned. Now I just feel like I'm soaking everything up like a sponge and it feels great!

E.T., Toledo, OH USA

## God Got Her Attention!

Home again! After a month in Dothan, AL, where I renewed the fellowship with my precious older daughter and spent a delightful time playing my role as great-grandmother, I am back home much better for the time.

I called for messages only once, answered only urgent emails, etc., baked Jesus bread and cooked for the family, caught up on ironing, taught them how to iron and just rested. I am finally learning in my "old age." Caught up on reading, studying the book for the seminar this month in Georgia—a phenomenal experience and one that will have very long-range effects on my health.

The church has seen tremendous miracles in the health of members who have attended this 2–week experience. Henry Wright has established a ministry teaching what the King James Bible (he only uses it and has convinced me finally that the NIV has significantly changed much in the original Bible and thus must be suspect) says about God and diseases. Basically, about 80 percent of our illnesses have deep and sometimes unrealized spiritual roots which, when dealt with, bring health and healing.

They have been 100 percent successful in seeing healing in an amazing and growing group of people suffering from MCS/EI, which is Multiple Chemical

Sensitivity/Environmental Illness. I had spoken with a lady at the church who had first heard of this ministry. She began being healed when she attended but then "walked out" the rest of it over the next months. She said after a year of applying the principles, she was normal.

I was amazed how many of the approximately 100 people there in January who were suffering from this. Their theory: it is an anxiety disorder stemming from broken human relationship(s) and resting almost completely in fears. Allergies, simple and complex, are also, for the most part rooted in this. The immune system is compromised, and the symptoms evolve.

They give us the Scriptures to study and work through, allowing the person to reach the realization of where their particular root cause could be lurking, then leading the person through recognizing, repenting, releasing the person from these through building their relationship with God the Father and allowing the Holy Spirit to bring the healing. I was really suffering from the allergies that are always particularly bad, supposedly due to the farms surrounding. I literally kept myself awake a lot coughing and suffering from scratchy, tickling throat, couldn't even sing at church from the congestion.

After a couple of days in Georgia, as I began seeing the wisdom and Scriptures, I found that I was perhaps coughing once or twice during the night. I was able to sing in worship like days of old. I still feel some problems, but nothing like all the time so I am "walking out the problem" and praising the Lord.

Osteoarthritis, which has stolen 3 inches from my height, was destined for death for one lady who was Jewish and 60 came almost bent over. She made sure she didn't have to accept our Jesus in the beginning, and Henry Wright used her own "Bible." When she returned home, her physician did a bone density test and told her she had the skeleton of a 30-year-old woman. By the way, she had changed her mind about Jesus.

More than one came who were not born again, and some were healed as they said that God can work when He decides to on whomever and whyever He wants. Of course it would be hard to leave without Jesus, and they said it rarely happens.

A number of people were there who had been before, and some had come several times. The worship is fantastic. Our day started with the most anointed praise and worship. The Holy Spirit was so strong, and the peace and joy was wonderful.

Doctors are sending their patients from all over the country, even doctors who do not believe. One lady had been there who had a horrible cancer over a lot of her face and had been told there was nothing that could be done medically. She looked like those people who have hideous birthmarks. There were people there who had witnessed it. (By the way, they do not lay hands like you see so much and people are healed on the spot. They believe that if the reason has spiritual roots, the real disease is the root and must be dealt with.) On the last Friday, the whole cancer literally fell off, leaving her face needing to restore itself much like a burn healing. After a period of time, her skin was healed and she was renewed. Her doctor could not believe it but had to. I saw a video with her cancer and without.

One dear lady came with a face that made her look years older. A service dealt with the fact that fathers had not shown love and nurtured their children, and thus gave them the root problem many had not understood, thus hampering their relationship with God the Father. The men who ministered simply hugged them and held them while they worked through the realization of the depth of damage done to their personality. God had one of the sweetest husbands of a dear lady be her substitute for her father. They just let the lady decide how long to hold onto this caring friend. She cried as though her heart was split in two for 45 minutes, and when she was finally through she turned around, and I tell you she had dropped 10 years off her face. The rest of the week she glowed and had solved much of her base problem. Then she started growing in her love and trust of God the Father. It was awesome! Interestingly, the man told me he was blessed as much as she. He had intended to go when the men went up for the same purpose.

The week was very intense, and frankly I was exhausted, which helped sleep when it came. We were like teenagers developing friendships, which should be very delightful among our dorm mates. The food was excellent and inexpensive. It was a lot less expensive than one month's medicine bill.

Everyone wants to return because it was such a pleasant time and very spiritually refreshing. The Friday night church service was wonderful. Then Saturday we were separated into very small groups and were ministering one to another. We have long prayer lists. I cancelled my flight and drove home with a lady from Temple and one from Austin. The one from Temple had been in my dorm. Her husband is a pastor, and she was lovely. We had the neatest trip, leisurely and enriching personally and spiritually.

The 2nd week they always have is actually teaching us how to teach this when God presents an opportunity. I didn't have that opportunity and hopefully will be able to go back after the next semester, but I understand there is a ministry that has started here. I plan to volunteer and take part in it since they use the principles and research that is ongoing. These people emphasize that God promises health and not just management of illness that the pills we take generally do. They do urge you to work with your doctor, however, and not go off half-cocked, throwing away your medication. However, a number told me that as they were healed, the medication was eliminated one by one and that is what I am praying for. I told my doctor that I could not believe that some were working against others, there are so many. When I take the morning bunch, I haven't room left for breakfast, which they tell me is so important.

They have a telephone ministry, and they tell us that people are healed without ever having attended the seminars. A few are healed once they read the book and grasp hold of the concepts, allowing the Lord to heal them without it. Tapes are available too for those who cannot come for whatever reason. They aren't trying to build a closely held secret group. While it is copyrighted, they urge us to share with others the principles, and that is why the training.

When I think of the people spending months and years going to counselors and huge amounts of money doing it, I felt as though I had been turned inside out, and during some of the sessions I would think, "oh, this one will be a breeze as it won't reveal much about me." Then all of a sudden I would see and understand areas that needed work. I was only on page 60 (I am a fast reader) and said, "well, I found myself there." By the time I finished the book, I saw myself in a number of places.

I'll tell you when I asked the Lord to reveal to me those I might have at least a root of unforgiveness and bitterness (not me) toward, the list was long and some of them I couldn't even remember their names. The Lord just had me write down their location when it happened. Do not try this unless you want to be stripped naked! And fear? They said that it was the root of most problems and there are 4000 plus different kinds of it. Wow!

They have only seen one person with epilepsy not healed. I thought it wouldn't be healed, but they assured me it is. Chronic fatigue syndrome is also 100 percent on their healed list. People have been healed of a lot of different types of cancer, etc. etc. etc.

They attribute this to their belief that most Christians do not take sanctification as seriously as they should and want to live under a cheap grace. They say a lot of healing is conditional on obedience, and freedom comes from a degree of responsibility. True repentance brings about sanctification. Basically it boils down to their teaching that in salvation our spirit is saved, our soul is being saved, and our body will be saved as we progress through sanctification. It makes sense. As they said, over and over, we do not heal. They urge us to develop a deep and close relationship with God the Father through the stripes of Jesus on the cross that were to heal our diseases and allow Him to heal us with knowledge followed by obedience.

I'll tell you this—I feel better than I have for a very long time and know that I have more work to do and God intends for me to be able to do it. He just had to straighten out some things. No more short prayers. I am getting serious about things.

B.K., Garland, TX USA

### *Creative Miracle in Foot!*

Some two years ago I first injured my left leg and foot, breaking the bones in the instep and causing damage to the nerve plexus in my leg. The medical opinion was that there was very little that could be done without surgery and casting after the swelling had gone down. I decided to leave it alone as it worked, although it was somewhat painful. Then about two weeks later, while purchasing a "solid core" door, I lifted the door to the counter at Home Depot to check out. It slipped and fell on my left foot, breaking the three toes on the outside of the foot causing them to be crooked up and misshapen. Again the remedy seemed to be worse than the malady, so I chose not to have treatment. The disability was no greater than before. Many years before all of this, I had injured the large toe on this foot, causing it to be immobile.

During the first day on my second visit to Pleasant Valley, the Lord spoke to me that He was going to reconstruct my foot, and I shared that with the assembly. On Wednesday of the first week while in class about disliking one's self, my foot began to heat up. I took off my shoe to see what was happening, and the Lord was remolding my foot. The toes were straightened, and the bones in my instep were healed and restored to normal. I also discovered that my big toe was functional! It had not moved in many years! Thank God the foot was back to normal. I could dance in the Lord and jump and praise Him on two feet again, and all is well with that foot today. Isn't our God great?

B.V.N., Duluth, MN USA

## Incurable Cancer Eradicated

Through my husband's infidelity I contracted condyloma. I was totally unaware of being infected. Eight years later, while at the doctor's office for a kidney problem, he did a pap smear. The pap smear came back positive for cancer. In fact, the doctor had never seen a pap smear so bad. I had surgery immediately.

A year later I had bleeding in the bowels. Treatment brought no relief. Finally I had to have surgery again. This time they found four clusters of the condyloma. While they removed those, they said there was no hope. They would keep coming back until my whole system was infected. It was a death sentence.

The surgery left me greatly debilitated. I was in constant intense pain. I continued to bleed.

I came to Pleasant Valley Church as a last hope. I was healed, totally healed. In fact, one doctor who I saw two years after surgery said he saw no evidence that cancer had ever been there. Recently I visited my first doctor. She said she had never seen someone in my condition healed. She could not believe that there was absolutely no trace of the disease there. I give God all of the glory!

K.R., Anchorage, AK USA

## MCS/EI Healed!

I was diagnosed with MCS/EI in 1983. I had never heard of it before and didn't know what to do because most physicians do not treat it. I went to two clinical ecologists in another state but nothing they did ever helped—I only got worse. Because of the restricted diet I was on, my weight was down to 73 lbs. I had to remove the carpeting from my home, sold some of the upholstered furniture, cut off the gas heat and bought electric ceramic wall panels for heating, etc. I lived in a large city, and the doctors suggested that I move to a less polluted environment to take the load off my body so that it could heal. I stayed in an "EI safe" home in CA for a few months and then finally had to sell my house and move to Texas.

I lived in Wimberly, Texas, for 1½ years in a "safe" house with a couple who also were dealing with MCS. During that time I went to Mexico twice for their live cell therapy that was supposed to help the immune system. Nothing helped me and I was still allergic to everything—food, chemicals, clothing, exhaust fumes, perfume. As my last hope, I went to the environmental clinic in Dallas for help. I moved to an area outside of Dallas where people with MCS went to live because they couldn't live in the normal world. My "home" was a 20-ft Airstream trailer that was gutted and lined with foil tape. All I had inside were a few clothes I could wear, a cot to sleep on, and a metal folding chair. The kitchen and laundry facilities were in a separate building. The environment I lived in was one of sickness, negativity, hopelessness and depression. I lived that way for 8 years.

During that time I heard of a doctor in Baltimore who was having some success with this illness, and I went there twice in hopes he could help me. I spent a lot of money with no results. I tried to get neutralized to different substances but had no success with that. Because my weight was so low, I had a subclavian catheter and had to hook myself up to IV feedings; that was no help either. In fact, it made me very sick. Everything I did made me sick. I was very depressed and hopeless. I went to chiropractors, did energy testing, tried to take vitamins and homeopathic remedies, etc., etc. My last big attempt at trying to get help was in going to Los Angeles for 3 weeks to a New Age chiropractor, where I spent $10,000—with no improvement. After that I told God He would have to heal me because I was finished throwing money away. I would rather give any money I had to Him.

I contacted a few churches in the area during those years, but no one had ever heard of such a condition and didn't know how to help me. I had a hard time with this illness also because all my life I believed that everything that happened to a person came from God—good and bad. Why was He punishing me this way? Why was He angry with me? My family had just about given up contact with me and now God had deserted me. The emotional pain was as bad as the physical pain. I used to walk on the road and behind the trailers near gravel pits, where I could be alone and no one would see me, and I would cry out to God for help. Sometimes I would even kneel in the dirt and cry and beg Him to help me. I felt so alone.

At one of the churches I had called, the person asked me if I had ever been through deliverance. I didn't even know what that was. She told me to come there and they would pray for me, so I did. I hired someone to drive me to Dallas to the church (I couldn't even drive anymore because of all the reactions I had), and a group of 4 people talked with me, I repented of some things, and they prayed for me. On the way home I remember feeling so warm, like a blanket was wrapped around me, and I couldn't stop smiling. I started reading my Bible every day after that and started to feel some hope for my life.

Ten days after the meeting at the church, I was reading my Bible outside and went to my trailer for some water. My foot slipped on the step of the trailer, I lunged for the handle but missed it, and my body went down on my right side onto the concrete. I lay there and couldn't move and couldn't even feel my hands and feet. I called out and someone finally came and found me. I declined going to the emergency room—because of fear of the chemicals in the hospital and because I really thought my injuries were minor, so someone carried me to my cot. After about 8 hours my right leg from the knee down was three times its size, hard as a rock and a funny bluish-gray color; the pain had become unbearable.

I finally had to call an ambulance to come and get me and then spent a week in the hospital while the doctors tried to decide what to do with me. The top of the tibia had been crushed, the fibula was broken, and I had numerous cuts and bruises on my body. The EI doctor said I couldn't stand to have any surgery or to have any materials put inside my body; the orthopedic doctor said the only hope was to have surgery. I left the hospital a week later in a full-leg cast that I had on for over 2 months. The pain I experienced was the worst I have ever had because I could take no medications and I was in constant pain.

During the healing process, I used a wheelchair and a walker for over a year; the healing came very slowly. The days I was in the cast I couldn't move out of my trailer, and the loneliness, frustration, and anger at God grew. I also couldn't get out of my trailer to the building where the kitchen was to fix my food, so I had to rely on others to do it, and sometimes that didn't happen for a long time. I felt like I was so alone and starving. Why had this happened, especially since I was starting to have some hope?

I never had thought much about God and healing. A person who had also come to stay in the EI housing area had told me that the chemicals weren't the cause of the illness; it was the devil and evil spirits. I dismissed what she said because I didn't understand it at all. She later died, so that confused me more. A church group used to come to the housing group and read the Bible, pray, and sing—but I couldn't see what good that would do, and I resisted attending when they were there. I was angry with God and couldn't understand why He wasn't helping me.

One day I was standing outside talking with another person. A friend passed by on her way to the trash container, turned around and handed something to me. She said she wasn't interested in the letter; it was probably from some church that wanted her money but that I might be interested. It was a letter from someone who was in contact with Pleasant Valley Church; she gave a phone number that she could call if she was interested in getting help with MCS. That was 2 years after the accident with my leg, and I had since given up hoping for any medical help. I had told God I was waiting for Him to help. I wondered if this might be what I had been waiting for, so I called the number that night. I spoke with 2 people who gave me hope that I really could be healed because others had been and God was no respecter of persons. I cried all night because I felt that finally this is what I had wanted. I spoke with someone on the phone weekly for 8 months and then finally had enough strength—physically, emotionally, and especially spiritually—to move to Georgia.

My healing did not happen overnight, nor was it easy. I had to really begin to look at my life, issues that I needed to deal with, and to learn who God really was—especially God the Father. He is good, He is love. I had a lot of anger built up, a lot of rejection, lots and lots of fear. I had lived in fear and avoidance for so many years and now had to reprogram my thoughts, words, and actions to agree with God's. It was hard work but so worth it! I now live in a normal environment, eat food, wear nice clothes, drive again, and am not afraid of everything! Praise God. And my leg—the last time I had an x-ray of the tibia, it was perfectly formed, no traces of the jagged bones that had been there! I never thought I would ever be able to live this way again. God is good. Never give up or think anything is too hard for God.

P.K., GA USA

## *The Joy of Relearning!*

Have you ever done something one particular way for many years and then had the experience, as I have, of discovering that the way you were doing it was wrong? Have you ever tried to help with a task and found out that your well-intentioned efforts actually hindered the project's completion? Yes, I have also done that, more often than I care to recall! Have you ever had the joy of re-learning something in a way that simplified it so much that you just couldn't believe it? Well, let me tell you about a book I recently read and a seminar I recently took that were just like that. Both the book and the seminar are entitled *A MORE EXCELLENT WAY*™.

You may recognize that phrase as the end of 1 Corinthians 12:31. And the book and seminar deliver just that. People are coming from all over America and even from around the world to discover that *More Excellent Way*™. There were 190 people from all over America (New York to Florida, Minnesota to California) and even one person each from Canada, Mexico and Israel at the seminar I attended. The book may be ordered from the web site www.pleasantvalleychurch.net. You can even sign up for two seminars on this site: the first is called *For My Life*™, and the second is called *For Their Life*™, which, while not grammatical, is very descriptive!

I know there are literally all kinds of crazy things "out there." Let me try to put your minds at ease a little. I am a Christian for starters, so you can erase fears about New Age, cults and crazy stuff. I have twelve years of higher education and three degrees, a BS Ed, MS Ed, and a DMD (doctor of medical dentistry). I taught first and second year physics, chemistry, first and second year biology and general science for five years, and I have been a dentist for twenty-six years. I have attended many, many, many religious seminars and many, many, many dental seminars in my day. I can be fooled, but not easily! (For instance, I was taught and believed the theory of evolution until I started working on my MS Ed with a National Science Foundation grant through the biology department at the University of Georgia in 1971. In one biology course, I realized that everything I had learned in physics, chemistry and mathematics totally negated what they were trying to tell me in biology about supposed evolutionary theory. I realized that evolution never had and never could have happened. I pondered the alternatives and realized that the only alternative that made any sense was that the Bible was true from Genesis to Revelation, no exceptions. So believe me, I have a *rational* faith in a *rational* God, and I do not like funny stuff.)

The *For My Life*™ seminar gave insights into the spiritual roots of many diseases. It also gave me insights into practical Christianity. There are many things that marked the lives of the early Christians that make us think of them as very, very extraordinary. They gave up ALL things for the gospel. They followed Jesus faithfully unto death. They actually DID the things Jesus taught them to do! But today we are surrounded by what I call almost-Christians. They almost believe Jesus. They almost follow Him. They almost follow the beatitudes. They almost obey the Scriptures. They almost forgive their enemies. They almost, almost, almost. And you know what? I have followed their examples a lot, to my dismay. This seminar doesn't hammer everybody else, but it sure did open my eyes to what I see in the mirror. And it showed the logical connection between many spiritual roots and different diseases. Doesn't it make sense that if my life truly moves into ALIGNMENT with God's Word, I should see the promises of Scripture opened up to me? Now I am not talking about faking alignment with the Word so I can test God or deceive Him (ever try that?) into "blessing" me. I mean aligning with God's Word until it KILLS ME to the flesh, until the carnal man is dealt a death blow. I do not mean playing church any more. I mean a total conversion of my mind, will and emotions, body, soul and spirit. I believe that is what characterized the early Christians. And this seminar was a very refreshing breath of fresh air, fresh spirit, in that regard. Please GET the book and ATTEND the seminars. You owe it to the Lord Jesus Christ of Nazareth!

B.C., Jasper, GA

## Testimony of Praise

Thank you for the personal touch of an e-mail thanking me for a monthly contribution and a sincerity of concern for my care and well-being and an invitation to express what Pleasant Valley has meant to me.

Actually, I requested to be on your newsletter just recently, and as I opened one, I seemed to hear the Holy Spirit interceding and letting me know that I was to be a monthly partner. It did take me by surprise in that I have not really been very involved with Pleasant Valley, even though I have heard glowing recommendations and testimonies, have been to hear Henry Wright until hours in the morning, and have read his book and heard a tape. I have sought and followed Jesus in any way I knew.

Anyway, my testimony is this: I said, "Well, yes, Lord, I will be a partner if that is what You are calling me to." Within the next few days, I ran into a friend that I had not seen in about 20 years. When we began to talk, it was as a divine meeting. She had gotten back from Pleasant Valley and had been healed in such incredible ways that it just seem to go all over me! She had been so healed that she had been able to cancel her surgery. We have met, and she has ministered to me. I am receiving something very special from the Lord in all this. We are keeping in touch.

I wanted to let you know of this testimony because I have been believing how important it is to be sowing into the right ground in His kingdom in whatever way and times He should show. I do think I'm reaping something from all of this. Also, I thank you for your prayers that you said that God would anoint my heart in how much to give. He has clearly done that as well.

Again, thank you so much for your heart of love and concern for me and for encouraging me to share my testimony with you as a praise to Him.

L.N., Fayetteville, GA USA

## Psychosis Gone after Prayer

We have seen the Lord do some pretty awesome things here the past couple of weeks, but He blessed me with a special one yesterday. I had admitted a Hispanic man about 52 years old who had frankly become psychotic over a one-week period of time. When I entered the room Monday on rounds, I realized that there was no objective medical reason to this man's insanity. He had indeed had 2 small strokes— one distant and one more recently according to the CT scan, but this did not account for what I was seeing. He was unable to speak and had not spoken in 15 hours. He was writhing in the bed with agitation. He would not respond to the family or me at all. I began to sense that the Lord wanted to show His power here, so I asked the family if they went to church. They are Catholic. I then asked if I could pray for him. They said yes. I then began to ask for the Father's peace for the family and for His presence in the room. I then took authority over the spirit of insanity and fear and cast them out. He immediately quit writhing in agitation. I left and returned in the afternoon. The family told me that as soon as I had left the room that he began to talk. He is now lucid and speaking quite normally today. I explained to the family that this is a miracle of God and that Jesus had healed the man. Medicine had not done it. They do not know what to make of it at this point.

P.S., Greenville, TX USA

## *Felt the Love*

I just wanted to let you know that I miss all of you so much. When you allowed me to sing my song, I thought that my heart would burst with love. I have never felt the acceptance and love of God so strong in a place by so many people in all of my life. I came home a brand new woman, and of course I am walking it out. I talked to my husband, and he is going to try to come for the January class along with (possibly) my son and his wife.

Please let everyone know that I appreciated everyone so much…the true love of God to the body of Christ. I cannot fathom the love that I feel for this ministry. I have never wanted to support a ministry so much in all my life as a Christian. As a matter of fact, I have never really wanted to pray for, build up and support any ministry like this. And I wanted you all to know…from whoever is reading this e-mail to whoever comes into this church to minister, that I will be covering you in prayer and support to the best of my ability.

I hope to see all of you again soon! I am back now in New Jersey, and the Lord had allowed me to walk out a fear of flying. My trip back on Sunday was flying into a storm that was over Philadelphia. During the turbulence, which was pretty shaky, I thought of the wonderful teaching on fear and…I told the devil to "book it"…and he did! You have to face the fear. Well, I'll be flying back to see you all as soon as I can.

J.S., NJ USA

## *Hypothyroidism, Hypoglycemia, TMJ GONE!*

I attended your *For My Life*™ & *For Their Life*™ seminars starting February 9, 2003. I was one of the "Canadians." Being quite a shy person, I did not feel comfortable getting up front and speaking about what was happening to me; however, I thought it is time to start letting you know what's happened so far. I came to Pleasant Valley with food allergies, MCS, Chronic Fatigue, Leaky Gut, muscle pain, Hypoglycemia, Hypothyroidism, systemic Candida, Rheumatoid Arthritis,

Osteoarthritis, Osteopenia and TMJ. Because of the systemic Candida, I had not been able to eat fruit or any sweets for the past 3 years. If I did, I got headaches that lasted for 3 days. I took fruit back into my diet on Wednesday, February 12, and have been eating 3–5 servings a day with NO headaches. By February 26, I realized that the "hurry up" spirit was gone, and I had a peace and calm I had never experienced before. I have even become a less aggressive driver! By March 11, I realized that the hypoglycemia was gone. On March 25, I had my TSH blood level checked, and it was 2.5—smack in the middle of the normal range—and my doctor says I can start reducing my thyroid medication. This is significant for me because one year ago my body had reached the "exhaustion stage." I was flat on my back for one month, and my TSH was over 150. The lab charts only go to 150 and mine was above that, therefore immeasurable. Even on Thyroid medication, it had never come back into the normal range. In fact, it has not been in the normal range for the past 10 years, at least. Over the past few weeks, the TMJ has gone, and the chemicals do not seem to be bothering me; however, I haven't done a real test on that one yet. My energy level is much better, and I'm getting my life back bit by bit. I would just like to say, "Thank you for giving to the Lord; I am a life that was saved."

I know God has a work for me to do in this area, and I am up to the challenge!

Many thanks to you all,

F.R., Delta, BC Canada

P. S. Thank you, Henry, for having the courage to take on this huge job. I have been looking for Christians who could help with autoimmune problems for the past 8 years. I could find none. I worked with people with these problems for 6 years and there were only New Age options that I could find. I come from a medical background, and my illness started in 1980.

### Repentance Gets Results

Thank you all so much for the wonderful ministry I received at Pleasant Valley Church last week in the *For My Life*™ session. I can't even express what all the Lord did and I'm sure will continue to do in the future.

When asked, I've said your ministry is a "class act"—very professional. Your ministry gets results when there are very few that get results nowadays. I think the missing link in ministry today may be ongoing "confession of sin"—repentance. I know that I have a fuller understanding of repentance and the very real Satan.

S.P., Peachtree City, GA USA

### Gloriously Healed!

Greetings! Many of you recently received a letter from my sister describing the Lord's healing in her life, and I want to join my voice with hers in honoring our Physician! *I also have been healed.* Truly Jesus is faithful to seek out the sick and needy so He can bind up their wounds. He *is* a God who keeps His word. He gives us our heart's desires in this life as well as in the life to come.

Many of you have helped relieve our burden during these years of physical stalemate through your thoughtfulness, prayers of faith, and practical acts of love….That is why you are receiving this letter. Besides wanting to share the awesome news with you all, I wanted to thank you for standing with my family and me during some pretty lonely and confusing times. You probably do not realize how important that was.

There are also those among you who are my friends from the world of chronic illness. We've been there for each other, we truly know what the other is going through, we've shared a very difficult season of waiting. I want you especially to know how thankful I am for your friendship. What a special joy I have in relating this new season of my life to you with the anticipation of sharing it as well.

I want to say up front that I understand what it means to hear many different, often contradictory paths and promises of health and healing. I've experienced what it means to repeatedly pursue those promises only to come up short somehow, to find less than was promised and hoped for and sincerely believed for. So, it is not lightly or prematurely that I write my testimony.

I believe truth has to stand the testing to be true. Truth will weather the test of time, knowledge, and godly discernment. A good tree bears good fruit. The basis for the healing that has touched my sister, brother and I, as well as many friends, has stood these tests.

For those who aren't familiar with my history, I began to experience a loss of health at the age of thirteen, in 1984. When I began to have reoccurring bouts with Mono and bronchitis, my parents realized there was something wrong with my ability to resist illness. I also started to experience unexplainable fatigue, pain, confusion, and other symptoms not in conjunction with these illnesses. My parents brought me to many doctors and specialists who administered a myriad of tests, trying to understand what was causing my symptoms. I was a creative and active young girl; what was happening to me physically was not normal, but no one could come up with firm answers. I received all kinds of diagnoses, including rheumatoid arthritis, depression, hypochondria, chronic viral infection, then finally, Chronic Immune Dysfunction Syndrome. This last diagnosis fit the bill, but while it was a relief to know what illness I had, the sobering fact was there was no understood root cause or cure for it.

As the years progressed, so did my physical problems. Despite many treatments, diet and lifestyle modifications, I developed other diseases and symptoms: food allergies, increased hypoglycemia (a major factor in CFIDS), chronic and extreme sleep-related disorder, non-inflammatory muscle pain, IBS, thyroid dysfunction, and especially, Multiple Chemical Sensitivities (a.k.a. Environmental Illness). Between the prison walls of CFIDS and MCS/EI, I lost my entire adolescence and young adulthood. And my brother and sister began to fall sick with the same illnesses six years after I did.

When all was said and done, the treatments, diets, and altered routines made it possible through some alleviation of symptoms for us to keep going. But it became apparent as the years progressed that nothing was bringing significant restoration. All that our efforts amounted to was disease management, not cure. Instead of climbing the slope to recovery, we found ourselves caught in a cycle of survival that basically had the effect of making illness the definitive element of our life.

To come out of the quagmire of CFIDS and MCS/EI is to come out of a prison  house, and that is exactly what the Lord Jesus came to earth to rescue us from! "I will keep you and give you as a covenant to the people, as a light to the Gentiles, to open blind eyes, to bring prisoners out from the prison, those who sit in darkness from the prison house, I am the Lord, that is My name, My glory I will not give to another..." (Isaiah 42:7–8)

Before I go any further, here are some ways the Lord has set me free: Instead of waking up tired, I wake up with a full day's worth of energy. I do not have to plan my life in minutes anymore, I can plan weeks and years ahead. Instead of a hike to the mailbox, I can hike a mountain trail. Instead of having to eat expensive, alternative foods to avoid allergic reactions (to wheat, soy, nuts, dairy, sucrose, additives, eggs, etc.), I can eat anything without a reaction, the way God created my body to. Instead of being isolated by allergies to even extremely small amounts of chemicals found in public places, I can go wherever I want without fear of reaction. I can go to school, church, peoples' homes again after over a decade quarantined because of illness. I can drive significant distances without fear of memory loss, confusion and panic attacks. My chronic sleep problems are gone; I no longer have months at a time where my daytime is in darkness and my nighttime is keeping the sun behind the shades. "Who walks in darkness and has no light? Let Him trust in the name of the Lord and rely on his God!" (Isaiah 50:10).

Can you imagine what it is like to read the Bible and not have to "spiritualize" my illness above all of those passages about healing, about God's desire to heal, clearly spoken and demonstrated through Jesus? Can you imagine the relief to finally understand a little bit WHY, when for years I and my family went to God for healing, with tears and faith and anointed oil, I was *still not* healed?

When I described how my family and I pursued healing from the medical and alternative medical community, there was a parallel spiritual pursuit too. I was raised in a Christian family, I accepted Christ when I was six years old. My parents, three other siblings and I loved God and served Him as faithfully as we knew how. My parents asked the Lord to heal their children—they prayed, they fasted, they did battle for us.

I prayed and asked my God for healing. I remember praying, "God, I can't stop hoping in You. You are all I have. I know You are going to answer my cry, Your Word says You will. I've heard of people healed, even people with the diseases I have. Jesus healed all those who came to Him. You do not have favorites. Please heal me." As time passed, I continued to hold on to this hope: that God would give a doctor somewhere the wisdom for a cure, or I would have a miraculous healing. I couldn't imagine He would heal me any other way.

Months turned into years, and I continued to pray. I prayed from the depths of my heart. I prayed in sincere faith. I claimed Scripture promises. I waited for His perfect timing. My parents and family continued to pray. Several churches prayed. I was anointed with oil and prayed for by the elders of our church (James 4). I went through spiritual warfare books and prayers. I listened to songs and sermons and studies. I claimed, I stood, I rested, I worked, I resisted, I watched, I believed, I hoped, I persisted, I sacrificed, I submitted, I died to my flesh, I waited....

No healing. After years, the questions come: "God is love, He says He will answer my prayers, He says, 'I am the God who heals you...,' so why doesn't He answer my and others' prayers for healing?! What do You want me to do, Lord? What am I missing? Is this a great test, the great trial of my life, my cross?"

Anyone who has gone through it will agree that it challenges a believers' faith deeply when God doesn't seem to answer their prayers for healing.

No Christian can live with these difficult circumstances without in some way making a resolution about God's role in them. It raises questions that have to be answered, and will be, either consciously or in the secret places of the heart. Sometimes the right answer, though, is to keep listening for His answer.

After years of waiting and doing all I knew to do, I concluded that God must have a special reason for not healing me. I decided I must be one of the chosen ones like Paul, whose answer was to be, "My grace is sufficient for you." I decided that, while I still believed God could heal, this illness must be for my own good and God's glory. It was a blessing to me, to make me rely on Him more, which it seemed to do....My illness and the torment of it was to make me more like Christ, to make me like Him in His sufferings. Though I was dying daily on the outside, I would be increasingly renewed on the inside. All this was Scripture, and I applied it to me. The pieces fit. So my spiritual world was in order again.

I never perceived that it was ME, not God, doing the ordering. I didn't remember that my enemy, a liar who steals, kills and destroys, knows how to quote Scripture. In light of God's seeming silence, my flesh, dressed in religious reasoning, with the Enemy's help, found some stones I could turn into bread. It was the only way my world made sense again. But, "Let God be true, but every man a liar!" "Trust in the Lord with all your heart, and lean not on your own understanding; in all your ways acknowledge Him and He will direct your paths." (Romans 3:4, Proverbs 3:5)

The way the Lord brought me and my siblings, and many others to healing from otherwise incurable diseases is simple; please understand that. It is what the Enemy of God enmeshes us in that is not simple. "But I fear, lest somehow, as the serpent deceived Eve by his craftiness, so your minds may be corrupted from the simplicity that is in Christ" (1 Corinthians 11:3).

I want to expose the lies I fell into, so that I can comfort others the way God has comforted me. It was lies that brought our bodies to a point of breakdown, and it is simple truth that set us free. My brother, sister and I walk in healing after years of incurable illness, and it is because the Lord is the same yesterday, today, and forever.

There is no change in Him. His words do not come back to Him empty; they accomplish the purpose for which He sent them.

Listen to the hope in these words!

> **⁴Surely he hath borne our griefs, and carried our sorrows: yet we did esteem him stricken, smitten of God, and afflicted. ⁵But he was wounded for our transgressions, he was bruised for our iniquities: the chastisement of our peace was upon him; and with his stripes we are healed. Isaiah 53:4–5**

> **²Bless the LORD, O my soul, and forget not all his benefits: ³Who forgiveth all thine iniquities; who healeth all thy diseases; ⁴Who redeemeth thy life from destruction; who crowneth thee with lovingkindness and tender mercies; ⁵Who satisfieth thy mouth with good things; so that thy youth is renewed like the eagle's. Psalm 103:4–5**

During the summer of 1998, a good friend of mine, also a long-time sufferer of CFIDS and MCS/EI, went to a seminar hosted by a Wycliffe mission center. Henry Wright was scheduled to speak about "Spiritually Rooted Diseases," and she wanted to hear what he had to say. A couple years earlier a woman who had been healed of MCS/EI sent her a tape by Henry Wright, who taught that this illness, as well as CFIDS, were spiritually rooted diseases, and if treated accordingly, were curable. She threw the tape away, as I would have! We had heard so much to the effect that our illnesses were all in our heads, and this seemed like a religious version of the same tune. And, being raised in the church from childhood, this sounded a little off—certainly nothing she'd heard of in Sunday school! However, as she heard more about what this man was saying, her spirit and a personal examination of Scriptures bore witness with it.

She called me after the seminar was over to tell me about it. Honestly, I was skeptical about the whole idea that my disease had a spiritual root. I had a good relationship with God, I had fruit in my life, I felt my prayer and praise life were great, I grieved over my shortcomings, I helped people around me as I could, I was a mature Christian, and I was suffering in God's will. And this guy is going to lay another burden on me by telling me I have a spiritual problem? I do not think so. I will tell you, what broke my skepticism was not what this man said, but what God did through it for the health of my friend.

She was worse off than I was in both diseases. She had nearly died several times from throat closure, and experienced severe muscle weakness and collapse in allergic reaction to chemicals and foods. She, as I did, had to use an industrial strength, chemical filtering face mask nearly anywhere outside her home. The final night of the seminar, Henry Wright led those who were sick in prayer, encouraging them to repent before the Lord of those things that were demonstrated as being a spiritual factor in their illness. She told me she prayed and was prayed for that evening, and then she took off her mask—in a room full of chemically saturated people, carpet, and chairs—and was fine.

I could not argue with that. I knew her too well to deny that was a major change. Nor, as she continued to speak, could I argue with what was bearing witness in my own heart. This man taught that God knows how our bodies are wired together, that He created us to be very chemically responsive to what is happening in our spirit-man. For example, he explained, when a person panics, their cerebral cortex sends signals to the hypothalamus gland—the brain of the endocrine system. It in turn sends out impulses and chemicals that make the body respond with a faster heartbeat, slower metabolism, an adrenaline rush, dry mouth, shaking knees, etc. This is called a "fight or flight" reaction. Normally, this lasts only a few minutes. However, when a person is in bondage to fear, when stress and anxiety are a way of life, their body is going to respond very negatively. You weren't wired to remain in *constant* "fight or flight," and many serious illnesses are the result of just that.

Henry Wright went further on to say that fear is in fact a sin, not simply a "negative emotion." How many times in the Word does God say, "Do not fear"? We are not to be in bondage again to a spirit of fear....Fear, stress and anxiety are not emotions we need to "manage" but sin we need to repent of. Only then can we be free of it. He observed that when people repented of those sins, turned away from them and were cleansed from spiritual bondage, their bodies started to return to health.

Through the Word, pastoral observation and education by the medical community, he discerned that not only did the sin of fear have a physical consequence, but also sins like self-hatred, unforgiveness, jealousy, rebellion, double-mindedness, bitterness, anger, rejection, occult involvement, self-condemnation, etc. Generational sins, and traumas like abuse, and failure of a man to be a godly leader in the home also manifested in the physical realm.

With this discernment he was seeing people with a myriad of incurable diseases completely healed. He wasn't operating in the gift of healing—people were simply responding to a revelation of truth about their lives, repenting, being set free from spiritual bondage, and their bodies were returning back to health as a result.

After my friend's call, I sat on the sofa with a growing conviction of the truth in what I just heard. I never would have called myself a fearful person, but the practical reality is that I was. I functioned daily in a gut belief that fear, not the Holy Spirit, gave me foresight, and made me alert to details that I would not notice otherwise. Fear was looking out for me, because, let's face it, God failed to protect me and those I loved one too many times. The same with bitterness. After wiping away some religious denial, I had to admit I believed God wasn't just when it came to standing up for me; I needed a wall against people who hurt me, and Bitterness was a better defense lawyer than God. I discovered I was bitter against God, myself, and others. That was another thing Henry Wright pointed out: disease is often a result of separation from God, yourself, and others. When it comes to healing, bitterness has to go. It is the sin God said would open your life to spiritual torment (Matthew 18:35), and where you find spiritual torment you will find physical torment. He just didn't create us—spirit, soul, or body—to function in unrepentant sin! (1 Thessalonians 5:23).

So, that night, overwhelmed with a deep and refreshing conviction, I let go of all the things I knew I had turned to instead of God, especially those things Henry Wright said were at the root of my illnesses. I really felt like a infant, helpless, dependent for my very life; it was a frightening feeling. Hope was starting to awaken in my heart again, hope that I could be healed—truly, finally healed. It was too good to be true, too simple. Fear and other spirits of Satan's kingdom fought over my thoughts and emotions. I had been disappointed too many times! But God did not let me go, and hope grew into single-hearted anticipation that He not only wanted to cleanse my heart, He wanted to heal my body, too. The new refreshment I felt in my spirit testified that indeed something big was about to change.

It did. Three months later I began to see changes in my energy, in how I felt all over. I could think clearer, I could breathe more comfortably, I could eat small portions of once forbidden foods….I began the process of "walk-out," taking back the abundant life God promised me, with the Holy Spirit, and help from the family of God. (Tapes from Henry Wright's ministry helped tremendously.) Within six months, I was 80 percent well, and after a year, 100 percent well. The pain of fourteen years of life-devastating disease is now just a memory! God is good!

I first wrote this testimony during the fall of 1999; it is now 2004 and I remain in total healing. My brother was healed soon after I was, and God healed my friend and my sister during a stay at Pleasant Valley Church in Thomaston, GA. Other friends were healed by simply responding to the Holy Spirit as He spoke through our testimonies. God has no formula, but His truth remains the same.

I had so many questions about things, and no doubt you do too! Please feel free to contact Pleasant Valley Church. They have many resources available, including awesome ministry and training programs. Thousands of people—the sick, doctors, pastors—come yearly from across the country and around the world to partake of this awesome grace of God in discernment for healing. Some examples of disease that God is healing through the ministry: Asthma, Allergies (food, particle, chemical), Anorexia, Bulimia, Cancers (including breast and Leukemia), Diabetes, High Cholesterol, Heart Disease, Blood Pressure disorders, Crohn's, Panic Attacks, Addictions, Fibromyalgia, Rheumatoid Arthritis, Arthritis, Sleep Disorders, Spiritual Oppression, Depression, Manic Depression, Schizophrenia/MPD, OCD, ADD/ADHD, Scoliosis, CFIDS, MCS/EI, Lupus, Some Virus Related Diseases, Osteoporosis, Epilepsy, MS, Cysts, Parkinson's Disease, Skin Disorders, Migraines, Hypo- and Hyper-thyroidism and others. Creative miracles also take place at Pleasant Valley Church as they operate in all the gifts as a home church for the area.

The ministry notes on their materials and carries out in practice that they "Do not seek to be in conflict with any medical or psychiatric practices, nor do we seek to be in conflict with any church and its religious doctrines, beliefs or practices. We are not counselors, but ministers, administering the Scriptures in line with 1 Corinthians 12, Psalm 103:3, 2 Corinthians 5:18–20 and Ephesians 4.

We are not a part of medicine or psychology, yet we work to make them more effective, rather than working against them. We believe many human problems are fundamentally spiritual with associated psychological and physiological manifestations."

It is my hope that the changes God has brought to my and so many other lives will bless you too. Good news spreads quickly and keeps spreading! It is so awesome to praise Him with you!

P.L., Central, SC USA

## No More Colic

When the baby was born, they brought her home, and she began to have that all night colic stuff, and they couldn't sleep. They even put her in a clothes basket on the dryer one night and turned the dryer on, hoping the vibration of the dryer would make her go to sleep. They were frustrated. The daughter had inherited a spirit of fear. That is the iniquity of the generations, a familiar spirit, a fear of abandonment....They dealt with it and she slept seven hours. And they slept seven hours, too. She never had colic ever again. When they had another daughter, the first thing they did when they brought her home is that they set her before the Lord by faith, the Father, and they broke the power of this iniquity that is traveling in her also, and that child never had colic one time.

S.H., GA USA

## Tumors in Breast Disappeared

If you sow and have bitterness against your mother-in-law, do not be shocked if tumors appear in your right breast. And if you have bitterness against your mother or one of your sisters, do not be surprised if tumors appear in your left breast. Or if you find tumors in both breasts, do not be surprised to find that if you have bitterness both against the sister or a mother and mother-in-law or another female, maybe in your church or where you work.

We have seen for a number of years the connection between bitterness and breast cancer. A lady who attended the seminar to the Wycliffe Bible Translators in North Carolina, from which the transcript became the book *A More Excellent Way*™, sat in the audience with tumors in both breasts. She had bitterness against her mother and she had bitterness against her mother-in-law, and she sat in an audience and didn't come up to me. We didn't have a day of ministry. We just taught for three days the principles. And she left that conference. Never said a word to me. She went back to her home with something called conviction. Conviction is the work of the Holy Spirit. Condemnation is a work of the unholy spirit. Whenever you feel condemned, it is the enemy; when you feel convicted it is always the Holy Spirit.

She went home with the truth. And the truth pierced her because she had the bitterness issues. Talking about left breast, right breast. I have doctors that have been impacted by our teaching on cancer who have been doing case histories with their patients and going back and reviewing the pathways of case histories of those females to see if they had bitterness in the area that I see it. And sure enough, they have seen it every single time. But here's what they have discovered: tumors that form in the right breast is bitterness between that female and another female that is a non-genetic family member like mother-in-law or some other person maybe or of the women in the church or something. But tumors that form in the left breast are against a genetic female like mother or sister and they have found that 100 percent of the time.

So this lady in North Carolina began to recognize that bitterness against her mother and her mother-in-law was sin. She recognized that bitterness was a sin. She repented to God for her bitterness. And in her heart these words formed, "Go to your mother and deal with her."

So she made an appointment with her mother and repented to her mother for her bitterness and made peace with her mother, and when she was re-checked by her doctor, all tumors had left only one breast.

She went to God in her prayer time and said, "God, how come only one breast?" And in her mind's eye these words formed: "Because you have only done half the work. What about your mother-in-law?" When she made the appointment with her mother-in-law, she went and confessed her bitterness as sin and repented. When she was re-checked by her doctor, all tumors had left the other breast. And she has been tumor free for five years. I know her well.

M.B., NC USA

### Chronic Constipation, Insomnia Healed

We attended your *For My Life*™ and *For Their Life*™ seminars in April, 2003. We are from Oregon. I want to thank you for working so hard to care for thousands of hurting souls. We were very much blessed and, suffice to say, I had to change some of my old theologies after attending your seminars. I was plagued with chronic constipation for more than twenty years. All of that left in the first week of the seminar and has never returned. I was battling serious insomnia, and during that first week, my sleep returned, and I have never lost it since.

OR USA

### Many Healings!

I want to thank you for your ministry. I have been teaching the principles of your ministry at our church and we have seen the following things healed in our church: allergies, asthma, arthritis, flu/virus/bacteria, breast cancer, and scoliosis— the lady grew one inch! Praise God!

Pastor, IL USA

### Allergies

Recently your church advised one of our families regarding their son's and daughter's allergies. Our pastors are very encouraged by your ministry. God has given them a revelation regarding the endocrine system. Your understanding is much greater than ours and has moved us on in our understanding. If you ever want to visit England, we would be more than happy to host a conference in England.

England

## *Praise God, I'm Pregnant*

A few months ago I called your church, and you returned my phone call and spent almost an hour on the phone with me. I had been struggling with infertility, allergies, hypoglycemia and a sluggish thyroid. I had been trying to get pregnant for two years and had spent the last four months on fertility drugs. My infertility was "unexplained" according to the doctors. After our talk, I went off the fertility drugs.

**PRAISE GOD, I'M PREGNANT**! I have been working on freedom and my life has changed dramatically for the better and God healed my infertility! I just want you to know how much I appreciate your phone call and prayers and how joyous we are over God's miracle in our lives.

J.B., Matthews, NC USA

## *Face Cancer Fell Off*

Do you think self-hatred is sin? Nobody prayed for her. She came to our program. She heard the truth. If you know the truth, the truth shall make you free. Self-hatred is sin because it calls God a liar. You think God is greater than you?

She sent pictures just before she came to our *For My Life*™ program in Georgia a couple of years ago with cancer of the face. Her eyes are dark with anger. Thirty days later in the final stages of her face healing, see her eyes, how sparkly they are.

She came to our program with cancer of the face. She hated herself. When she looked in the mirror, it did not say that she was the fairest of them all. And where she looked is where Satan put the disease so that she could be convinced. In our program, *For My Life*™, when we got to the section on self-hatred and in fact, self-hatred is a sin unto death because it produces diseases that are unto death. When she recognized that self-hatred was a sin, God opened her heart. She went from *logos* to *rhema* quickly.

She was staying at one of our retreat cabins and when she called self-hatred sin and repented to God for hating herself, that evening the cancer fell off her face onto the floor. God forgave her.

J.S., Shepherdstown, WV USA

## *Thank God, I Can See!*

Can you send me any information about hearing and ears and the spirits behind this? I have taken authority over the spirits behind the eyes that you sent to me, and last week when I was driving for the first time afterward, I realized my eyes were strained with my glasses on. I lifted them up to see a milepost sign and could see it clearly without the glasses, but when I put the glasses on, I could not see as well, and my eyes were strained. When I got into town, I tried this a couple more times before taking my glasses off. I could see better without them! Thanks!

J.B., USA

## *Hodgkin's Disease and Infertility*

...a few things I will tell you that have led us to being able to conceive a child.

I am an emotional, physical, verbal and sexual abuse survivor. I never in a million years thought I could ever get past these awful events in my past. I have had multiple illnesses that included asthma, allergies, infertility and Hodgkin's disease. I have been working with the help of your book, *A More Excellent Way*™. I am now free and clear of all of the above illnesses. I never thought I could have this kind of peace and joy in my life. Being pregnant has been one of the greatest blessings of all, after being told by doctors that I would never have children due to the radiation I received for the Hodgkin's disease. I believed them, and went on my way until I truly found out how wonderful God is, and how hanging on to the past was so binding, and how idle words can be such a curse. Thank you for your ministry and for being obedient to what God has asked you to do.

K.

## *We're Having a Grandbaby!*

I first heard of Henry Wright from two men who had received healing in Georgia. Truly I really thought nothing of it till I heard about the Detroit Conference this year. The Holy Spirit quickened me to attend. While there, I talked with Henry about my daughter-in-law. She had trouble conceiving and eventually miscarried.

After getting her the book and sending the conference tapes to her, she did the following…She quit taking all the drugs. Thirty days later she had her first period ever without the use of drugs. She had her next period again after 28 days. Yesterday, she announced that she was again pregnant. She is sharing the material all over Malibu.

Thank you for your obedience.

T.M., Cincinnati, OH USA

## *Free of the Curse!*

It has been almost 3 months since I was there, and I want to thank you for all you did for me during my 3 and ½ week stay. Never before have I experienced so much love from anyone outside of my immediate "Christian Family." The friendship that I received from the fellowship and the women I lived with will stay tucked away in my heart for my lifetime.

The good news is that I am healed, not just in the faith, but also in the body. Whatever disease Satan tried to put on me, whether Crohn's disease or ulcerative colitis, his plan failed. Not only am I fully and completely healed from the disease, but I am also healed from the spiritual bondages and generational curses that I carried for 50 years of my life. I have been giving my testimony about how I was released from the torment of the "Unloving Spirits" from the very first time that I learned of their existence and how they convinced me to believe that was who I was. I will continue to help others in their search for truth, giving the glory to God using the knowledge that I received while staying at your ministry.

S.W., Vero Beach, FL USA

## *Thanks To You, We Have Our Daughter Back!*

God has given our family a wonderful praise to share. Our 11-year-old daughter, who has had allergy headaches since age 4, fibromyalgia from age 8, and migraines since age 10, has been totally and completely healed by our Lord!

The information in Henry Wright's book, *A More Excellent Way*™, states that fibromyalgia can be triggered by a spirit of fear in the realm beyond consciousness. Someone with FM may not feel covered, protected, nurtured, or secure. The fear is something that threatens you and is enough to keep you awake all night.

I approached my daughter and asked if there was anything she was afraid to tell me. There was one event that happened when she was four that she knew was wrong. Week after week, the other child involved in the incident would reinforce the fear and remind her not to tell. She knew she should tell us, but believed Satan's lie that her parents would not love her anymore.

Once she confessed the fear and forgave this person, she slept that night without fear! Over the course of a month, as she slept her body began to heal. The muscle pain is completely gone, and her ever-present allergy headache vanished. The twice-a-month 4-day hormonal migraines also disappeared, and the foods and odors that triggered a migraine no longer caused one!

One of the dearest moments for me was two months after all this had happened; my daughter smiled and said she didn't have a migraine. She had eaten food dyes for the first time and experienced no pain. She loves to decorate cakes. She is now able to decorate and eat her cake creations and do anything else He has planned for her. She is no longer limited by a chronic disease that God never intended for her to have. We praise God for being faithful to His Word and for the knowledge you shared with us!

V.B., Houston, TX USA

## *Healed of Lactose Intolerance*

I had had stomach pains, cramps and diarrhea for several weeks. My Mom and I finally went to the doctor and while we were in the waiting room, my Mom found an article on lactose intolerance, and she thought that the symptoms in the article were a lot like the symptoms I was having. We went in for the appointment and the doctor said to stay off all milk products for one week. When the week was over, I had a full glass of milk and ran to the bathroom and experienced all the symptoms in about 5 minutes.

Then I met a lady at Pleasant Valley Church, and she prayed a really special prayer for me, and I began to use that same prayer every time I would have milk products. I would have cereal and milk, trusting that God would take care of it and **HE DID**! Since then, I have been eating tremendous amounts of dairy with no problem. So thank You, God!

D.S., Woodstock, GA USA

### No More Migraines

I have been healed from 25 years of chronic migraines. The healing was a direct result of what Henry Wright had to say in *A More Excellent Way™!* Please share this blessing with whomever would rejoice with me.

A.O., Tyler, TX USA

### Healed of Chronic Fatigue Syndrome

I attended your recent conference in Houston, Texas, and was miraculously healed of 10 years of Chronic Fatigue Syndrome. No more sleep disturbance, no more headaches, no more esophagitis, no more fatigue or afternoon naps! God has really been using this greatly! I gave my healing testimony to the church we attend at a healing service. It was wonderful to have a clue as to how to pray for people. I told my doctor that I was healed at a spiritual healing conference, and she said I was the third person in her practice to have been healed of CFS through spiritual means and that she was very interested in getting more information. I gave her a copy of my notes and a video of the Sunday morning sermon you did, as well. My pharmacist is also interested in more information. I want to thank you so much for heeding God's call and letting Him use you to help His people find healing!

P.B., Houston, Texas USA

### Healed of 13 Diseases

Because of your personal commitment to help me get well, because of countless hours of teaching, patient and loving ministry, because you have a heart to go after lost sheep and pull them up out of the pit of destruction, because you have a heart that reaches out to suffering people, because you understood how to approach a person with an anti-Christ spirit, because you love Jewish people and the foundations of the Christian faith in Judaism, because you knew how to disciple me without preaching salvation with a big drum, because you showed me that the Bible applied to my life on an everyday basis, because you gave me the respect I needed to receive in order for me to listen, because you and your staff are the first Christians I ever saw apply the Word of God, and because you and your staff do not condemn people who are sick or who are non-Christians, because your prayers and your staff are the first prayers I ever saw God respond to, because you have such an extensive knowledge of the Word of God and can explain human being's situations through Scripture—I am healed of:

Devastating Multiple Chemical Sensitivities/Environmental Illness

Hypothyroidism

Extreme hypoglycemia

Leaky gut / malabsorption

Extreme food allergies

Electromagnetic field sensitivity

Chronic fatigue

Nightmares

Depression

Central Nervous System damage

Neurological Dysfunction

Injuries on hands healed (had not healed for 3 years)

Knees healed (would slip out of alignment for past 2 years)

I looked like a person whose entire life had been destroyed, and it seemed that I would be dead soon. I missed my daughter's college graduation because I was too sick to travel. When she dropped me off at Pleasant Valley two years ago, she said, "I expect you to be at my graduation from law school in three years." Henry, because of your work, I will be there.

I have been given back my life. I now have the opportunity to experience God's abundance as I go forward, walking in the Word. I am excited about what God has in store for me. I am excited about being in relationship with God throughout the rest of my life. I am excited and relieved that He is in charge of my life and I do not have to figure it all out. I am excited that He has a plan for my life and that there is work for me to do for Him. I am so relieved to have a focus that is not based on human strength.

Thank you for introducing me to the true God. I searched for Him all my life in all the wrong places. I am so happy.

P.J.B., Broken Arrow, OK USA

### Set Free From Allergy to Sugar

I suffered from an allergy to sugar for the past 3, almost 4 years. I would get terrible migraine headaches if I ate anything with sugar in it. Believe me, just about everything has sugar in it. I was so limited. I had to read the labels on everything before I would dare eat it. I was in a sort of prison that was a lie from Satan. I lived in fear that if I ate something I enjoyed, I would be sick in bed for two days with a terrible headache. I'm not talking just about sweets, I'm talking about everyday food, like yogurt, spaghetti sauce, cereal, almost every kind of drink except water, simple things you would not think are full of sugar. It was very confining and miserable. Friends would say, "Oh, I couldn't do that," and I would have to eat it and put up with the headache.

I spent thousands of dollars going to doctors. The only thing the doctor could do was prescribe Imitrex for the pain, which I took for 3 years. Then I read your book and saw what a lie Imitrex is!!!

Well, all of that history to tell you that the Lord has healed me! I have been eating everything and anything I want for the past 4 months! I do not even look at the labels. I have been set free from that allergy and from the lie of Satan. I am so excited that I am free to enjoy all the food that the Lord has provided and without fear.

I want to thank you and your wife so much for coming to Alaska and spending so much time with us. I want to thank you for your dedication to teaching God's

Word and precepts. Thank you for your faith that was contagious and helped to build my faith even higher. Thank you that you allowed your tapes to be printed so I could read and study. Thank you for exposing Satan for what he is and teaching us that we can be free—that we do not have to live under his oppression and the sickness that he bestows on people.

C.S., Valdez, AK USA

### God is Still Doing Miracles!

This is an amazing true story about how I was miraculously healed by the Lord. It is well worth taking a few minutes to read about how God is working. I believe it will encourage you.

Some years ago I was involved with Broadway, playing the part of John Lennon in Beatlemania, and also recording as a solo artist for Atlantic Records. With my career going the way it was, a lot of people would think I was in the midst of fulfilling the American dream, but in actuality, it was a very stressful time in my life. My mother died from cancer, and then my father was murdered shortly thereafter. Little did I know that it would all take its toll on me some years later.

It was a friend who led me to the Lord back then and helped me to break free from secular music, and learn to live my life for the Lord Jesus Christ. I will always be grateful to him for sharing Jesus with me and for being such a good role model to me. Anyway, I was out playing here and there doing concerts and ran into some difficulties a few years ago. Somehow I managed to come down with a heart condition. We are talking serious stuff here. I discovered that it also ran in my family tree, but having been an orphan now for a number of years, I did not know anything about this at first. The Bible talks about blessings and curses, and the sins of the father being passed on to the third and fourth generations. (Exodus 34:7, Deuteronomy 28, 2 Timothy 3:16, and Galatians 3:10–3:29.) I will tell you that I did not grow up in a Christian home.

I was sent to see a cardiologist after a week in the hospital in the fall of 1999, and the future looked pretty grim. I had just acquired a young 3-year-old Tennessee Walking horse, as I have been an equestrian most of my life and am as passionate about horses as I am about art and music. I was told I would never ride again. Soon I was put on some very dangerous medicines that actually have caused sudden death, the very thing they were supposed to prevent. Being a believer, I desperately ran after the Lord. Hebrews 11:1: "Now faith is the substance of things hoped for, the evidence of things not seen." I was at a church service in Dallas, GA, about that time. My friend who was a pastor there prophesied over me, and told me the Lord would heal me and I would receive a miracle and live a long, healthy life. He helped me understand that the Lord wants to heal us, but we still have our part to play. I mean, not everyone gets saved, and yet the Bible teaches that God wants to save all of us—that none shall perish. Of course, you can see God wants to heal all of us as well, but we still have a part to play. We have choices to make. How many times in the Bible did Jesus say to someone, "Your faith has healed you"? So faith must have a part in getting one healed. Without faith we cannot even be saved. You are saved by faith! (If you have not yet been healed, I am not saying that maybe you do not have enough faith, because God gives us all a measure of faith. Faith can increase, however. "So then faith cometh by hearing, and hearing by the Word of God" (Romans 10:17). Also, "As a man thinketh so he is." So I came to that place where I had to ask myself, "Whose report are you going to believe?" I sought after the Lord Jesus day and night and discovered in Hebrews 13:8 that God is the same yesterday, today and forever. Malachi 3:6—He changes not!

So, I got to thinking, "When did He stop doing miracles?" My Christian friends all prayed for me, and the lead singer told me his dad had prayed for a blind man once back in Australia and he received his sight. My good friend of AIM (Adventures in Missions) encouraged me in the Word and also showed me amazing reports from around the world where the Lord was still doing miracles, healing people and even raising some from the dead. He got me to read a book by Jack Deere, *Surprised by the Spirit*, and in it I found stories that also helped build my faith. There was one story of a young boy who had been dead over six hours, and an evangelist from North Carolina was used to pray him back to life with many witnesses. Yes, this happened in our lifetime. Read your Bible and see for yourselves. It talks about casting out evil spirits and raising the dead (Mark 16 and Matthew 10:7–8 KJV). After the Holy Spirit came upon them, even the Apostles did these things. As believers we are told "this and greater things shall you do!" Many Christians just do not study the Word for themselves but trust their pastor instead to think for them, which actually puts extra burdens on the pastor. No offense, but they are still just men too, and in Romans 7, Saint Paul admits the things he wants to do, he does not always do, and the things he does not want to do, that he does, because of the evil that dwells within. All of us have fallen short of the glory of God. What I am trying to say is you need Jesus Christ to be Lord over all of your life—every aspect of it. So make sure all the thoughts you have line up with what God says. Think holy words always!

I started looking for the Lord in a number of churches and ministries and as He said, "Seek and you shall find!" Eventually I ended up at Pleasant Valley Church in Thomaston, GA. After receiving ministry there, I was healed of a so-called incurable heart disease! Then in July 2001, I was there for a church service just a week after I was ordained as a minister, which was also the same day I was taken off heart medicine. I was asked to share my gifts of music in that service, but instead of doing so, I began to have heart trouble, of which I knew I was already healed. My doctor, who to me is the best doctor in the world, was with me at the time. I recall her taking my pulse and looking very concerned, but saying, "We have tried medicine, now we must just trust the Lord," and she kept praying for me all through this time.

After the service had ended, I was talking to Henry Wright and his staff and I suddenly started to pass out. Actually, I was dying right there on the altar of the Lord. My doctor was taking my pulse. For two and one half hours it had been faint and irregular and was at this moment completely gone! All I recall was hearing Henry Wright say, "I know how to deal with this." Henry prayed at this time, apparently casting out a spirit of death. I recall my doctor telling me how astonishing that was because she had her finger on my pulse and it was non-existent. The instant

Henry Wright prayed, my pulse came back so strong and healthy that it pushed her finger off, which had never happened to her before in all her years of medical practice and ER duties.

It is impossible to have no pulse and then suddenly have a normal healthy one. A staff member who is a nurse was taking my pulse on the other hand and had the exact same experience as did my doctor. The Bible tells us, "Nothing is impossible with God!" In a tape series called "Spirit World Realities 2002" he mentions this story and goes on to say, "What should we have done, called 911? It would have been too late." We called on the name of Jesus, and I am alive and well today!

Henry Wright is one of the most Christ-like men I have ever met in my life. I believe he operates in all nine gifts of the Holy Spirit. I am eternally grateful to him for the work he does in ministry to teach the truth and set people free. I believe perhaps thousands of people have been healed of all sorts of terrible diseases by the Lord through this ministry all around the world. I would strongly suggest you take a look at the book, *A More Excellent Way™*, written by Henry Wright.

A few months ago I was preaching at a church, and my doctor drove over four hours both ways just to help me testify to what I have just shared. When she shared her side of the story at the end of the service, she went on to say that indeed, it would have been too late to call 911 and that I had already been on last ditch medicine. There was nothing anyone could have done to save me. I ask you, do we serve a living God or what?! All praise be to my Lord Jesus Christ! I thank Him every day for my now good health, for allowing me to still be here to watch my children grow up in the knowledge of the Lord, to be here for my wife, family and friends, and to ride my horse again, to make music and art unto the Lord and serve Him through this ministry. Alleluia!

C.M., Canton, GA USA

## Healing of Hepatitis B

I am writing to you to express both my gratitude to God and to many of you for your help during the past year. The intent of this letter is to acknowledge the power of God at work to restore His people.

This is currently a very significant time for me because I became very ill around this time last year. I contracted Hepatitis B, which was thought at first to be fibromyalgia or chronic fatigue syndrome. I lost 50 lbs. in 2 months time. I could not walk up the stairs of my house. Needless to say, I was in bad shape. My life came to a screeching halt. I could not believe that this was happening to me. Yet it was, and at the time I could not stop it.

So I did what most of us do. I consulted the help of the medical community. I thank God for their help and support. I am especially grateful for my friend who is both a man of God and a wonderful practitioner. He and another doctor were used by God to get me out of a serious crisis.

However, I knew there was a deeper work going on in my life. Although some of my symptoms began to subside, there were some that continued to oppress me. I could not shake them, even with superb medical assistance. There was a spiritual work that needed to be addressed.

It was about this time that I discovered a book called *A More Excellent Way*™. The author, Henry Wright, has spent about twenty years researching why certain people do not recover from various illnesses. What he discovered, and what I found to be true, is that many times there is a spiritual root that must be addressed in order for healing to take place.

The truth that I found in this book restored my hope that God was able to meet me in my pain. Henry addressed the issues of diseases and their spiritual roots in a very direct manner. He presented truth with a solid foundation according to Scripture that made me aware of the real issues in my life, unlike all the other stuff I have been and was being told.

Some said that they had friends who had the same illnesses and their friends were "OKAY." Others said I did not have enough faith. Some said I was not using the RIGHT doctor. Many said that I just needed to accept my pain and learn to manage my life, as if this were God's plan for me. There were those who blamed the Devil. Others gave up and went back to their busy lives, which I understand because the lives we create are very demanding.

Please understand I condemn no one for what they believe. However, it is a very different ball game when you're the one who has sustained an injury that could knock you out of the sport for good. I found that it is easy to throw out opinions, but when your life is on the line, it is an all-together different matter.

I so desperately wanted truth. I wanted someone to sit me down and share the hard-core realities, no matter what they were. I believe that I found the essentials that I needed to set in motion a process of restoration that only God could design and provide. Most of this information came to me from Henry Wright's ministry in Thomaston, Georgia—Pleasant Valley Church.

What I learned from Henry Wright saved my life. I know that. I attended a 2–week program that they hold monthly at their church in Georgia in June 2002. It began the process of healing that I deeply needed. The spiritual issues that I was facing, I learned how to recognize them and rightly deal with them.

I learned some crucial things about my life. I learned that I had opened the door to much of what I was suffering because of the way I was living. I had forgiven many people in my life, but I had not forgiven myself. I had some bitterness about life that I was holding on to. I had made fear and drivenness my friends. Any time I had a project to do, I drove myself until I collapsed. These are the foundational issues that I needed to deal with.

As I have dealt with these issues and others over the past year, I have become more spiritually free and physically healthy. My doctor told me that my blood is clean and that my liver is fine! I now am sleeping through the night, as opposed to getting as few as two hours a night. My body is practically pain free. All of this new information came from my last doctor's visit, which she described my body as strong and my immune system operating the way God created it to.

I am sharing this with you with hopes and expectations that, if any of you or someone you know needs the same help, you can find it.

Finally, ultimately God deserves the glory for my healing. God made a way to restore me. He does and still is in the healing business. He is my healer and deliverer. I acknowledge that the life He has given me is a precious gift for which I am forever grateful. May His Name be praised!!

P.F., GA USA

## Blood Sugar Dropped and Blood Pressure More Normal

I returned Saturday evening after two weeks at Pleasant Valley Church in Thomaston, GA. Check it out on the net www.pleasantvalleychurch.net. What a revelatory adventure! It was like taking a semester of college in a week! So much revelation. So many aha experiences!

I arrived a week early! It was definitely a God thing!

So much heaviness has been lifted from me. The brain fog is gone. My blood sugar has dropped so much that I was able to drop my oral meds and reduce the insulin. My blood pressure med is halved. I do not need the nitroglycerin for my heart. It is not racing any more. I am off prednisone. I do not need the Nexium or Bextra anymore either. I replaced the Darvocet with Alleve. I sleep like a baby. Plus I lost ten pounds.

PVC isn't anti-doctor. They do not tell you to throw all of your medicine away. Mostly you have to listen to the Holy Spirit and not be presumptuous.

And church. These folks know how to have church. No showmanship! The focus is on the Lord and is directed by the Holy Spirit. The church ministers to the church. There are no cliques. In fact, after the Sunday morning service, they have lunch together, because they believe fellowship is so important.

D.D., FL USA

## Chronic Fatigue and More—Healed!

**For whosoever will save his life shall lose it: and whosoever will lose his life for my sake shall find it. Matthew 16:25**

The past four years I was dealing with chronic Environmental Illness, which almost took my life due to severe nutritional deficiencies. My immune system had been weakened to the point where I was allergic to all foods and my body was unable to withstand the environment and being around people without getting sick. This was triggered by your average everyday exposures such as fragrances, carpeting, and laundry detergents. I ended up living in a world of isolation. The only people I really got to spend time with were the "helpers" I hired to do some of the simple chores in life that I couldn't do myself because of the chronic fatigue. For a year and a half my body was debilitated to the point where even just putting one foot in front of another was extremely painful. At times I had to be carried down the stairs, pulled out of bed, and it even hurt to lift a glass of water to my mouth.

There was definitely a lack of medical options since I would have such severe reactions to them, such as a seizure and heart arrhythmias. With several years passing, there were some improvements with treatment. However, after spending close to half a million dollars it became quite obvious that no man could fix me. God was the only One who could take this away from me. The more I leaned toward the Lord and put my complete trust in Him to heal me, the more spiritual healing I received. It was a big turning point for me when I realized that God wanted me well and that He had beautiful plans for me.

I started reading *A More Excellent Way*™ by Henry Wright. Simply by acknowledging some of the spiritual roots behind disease (such as guilt, perfectionism and addictions), almost immediately I regained my eyesight to the point where I could read for hours at a time. Prior to that, 15 minutes was about the limit since I was losing my vision. Believing that I found my answer, I hopped on a plane from New Mexico to Georgia to attend the very powerful program offered by Pleasant Valley Church, which focuses on sanctification. When I left for the airport that morning, I not only believed that God was going to get me there safely, but that He was also going to heal me. When I first arrived I needed to be on oxygen, lying down on a lounge chair in the back, too exhausted to even lift my head. Within 5 days I was off oxygen; within a week I was eating sugar; within two weeks I got all my foods back, within 2 and a half weeks I was driving again, going to the gym, and walking into stores. I am also off of the daily treatment program my body used to rely on to function.

The more I healed spiritually, the more my body was strengthened. I did my best to *keep my peace* by making *choices* that were from God. I stopped hiding and started *facing* all of the things that were making me sick, but this time I did it with complete faith that my body would be able to handle it. Doubt and fear do not come from God. He has a better plan for me than that. God is no respecter of persons (Acts 10:34). He wants to bless you too. Let Him bless you.

## MY WALK OUT (or) THE TOP TEN WAYS I OPENED MYSELF UP
## TO RECEIVE GOD'S GRACE AND HEALING

**For by grace are ye saved through faith; and that not of yourselves: it is the gift of God: Ephesians 2:8**

1. I put all my faith and trust in the Lord without any doubts about my complete healing.

2. I began reading God's Word to be the truth and only the truth in my life.

3. I stopped asking God to heal me and starting thanking Him for already doing so by sending his Son to die on the cross for me.

4. I stopped focusing in on my body/symptoms and put all my attention on God before anything else.

5. I started exercising my faith instead of just talking about it. I did this by facing all the stressors in my life with the absolute knowing that the Lord would take care of me.

6. I went through the sanctification process, taking responsibility and repenting for the sins in my life.

7. I laughed (when I could) and listened to praise and worship music morning, day and night.

8. I distanced myself from all the programming and bondage relating to illness.

9. I praised God for every victory, no matter how big or small.

10. I helped others by sharing my testimony.

C.C., NM USA

## Pain Free after One Week!

In January 2001, we took a vacation, spending time at a Christian retreat center called Pleasant Valley Church and Associated Ministries in Thomaston, GA. It was founded by Henry Wright. It was a wonderful experience! They specialize in dealing with the "spiritual roots of disease."

We have been dealing with a number of debilitating health problems over the last few years. We'd heard from a number of different people that Pleasant Valley Church had a wonderful program of Bible teaching that actually leads to physical healing as you apply biblical principles to your life. No "hocus-pocus or hyper-spiritual mumbo-jumbo," we were told.

Even though I was a skeptic, I decided to go.

What happened? I had been suffering with severe pain for years (three crushed disks in my neck from an on-the-job injury, arthritis in my neck, hips, knees, feet). After our first one-week retreat in January, I was pain free and am still pain free!

The question many have asked me is whether I am just one of the roughly 5 percent of Christians who get prayed for and God heals them immediately or if this is something more significant. The answer is: it is more significant. What we have gone through is part of the process of sanctification. Pleasant Valley taught us about how to get our lives in line with the Word of God, and the Lord has used this to radically change us and bless us. We will never be the same!

T.R., Eagan, MN USA

## Thyroid Cancer Gone

I had been diagnosed with thyroid cancer. I went through surgery and treatment, but I ran to my Father when I was first diagnosed, and He has walked with me through an incredible journey of discovery. Your ministry was part of my recovery.

Jesus came that we might have life and have life more abundantly, and Satan's job is to kill, steal and destroy that life. I am happy to say that I believe God showed me the root of my cancer, and I am well on the way to recovery. He has also promised to "complete me" or finish the work He started. I recently went back to my surgeon for follow-up testing. He said the cancer was back, and I would have to have more surgery and follow-up radiation treatment. I went back to my Father, who dealt with three other issues in my life. When the "official" pathology report came back it showed **No Cancer.** I know Jesus has healed me and part of that healing is restoration.

D.G.

## *Delivered from Bipolar Disease*

The Lord used you to get me healed/delivered from bipolar disease. I was raised in a strict religious (not Christian) home. My first recall of problems with depression occurred after being rejected by my high school sweetheart. We had dated for almost 3 years and planned to marry after we both finished college. When I got my "Dear Jane" letter, I was devastated, my grades dropped, I gained weight, and I turned to daily religious activities (not Christian). I dated a little and was very "proud" to be in a very small minority to be a virgin at graduation.

By then I was old enough to drink (legally), and my inhibitions left, and soon I was pregnant. Being afraid of my parents' reaction and sharing that fear with my doctor, the enemy used him to suggest that I did not have to tell them. In 1971 abortion was not yet "legal," so off to a dirty, secret place in an eastern city I went.

The shame of that horrible decision is what I have come to understand was the open door for the enemy. It wasn't until only recently when I took the responsibility and stopped blaming others or using the crutch that I was mentally ill that my freedom began. Praise God.

You see, starting in 1975 in Alaska and ending in Minnesota in 1997, I had been in mental hospitals a total of 8 times. When I became coherent after my first stay, some of the staff told me they had never seen anyone as bad off as I was, and they were certain I would be locked up in the back wards of a state hospital the rest of my life.

I have been off and on medications since 1975. But this time because by God's grace and love and the help of the teaching and ministry through Brother Henry, I believe the root(s) have been exposed. I took the godly counsel to taper off the meds with the oversight of my health care professional. July 17, 2001 she asked if I was ready to be off the Depakote completely! I floated out of her office. Praise Jesus.

Thank you again for being obedient to the Lord's call on your life to "Set the Captives Free."

Tormented no more and eternally grateful.

S.F., Alexandria, MN USA

### Astigmatism, MCS/EI, Bleeding Skin Cancer Healed and a New Heart!

I have learned so much and been healed from so much through the *A More Excellent Way*™ ministry that my agenda is to receive all that I can to learn to minister *a more excellent way*™ to others. I give testimonies, I share the books and tapes with the pastors and others, but I want to actually minister *a more excellent way*™ to others. Our class will be leaving for two months in the Philippines shortly after Henry Wright's visit, and I'm hoping that we will all have something special to take with us. I really believe that his visit is in God's timing and will be used for His glory, big time!

In addition to all the MCS/EI healings, deliverances, and creative miracles that I knew that I had received before I left Georgia, I have also received documented (from Kaiser Permanente) healings for a bleeding skin cancer on my face and astigmatisms in my eyes. The Father also gave me a creative miracle of a new heart at the end of August. The old heart was enlarged and must have been totally worn out from the MCS/EI reactions. And the normalizing and healing of my body, soul, and spirit has continued throughout the walk-out period. I believe that our Father has let me experience all this so that I can more effectively minister to others.

O.B., HI, USA

### Gallbladder Cancer and Connective Tissue Disease Healed

Do you have any teaching guides other than the book *A More Excellent Way*™? My husband and I are going to teach the book at our church in Lubbock, Texas, this year. We have gained much spiritual insight for our own lives. My husband has been healed of gallbladder cancer and I have been healed of Fibromyalgia, Connective Tissue Disease and Environmental Illness (MCS/EI). This book is what turned me around and showed me what was really wrong.

My sister sent the book to me. I could not go to church because of the smells of perfume that are in any crowd. We had to clean out all chemicals in our home. I went on a health diet an allergist gave me. We bought air filters and had the vents cleaned out on our heating unit and air conditioning system. I could hardly breathe. The story goes on and on. I would have gone to Dallas to the Environmental Center if we had insurance. I lost 25 lbs from 160 to 135 lb. Now I am off all medications except half of a sleeping pill.

This book brought insight to me that I had never heard of. I had much prayer, but *A More Excellent Way*™ truly is *a more excellent way*™. Thank you so very much for your spiritual insight. God's way is *a more excellent way*™! To God be all the glory! I praise the Lord that you have allowed Him to use you in the great way to bring truth to God's people.

My husband's testimony is wonderful, a true miracle. He stepped out on faith and stopped his chemo and radiation treatment and forgave. Gallbladder cancer is very, very rare. He has been free of cancer for 2 years now. To God be the glory!!

We want to pass this wonderful knowledge on to those in our church. We are very excited about what God is doing in our lives and what He will do in others. We know that there is much, much more we need to learn and be delivered of so that in turn we can help, by the grace of God, bring deliverance and healing to others. Thank you for being God's instrument.

B.H., Lubbock, TX USA

## The Long Journey Back From E.I.

Can you imagine what it was like to live five years homebound, disabled, and isolated *Back From Environmental Illness?* This is a story of God's power to heal broken hearts, broken relationships, broken bodies and broken spirits.

*Environmental Illness* or *Multiple Chemical Sensitivity* (also called E.I.) is a complex disease resulting from many different variables, the least of which is chemical exposures—the final straw that broke the camel's back. The illness is extremely painful and disabling and compromises the immune, neurological, gastrointestinal, and endocrine systems, and causes organic brain or toxic brain syndrome. For over twenty years, physicians, research scientists and congressmen have been trying to unravel this complicated disease, for which there is no known cure.

I felt that I would be healed someday. My traditional faith had not prepared me with the faith knowledge to believe that I could appropriate Psalm 103 for healing with a chronic incurable illness that defied medical resolutions. I believed the part that said "He forgives all mine iniquities," but the second part of "healeth all thy diseases" just didn't seem to apply to an illness that had drained me of all vitality and health for so many years. Although I believed that I would someday be healed, I did not envision that healing would come from God.

For five long, devastating years I had not been able to worship with my church because of the chemical barriers that made me ill. Out of my own heartache, I did an exhaustive study on "Environmental Illness and the Church: An Interfaith Study of Churches in America and How They Are Ministering to the Spiritual and Emotional Needs of the Chemically Injured." I thought the spiritual path to healing would come through worshipping with fellow Christians and the immune system would be strengthened through hugs, laughter, good feelings, spiritual uplifting and people contact.

Through years of trying to rebuild health, I became totally dependent on as many as 200 different allergy shots a month, a huge amount of vitamin and mineral supplements, and total removal of all chemicals in my home environment.

Environmental illness, for many people, begins in early childhood as a result of a broken relationship where the child does not receive proper nurturing and love. The majority of E.I.s carry a broken heart from early in life, unaware of the fears that stem from early traumas. A broken relationship later in life can also compromise a person's health. For others, events in life that the individual has not come to grips with can erect fences that present problems later in life.

For many, the illness seems to have been inherited genetically. If a father abused the child, his father was probably abusive, as well. And, so the path for spiritual separation from God began before the person with environmental illness was born. The majority of E.I.s are women, and biologically they are weaker. The majority were brutalized as a child or teenager—either spiritually, physically, emotionally, or sexually. The men with environmental illness are sensitive, caring individuals. The extremely stressful conditions under which most grew up weakened the immune system early in life, set in play the mind-body connection, and spiritual separation from God began early in life. Even though I was a Christian, I could never identify with our heavenly Father's love for me.

The majority of E.I.s were professional people who worked under stressful conditions, often as workaholics, still striving to win approval or acceptance through recognition that was lacking during childhood. We thought we performed well under stress, but most of us were sickly throughout life. Growing up under stressful conditions weakened our nutritional status and compromised the immune system, which later cracked from chemical exposures. Other E.I.s find that the triggering point for their collapse came following an extremely stressful period during their life.

Whatever the reason for the illness, the groundwork was set for Satan to enter this terrible illness. Environmental illness can be totally healed by God by healing the broken heart, the individual taking responsibility for the disease, or coming to grips with events in the past. Suffering cannot be explained away, nor can other "giants" like fear, bitterness, anger, and unforgiveness that stand against the Holy Spirit in us. Once chronic illness sets in, our attitudes keep us down, eat away at our peace of mind, and drain the life-blood from our faith. The more I talk with other E.I.s, the more I see separation from God from broken hearts or these other "giants."

It took five years for me to recognize the full extent that fear plays in environmental illness. The types of fears we are talking about are not your ordinary, easily recognized fears. Many of the fears originated from early traumas. The Bible uses the word "fear," but society calls it worry, anxiety and stress. The second step toward my recovery was coming to grips with the broken heart. The last thing that I was slow in recognizing was that separation from God and His works had allowed Satan to enter in.

For three decades before my health collapsed with E.I., severe allergies from airborne toxins and pollens plagued me. As a bank officer, tobacco smoke, fragrance, inks, news material, and many other chemicals in the work place continually circulated indoors in the large, energy-efficient office buildings where I worked.

Outdoors air pollution carried the toxic chemicals from nearby chemical industries. Carbon monoxide from exhaust fumes engulfed me as I commuted to work in Houston on freeway systems, parked in garages, and walked downtown streets.

Frequent building expansions involved new building products and industrial chemicals. Chemicals in new carpeting, paints, woods, wallboard, wallpaper, and fibers took their toll. In one expansion, the entire floor was gutted, and dust and debris covered my work area, despite the fact that plastic sheets suspended from the ceiling surrounded me.

Although I knew I was allergic to formaldehyde in personal care products, I was not aware that this industrial chemical was used to treat my clothing and everything in my environment and was robbing me of health.

Drinking water contained chemicals, too. Produce was adulterated with pesticides, often imported from countries with little or no pesticide regulations. Antibiotics and hormones contaminated our meat supply.

We dipped our dog and fogged our home for fleas on the advice of the veterinarian. Pesticides were recommended for flea outbreaks in the yard. Our yard was often commercially treated with pesticides and fertilizers. Little realizing the complications we were inflicting on our own health and that of our children, we all became increasingly allergic.

My rain barrel continued to fill until it finally ran over. At the age of 54, my health totally crashed, and I became disabled as a result of multiple variables and multiple chemical exposures.

In 1991, I suffered damage to the brain and central nervous system from adverse reactions to prescription medications. The endocrine system collapsed, the gastrointestinal system was affected, and I suffered retina and optic nerve damage. Not realizing I had a serious illness, we fogged our home with pesticides for fleas. We had no way of knowing the terrible devastation to mind, body and spirit that was to follow.

For six weeks I lay critically ill with an inflammation of the nerves, broken speech, and damage to the hearing. I was unable to walk except for a shuffle, and required assistance to the bathroom and with bathing. Alarmed over my deteriorating health, we purchased cemetery property.

My husband closed his engineering office and moved his business home to care for me. To provide office space, we added on to our home and brought new building products and chemicals into our environment. Six weeks later, water damage required major renovation to our home. A cleaning and restoration company further compromised my health by the use of strong dry cleaning solvents and other chemicals. Chemicals in our home environment caused burns around my mouth and nose. Little did I realize that those same chemicals were causing me to fall. For a long time, I was dependent on a walker or wheelchair for mobility.

My husband of 41 years was also struggling with environmental illness. The use of pesticides in our home and yard left him with chronic fatigue syndrome and other health complications. Fourteen months later, he suffered a heart attack following exposure to the dry cleaning solvents, coupled with the severe stress he was under.

For two and one-half years, my health was seriously compromised. I fell often and suffered many injuries requiring emergency room treatment. Physicians suspected multiple sclerosis, aneurysms in the brain, or intracranial pathology. Other physicians said that something serious was going on, but they didn't know what. Still others, in their apparent lack of knowledge of what to do, asked if I was unduly concerned about my health—or had I consulted a psychiatrist.

For two and one-half long years, we searched futilely for answers to an unknown illness and consulted 40 physicians in every medical specialty there was. My health continued to degenerate and I was slowly dying, losing 65 pounds from malabsorption and maldigestion. Every system in my body had collapsed, and I suffered severe bone loss and demineralization. Most of the time I was too ill to dress myself or pull up my bed covers. I often had a very limited range of motion with my arms. Transporting me by car became a major ordeal, where a bed was needed to support my painfully weakened neck structure. For three years, I couldn't perform small functions at home or drive a car.

I had become severely sensitive to chemicals. Loved ones found it difficult to visit. We were unable to visit parents, daughters, or grandchildren because their homes were not environmentally safe. Four years into illness found me still unable to tolerate grocery stores, department stores, parks and recreational areas, libraries, or my church.

Just when we needed spiritual help the most, we were isolated and held captive by the chemical barriers in our world. From the active, vibrant person who loved people, life and activities, I had become a virtual recluse in my home. Our church family and friends were at a loss as to how to minister to us.

Without loved ones, church family, or medical support, I felt despair and hopelessness, alone and forgotten. I was defeated by a horribly real, devastating illness. Unable to tolerate the air I breathed, the food I ate, and water I drank, I became totally dependent on God for every single aspect of my life as I searched for answers.

However, my faith alternated between despair, focusing on solutions for an illness I didn't understand and didn't want, and then grasping for God to help me.

Adverse reactions to all chemical-based prescription medications rendered me helpless to take any kind of pain reliever, including over-the-counter medicines such as Tylenol, aspirin, muscle relaxers, or any other medication.

When a pastor preached revival services in Houston recently, he asked, "When you became sick and were searching from one doctor to another seeking answers for health, did you ask God first?" That got my attention! I was desperately ill, and, of course, I was praying for answers and "Help me, God," but with prayers of despair. Before three years was over, we had searched every avenue of medical hope there was and were considerably poorer from the experiences. Our faith-limiting prayers always included, "God if it be Your will, please heal me."

During the time of serious illness, there was no one to help me through the crisis. Many who knew me just didn't believe there could be an illness that physicians in the Texas Medical Center couldn't treat; it seemed to matter little how ill I was. Others voiced concern that I had something similar to AIDS/HIV and wouldn't visit because it might be contagious. Others thought I just didn't want to get well. Still others said they couldn't visit because they wore fragrance.

I had been ill for four years and was in pitiful shape physically, mentally, emotionally and spiritually, when my sister called. During the previous four years, she had sent greeting cards, but I was indifferent. Her messages were always, "I can't visit because I'll make you sick." In September 1995, she called crying and said, "I want to come see you and help you." As I lay in bed sick with herniated discs in the back and neck, I was grateful to have someone come. I felt so alone and abandoned!

The sad part is that I had never known my sister. She was seven years old when I married. She had always seemed different from my other sisters who I was close to. Over the years, she had lived in other cities and had her share of problems, and we had not been in contact with each other. However, the difference between us was much more than that. I just didn't care for my sister. She was so totally different than what I perceived myself to be.

Have you ever noticed how God has a way of throwing your least favorite person in your path? God knew what He was doing because there was not one other person He could have chosen to reach me with a sickness of mind, body and spirit. He picked my sister because He knew she had been there, and she had been an overcomer through the power of Jesus.

What I failed to realize during those allergic years was that my health was weakening from more than chemical exposures. More importantly, I had failed to pull out the thorns and thistles that were separating me from a right relationship with the Lord. I recently asked God, "Why?" "Why had this horrible illness happened?" The Bible opened to Mark 4 and the parable of the sower where God's Word (the seed) is sown on different kinds of soil. This is the profound story about my life and the basic response I had toward the Lord in various ways. Some listen and then immediately reject. Others hear and respond well on the surface, but spin off when the going gets rough. Others grab hold and embrace what they hear, but by and by they get sidetracked as their growth is throttled by life's "thorns." There was Jesus' message for me! And, then there are those who hear, believe, grow, hang in there and reproduce healthy plants in God's vineyard.

My thorns represented the worries and cares of the world. Spiritual growth was choked out. Mark 4:18–19 says, "And these are they which are sown among thorns; such as hear the word, And the cares of this world, and the deceitfulness of riches, and the lusts of other things entering in, choke the word, and it becometh unfruitful." The thorns know nothing of peaceful coexistence with the life of freedom. Demanding first place, they eventually siphoned off every ounce of spiritual interest and emotional energy.

In Luke 21:34–35, Jesus said, "Take heed to yourselves, lest at any time your hearts be overcharged with surfeiting, and drunkenness, and cares of this life, and so that day come upon you unawares. For as a snare shall it come on all them that dwell on the face of the whole earth."

Although I was giving of my time in faithful attendance at church and spending long hours devoted to the business affairs of the church, my heart was losing its first love for the Lord. We got caught up in worldly possessions and then quit tithing. It had been several years since I had last counseled with people about their salvation and their relationship with Jesus. Yet, in all those years of working with the business affairs, I had a nagging voice inside that said Jesus wanted me for the people affairs of his church.

After I became ill in 1991, I became so chemically sensitive I could no longer attend worship services. I then began to realize how much my church meant to me. Four years into my illness, I reached the lowest point in my life. Living isolated from everyone I held dear, I was defeated! It had been four years since my loving husband of 40 years had seemed to vanish for me emotionally. I struggled trying to understand why he had grown cold and cynical and why he was so emotionally distanced from me.

I first thought he was just reactive to stress from being the sole financial provider and caregiver, from fatigue, from no one understanding our multiple illnesses, the closing of his business, and his own personal health problems. After all those beautiful years of a loving relationship, we had become abusive with anger, mood swings, accusations, and irrational behavior. He was unable to express why he no longer was a sensitive, compassionate husband. I had no way of knowing that he was grieving over the loss of a wife he couldn't fix—one who had been replaced by an ILLNESS!

In the process of my crusading two years to win disability status, and then another year on the Access to Worship study, I had also shut him out of my life emotionally. The worse our relationship became, the harder I worked to gain freedom from my prison. Satan's groundwork was easy, and we had been raised in a traditional faith that didn't put strong emphasis on Satan or the devil. We weren't prepared about how great the spiritual warfare would be to overcome an evil spirit world.

But, it seemed that an evil spirit had descended on our home. As I made each new progression toward wellness, his disbelief, frustration and anger would prevail, and I continued to slip further into despair. The only thing that seemed to prevail in our home and in our health was some form of demonic power. When I suggested this to him, he just became more livid with anger! In despair, I just kept crying out, "Why don't you want me well?" "Why won't you let me get well?"

Before my illness, we had never had any major quarrels. We were a family that did everything together. We played together, worshipped together, and enjoyed family togetherness seven days a week. We were both hard workers on our jobs. Then sickness entered in. And, suddenly, we found ourselves having to face each other 24 hours a day, under very difficult circumstances. I became intolerant to hormones, which caused buckets of tears. Suddenly, we were faced with the realization that he couldn't cope with crying, and he had a wife who had no control over crying. Then we discovered that in 41 years of a loving marriage we had never really been close in a sharing, caring way.

He wasn't the enemy! Through the power of Jesus and the love of my sister and her faithfulness in continuing to reach me, I began to see that there was an evil spirit world that had become embedded in our health, our marriage, and our home.

During my sister's visit last year, I shared with her the horrors of what we had been living through for four years. Before she left, she prayed with me. I thought, "What a beautiful prayer, what knowledge of Scriptures. I can't believe the transformation in my sister!"

I had been asking the Lord to heal me enough that I could help other people. It had been a year since my study was first presented to my church, and they had not responded in any way.

After my sister's visit, instead of going to sleep that evening, I began a beautiful three-day walk with the Lord. I remained in the guest room where I had been sleeping because of pain. For three days and nights, I spent the entire time in prayer, study of God's Word, meditation and singing. I did not sleep during that time. God walked me through His purpose for my life, and why the main three people I had encountered during those four years were a Mormon physician, a physician who was a member of the Church of Scientology, and a Jewish New Age physical therapist. During that beautiful three days, He told me that He wanted me to lead the environmentally ill back into the church before the second coming of Christ.

On the morning of the fourth day, I left my room and walked through the house. I instinctively picked up a salt shaker that was sitting out, and His words said, "You are the salt of the earth to bring light out of darkness." A pair of scissors was laying out, and as I started to put them away, His words spoke, "You do not ever have to fear for your life or want to take your life again."

I was to have been in Dallas for a medical appointment and confirmation of my housing reservations lay by the phone. His Words spoke, "You do not ever have to worry about housing in Dallas; all you have to worry about is your mansion in glory."

About that time, God began crossing my path with many of the people who have been healed through Pleasant Valley Church—letters and phone calls of testimony came to me from Pennsylvania, Maryland, New York, Arkansas, California and Sugar Land.

I called Henry Wright in Georgia and began interviewing him about presenting a seminar in Houston. His teaching ministry has been instrumental in transforming the lives of families with environmental illness, chronic fatigue, and many other diseases previously thought incurable.

We will be eternally grateful to your healing and deliverance ministry, which released me from the bondage of epileptic seizures and from the anger and fear that was destroying our health and home. We have found that exercising spiritual warfare against the enemy overcomes all reactions and symptoms of environmental illness.

I continued to interview Henry Wright and began to apply his teachings to my health. Over the past two months, I learned that only God can heal the broken heart that carried forward with me through life. An inner peace has entered my heart, and we feel a hedge of protection now surrounds our home and our relationship.

Recognition of areas in my life that were affected by fear were the most difficult to access. The fears we were dealing with were often unrecognized as fears, many stemming from tragedies of events beyond my control. Fear activates Satan the way faith activates God. It is totally destructive and cripples mind and heart. The Bible says that in the last days, men's hearts will fail them for fear. When fear was in operation, our lives were subject to bondage and torment. Satan did his best to destroy our testimony as believers in the Lord Jesus Christ. We weren't even aware that he had us operating in fear. By acting on the fear of sickness and disease, we could expect to be sick. As long as we fed fear into our spirit, we did not have the kind of faith power to take rule over the circumstances of our life. Fear was working against us to make us sick.

Once we could see how fear was affecting us physically, our health began to turn around. When we saw how we were affecting oxygen to the brain, the hypothalamus, limbic and pituitary systems, which in turn affected the endocrine, gastrointestinal, neurological and immune systems—we could apply faith, God's source of power. We had changed our entire body chemistry through Satan's power over our health with fear. He was working through fear to destroy our health and marriage.

When we were able to resolve our identity crisis with Jesus and place our total faith in Him, my husband was able to trust and believe that I was truly getting well. His tender loving feelings returned to me with emotional love.

Chemical sensitivities are diminishing, and I am now able to eat at restaurants and enjoy a few long forgotten foods. ALL symptoms of electromagnetic sensitivity have vanished. Fragrance scents now smell good instead of making me ill.

I have become bold in my witness for Jesus and bold in declaring that environmental illness is a demonic orchestrated illness, designed to destroy families and separate them from God. People with environmental illness, chronic fatigue syndrome, and all the other similar syndromes and peripheral diseases that go with these illnesses will never find healing apart from the spiritual path.

The real tragedy are the hundreds of families who tell me "I'm not very religious" or "I'm not interested in a spiritual outreach," as they desperately search for an elusive medical solution. My approach in getting their attention will now be "Forget the religious, forget the spiritual, do you want to get well?"

Our Savior's ministry was about salvation and healing! Psalm 103:2–4 says, "Bless the LORD, O my soul, and forget not all his benefits: Who forgiveth all thine iniquities; who healeth all thy diseases; Who redeemeth thy life from destruction…"

Our Omnipotent God is the same living God who lived yesterday, who lives today, and who is ongoing forever.

My story shows how AWESOME our God truly is. That He could use someone who was totally disabled, homebound and cut off from the world, wrestling spiritual warfare in a dimension I would have once thought impossible, and still use my life for His greater purposes is a revelation of His glory, power and might.

N.M., Houston, TX USA

## *Healed of Many Diseases!*

Here I was sitting in a wheelchair in Philly International Airport getting a pat down from some nice lady who, because of 9/11 had to make sure that, although unable to walk far and the pallor of illness under my eyes, I wasn't part of the terrorist underworld. I couldn't make it up my steps at home without searing pain in my thighs and breathlessness, no less be part of some nefarious plot to injure America. It just seemed so unreal to me. Here I was at 33 sitting in a wheelchair about to fly 600 miles to some church in the back end of nowhere when just going to the grocery store was a major event in my day. It required the entire day to be structured so I wouldn't get too worn out and be in too much pain beforehand and then schedule time to recover and lay down after I came home. Many days the mere thought of having to bring groceries in from the car seemed as though I was contemplating the energy it would take to write a doctoral thesis!

But somehow I had gotten to the airport. Bags packed. The back brace, the pain pills and all the other multicolored medications that kept things going, the heating pad, the special pillow, etc., etc. There is no "just toss things in a bag and dash out the door" when one has fibromyalgia. Days are comprised of mornings waiting until the pain and heaviness eases and finally the joints start to move again. This is somewhat akin to being the Tin Man from the *Wizard of Oz* every day. Then on to taking the pills and the vitamins, the most recent addition to the pharmaceutical war against my ailing body. A breakfast of unusually esoteric foods that were part of a diet that was sure to cure me. Spelt bread with coconut oil became quite a staple for a while, variations being the spelt bread toasted with cheese that was somehow made out of rice protein. I didn't even know rice had protein no less cheese potential; but anything to get better. This had the added bonus of being quite expensive; being ill is extremely costly. With 27 food allergies, a quick run to McDonald's just doesn't fly. Well, unless I only ate the napkin. I wasn't allergic to paper goods as far as I knew. I was allergic to eggs, milk, peanuts, onions, peas, broccoli, soy, shrimp, potatoes, apples, grapes, lemons. I stop there now, but the list went on. I was even allergic to oregano. Now, who in the world is allergic to oregano!? Even my doctor was floored when the results came back on this one.

In any event, and although eating, sleeping and walking were problematic and often surrounded by pain in one way or another, I was about to take a trip. It would turn out unlike any other path I had been down. In the past 20 years I had been to about 30 doctors in the effort to get well. Pediatricians, GPs, neurologists, internists, gynecologists, allergists of various specialties, urologists, osteopaths, orthopedic surgeons, homeopaths, rheumatologists, physiatrists, way too many chiropractors, endocrinologists, dermatologists, ENT's, dental surgeons, and even a podiatrist. There were also various pscolotrists, and therapists. Let's add to that yoga, aromatherapy, herbal and naturopathic therapies, internal cleansing, vitamins and special nutritional diets. Macrobiotic was definitely one of the dourest. I read and studied voraciously about different modalities and methods. I learned about how the body should work in an attempt to find out why mine wasn't. I hauled myself to libraries to find medical books and when I got too sick to do that, I sat for hours and poured over the internet. Searching, searching, and searching. I talked with web groups from people all over the English speaking world about the trials and tribulations of having a chronic and debilitating invisible illness. By invisible I mean one where you can't see the problem: if you are somewhat young and merely look very tired but the agony of each step is not apparent by, say, a cast or something. Many a person has been treated as though they were a lazy and deceptive person for needing a handicapped parking space without the wizened features of age to accompany it.

Eventually I came to realize that I needed the camaraderie and support of those who must be nearby as well as those on the internet. Surely if I was suffering so much I wasn't alone in this area. I started a chronic pain Bible study at my church. At last, a place where I was free to be real with the extent of my pain. I didn't have to sugarcoat it because it made someone uncomfortable; we could cry and pray together. We were free from those "healthy people" who just didn't understand—the well meaning people who prayed over me with such impassioned fervency because *they* needed me to be healed, they needed their prayer answered. The Christians I knew just didn't know what to do with me and my ongoing pain. They prayed sometimes but then it got old because I never got better. Mainstream Christianity is fast paced and very busy. There were things to do, events to plan for, after all. Sure Jesus healed the sick and it should happen today, but…and off they'd go back to their busy lives.

My world grew smaller even within the Christian community, down to those who suffered as I did. They understood. They knew what it was like to always be searching for a way to get better, only make any progress by increments. They knew what it was like to be left out because of pain-prohibited involvement.

I never did accept the "you just do not have enough faith" bit. I figured the God I knew wouldn't be so callous. But, truth be told, I had secretly given up any hope of getting better or that miraculous healings ever happened to regular people. Those things were things that happened in revivals in far away Africa. Maybe healings happened in the less sophisticated and more on fire churches in remotest Asia; a small band of persecuted believers reliving the miracles and passion of the first century church. However for this 30–something housewife living in middle-class America, I sooner saw miracles like, "Hey, isn't it a miracle that Macy's had my size!!" Sure, we heard prayers being answered. Joe finally got a job. Suzie had peace when she had to confront so-and-so. That type of thing. But no long-lasting dramatic healings of incurable diseases. I didn't see that. I figured I might as well accept it and focus my thoughts to just getting through the day or even that hour.

Sorrow and depression really caught up with me. I realized that I didn't want to live anymore, but there was no way out. Although our lives were ruled by illness and the havoc it creates, it still would have been worse for my husband and two children if I killed myself. So here I was stuck in a failing and painful body and things seemed to only get worse over time. Never being a Catholic, I had no hang-ups that suicide was a sin *per se*. Sure, a bad thing but I figured I'd go to heaven. Jesus forgave people who did really bad stuff, and after all, I just wanted to go home to heaven. I started to wish I got cancer or something terminal. That was my only way out it seemed. "How could I keep trying? How could I live like this anymore?" Every day was so hard, every hour was something to deal with. For example, if I had a migraine, which I very often did, I had to get the medicine in before it got too far and lay down. My thoughts went to *Operation: Find Cause*. Did I eat something I shouldn't have? Was it a food allergy? Or how about the weather? Was a new pressure system moving in? How about the pollen count or the dust in the house? Did they trigger it this time? I went through my mental checklist of possible offenders. Could it be another sinus infection brewing? Did I forget about the hypoglycemia and wait too long to eat? Am I upset about anything? Did that comment my mother made really bother me that much? Maybe I am stressed out because the house is a mess and I do not have the energy or ability to stand for 15 minutes, no less clean the house! Vacuuming one room was an accomplishment. Some days just getting dressed took 2 hours due to pain and fatigue. Most of the time I didn't even stand in the shower.

While sitting on the plane, tears in my eyes and a tissue clutched in my hand, I stared pointedly out the window. People were sitting quietly having their in-flight snack, and I was thinking about how I realized that every 20 minutes of my life I needed to make some adjustment due to pain or something. Sitting that way hurt my back so I needed to move. 20 minutes later a headache is brewing so that must be addressed before it turned into a migraine. 20 minutes after that it was time to eat something due to the hypoglycemia, but then what, considering the major food restrictions? Another 20 minutes, I had to take a pain pill because the roaming and shooting pains in the bones of my arms and legs started again. On and on it went. That was how I lived inside my mind. There was always a warning bell going off, always needing to put out the latest fire.

I knew I wasn't alone in this. I realized that God knew of my pain. I prayed and talked to Him all the time. So why didn't He heal me? I just figured I was supposed to learn something from this ongoing nightmare. I thought that somehow maybe my illness brought me closer to God than most people. After all I couldn't work or even be much involved in church events or my kids' lives, but I could lie down and pray and read the Bible. Most people always seemed so busy that just maybe I was blessed that I had the time for God and they didn't because they were able to run around. Now that I think about it, that seems pretty skewed with some arrogance thrown in there. In any event that was my mindset. I couldn't help out with my daughter's Girl Scouts or hardly help my children with their homework. Sitting for a while on the damp grass watching a little league game was excruciating.

I figured at least I can work on my inner spirituality. It a job you can do while sitting down quietly.

One book led to another or a workbook and so on and so on. I delved into how my personality type affected my pain and the misunderstood blessings of oversensitivity. I read about the struggles of those with chronic illness and did Bible studies on how God doesn't forsake us in our pain. I was always on the lookout for the link between my illness and God. How odd that just another book crossing my path made such a difference. Know my endless struggle when my mother gave me this book that described a pattern of certain diseases and their spiritual roots. He, like me, saw how the Bible says people can be healed but the church doesn't seem to have much success with that. I was interested. Very interested.

Flipping through the book, I looked up what was written about the diseases I suffered from. I looked up fibromyalgia, IBS, depression, allergies, UTI problems, chronic sinusitis, edema, asthma, hypoglycemia, migraines, back spasms and Hashimoto's thyroiditis. I was shocked. Here in just a couple of sentences this guy had me pegged! I thought maybe someone had been watching me. Fear, self-hatred, self-rejection and anxiety—the picture was me, that was for sure. But I never really told anyone about how deep my feelings of self-hate were. It is just not something that comes up in conversation. The fact was that fear was a part of my existence since childhood. I thought that was just part of life, and here this guy was saying that fear was a sin. Boy, was I angry! How dare this man write this? Fine, I realize it is unhealthy and stresses the adrenals and that, but a SIN? "Look here buddy, no kidding, I am afraid. If you had my body, you would be too. I have been betrayed by my own body. I never know when the next problem will strike. That is NOT a sin to be afraid in my position…that is reality!" Good thing this man wasn't in front of me; I might have hauled off and decked him! And then enjoyed it too!!

I put the book down. I felt personally rebuffed. Days passed. Fear is a sin, huh? Weeks passed. Ok, how is it possible that fear is a sin? I began to read more of the book and all the Scripture it cited. Yea, yea, I know, Jesus said all the time to fear not. I remember that, but wasn't that more like a suggestion? I mean the biggies came down from Mount Sinai, and I do not think there was a number 11. Thou shall not fear…was there? Ok, no other gods before Him. Got it, but I am afraid because horrible things happen and the only person I can trust is myself and deep down that sure doesn't make me feel better. So, does that mean by not trusting God I am putting myself above Him and in some sort of self-idolatry! No way! I have been a Christian for over 25 years!

During this time, my husband and I decided to move to Florida. My sister lived there, and when we visited, I realized how much better I would feel if it was warm all the time. We were living in Pennsylvania, and I was practically a shut-in from fall to spring. The cold weather sent every single symptom into overdrive. The depression for the pain, my seclusion and lack of sunlight became a deluge of misery every year. And every year my health was getting worse it seemed, with slight variations. Although the rest of my family was in Pennsylvania and all of my husband's family, we felt we should move south. My husband didn't even have a job to go to. We were really stepping out on faith that God would be providing.

I very slowly packed a box one day and thought about that book and the healings that they say they see. Could it be possible that I am not right with God? Could it really have something to do with my not getting healed all these years? My mother told me of a long time family friend who went to Georgia for one of their week long teachings about the spiritual roots of disease. He came home a man free of his many diseases, but more than that, he came home free from the emotional heaviness he always wore. That sounded pretty amazing to me. I mean to be miraculously healed of something, I guess, could happen. But I usually do not see Christians with real freedom in their emotions or spirits or however you want to classify it. I started to think, "Just what if I could learn about this stuff? Ridiculous. We are moving, it is expensive to fly, how could I even travel and sit somewhere? I need my sofa and my pills and all my stuff for when the pain gets really bad. And what about the food? How can I go anywhere? Would I lug my spelt bread and distilled water to Georgia? I couldn't even get through an airport on my own two legs! My husband would never go for this even if all these other things did work out. He would be on kid duty non-stop!"

Staring out the window of the airplane; somehow it had all happened. My husband, the kids, the money, my mother taking me to this church. If I had not felt really led by God, I would not have gone. But the idea that maybe things just weren't as I thought about healing propelled me. What else could these people have to say about God and healing? In most churches, healings and hype went hand-in-hand. I had a serious aversion to hype. I was assured that they were teaching and not a hyped-up healing service with temporary results. "Ok, God," I said. "I'll go and be obedient, but as far as healing goes, I just want to be able to come home and eat potatoes." That was it. I had 17 diseases and had just enough faith that it might be able to eat a French fry on the way home!

The people I met there had actually been sicker than I at one point. This was definitely a comfort since I was usually the sickest person in the room. But more than that, I learned so much. It was fascinating. Thankfully, I was able to sit in the back on the chaise lounge with the other obviously ill people. Even with all that sitting, I was riveted by what I heard: spiritual blocks to healing and spiritually rooted diseases and stories of real long-lasting changes in peoples' lives. It made the Bible come alive again. As the week went on, I went out on faith and ate some chicken. Now, I wasn't allergic to chicken, but it was dipped in stuff that I was allergic to: soy sauce and lemon. I did start to have some cerebral edema, but then it receded. That was the beginning of my healing.

I came home not knowing much else had been healed yet besides the food allergies. As days went on, I reintroduced more and more of the things that I used to be allergic to. Out of sheer joy I ate potatoes every day for a week and a half! French fries, mashed, tater tots, more French fries! That was wonderful, but I came home with much more than that. I, too, was free from the bondage that had encased my heart for forever. That was such healing. I met God in such a safe and beautiful way within my own heart. The physical healing came as a by-product of all that. I can't adequately convey what those people taught in a week, but I can tell you that God did a miraculous thing in my heart where the emotional pain had outweighed the physical.

We moved 3 weeks after I got home. I didn't have time to minutely self-monitor every advance in my healing. But by the time we packed up the truck, I was able to help! I walked up and down the steps. I carried boxes and ate pizza and cheese steaks with everyone else! I worked all day just like the "healthy people." It was amazing. We waved good-bye and drove off.

We stopped in Virginia in the Shenandoah Mountains to walk with the kids and our dog. I had figured that I'd do as much as I could, sit on a rock and then let them go on. That plan didn't pan out. I wound up hiking with them the whole 4 miles! And one part was a huge hill and I did it!! Not only did I do it, but there was no backlash from my body! No painful muscles, no headache from exertion. It was like I was a normal person!

About halfway through our trip, we got a call that our new house wasn't ready and it wasn't going to be ready for a month. Here we were driving down I-95 like the Clampetts from the Beverly Hillbillies. Our canoe was strapped to the roof of the car, stuffed with bags of laundry underneath; the kid's bikes tottering on the back window and the U-haul behind us sporting some extra accessories that didn't fit inside. Thankfully my sister lives in Jacksonville, and we could stay with her. We slept on the floor of her living room for 3 and 1/2 weeks. There was no special bed and none of the things that I had needed just a month before to cope with life. We were 10 people and a dog living in a 1400 sq. foot house. We had my kids, my sister's 4 kids and all of the neighborhood friends coming in and out of the house. It was Grand Central Station and not a quiet spot to be found. By that point I wasn't even on any of my medications. Since I didn't need the pain pills, I had forgotten about them. Somehow in all the chaos of packing, I had misplaced them. By the time we moved into our new house, I did it all without antidepressants, pain medicine, allergy meds, the thyroid hormones and the list goes on and on.

In fact I also went with my family to a water park! That was amazing. Since I had been sick from a very young age on, there have been many things I have never done. A water park was just a ridiculous thought before, with all those steps. Any amount of cold water would have triggered that bone pain, and forget about carrying that big inner tube! Well, I did it all and loved it! It was such fun!

My niece tried to teach me how to surf as well—another fun and new thing I could do without fear of pain. I now ride my bike all the time and walk 3 or 4 miles on the beach with my dog. I even got out the roller blades the other day! More discoveries happen all the time. I found out that I can swim. I knew how but never did because of the pain and muscles that felt as though they were starving for oxygen. But I tried it and found out I could. Everything worked the way God made it. How thrilling. My sister was at the pool with me at the time and just looked at me. "I do not think I ever saw you do that," she said after I went back and forth across the pool without stopping. And we even grew up with a pool in our backyard!

Sometimes people ask me if I feel all healed just a bit or even afraid it is going to come back. I do feel all healed. I also have days or moments when something will hurt or twinge; but those are the times I go running back to God, "Show me, Father, where have I strayed from You?" It is like having an early warning system. Warning, warning, beep, beep, beep, you have diverted from the straight and narrow path.

J.C., St. Augustine, FL USA

## Cancer Free!

Thank you for the newsletter. I am healed and whole, CANCER FREE. I so appreciate your ministry and the input that it has given me while I visited you, and the books and tapes available. With other resources and your training, I have finally come to understand what God wants of me to walk and live by faith to receive full wholeness. It has been a long journey, but after three and a half years of dealing with ovarian cancer, I am now free of cancer, and I know that this trial is over, PRAISE GOD!! I understand the fullness of the cross of Isaiah 53! Whole salvation....

Love and will always cherish you, your people and your church in my heart. You gave me the road to travel on to receive, and I will always share what I have learned to help others receive wholeness and the fullness of God.

B.C.

## Healed of Bipolar Disease and Fibromyalgia!

1. Ever since I was a little child, people knew there was something "wrong" with me in that I'd just sit, stare, and rock back and forth passively and not interact with other children. They suspected autism, but that turned out not to be the case.

2. Age eight (1984): I was diagnosed with severe ADD and put on medication. School performance did improve but I was still "weird girl" and experienced a great deal of rejection.

3. Age 15: We went to California to get my brain checked out. Doctor said I had one of the most messed-up brain chemistries he's ever seen and put me on new medicine.

4. Age 16: I was raped, lost interest in school, and did a lot of psychoactive drugs for the next few years.

5. In college: I cut down on drugs and began studying.

6. The learning problems and fear of failure kept me doing 60 hours of homework a week. Moreover, I began to abuse the amphetamines I was on by taking as much as I needed to get that speedy lift, which gave me the clarity I needed to get out of my otherwise foggy mind and the energy I needed to stay up all night and study.

7. I moved into my own apartment and left only to go to classes. I stayed away from men (namely emotionally) as I grew awkward around them due to their sexuality (which I perceived they were unable to control). Moreover I stayed away

from people in general because I always needed to study. My social skills began to deteriorate, and I grew terrified of people even looking at me.

8. I had severe ups and downs emotionally and ended up coming back to God, who began to get me back out into the real world, though I still spent far too much time on school work by myself as my brain never had predictable performances (and I'd always resort to more amphetamines). I still had no real steady group of friends, more or less anyone close, as I kept people at a distance.

9. Through my master's degree I improved greatly and became closer to God but still suffered from isolation and emotional ups and downs.

10. After my master's I came home for a year with hopes of pursuing a Ph.D. However, within the first month of being back (and quitting the amphetamines), I developed fibromyalgia and began to become tormented by the drugs I took in high school to the point where I thought I needed to be institutionalized, so I began intense counseling. Plus I joined a sexual abuse victim's support group to deal with my man issues. I grew mad at God.

11. By spring I was diagnosed with bipolar III (cyclothymia). They wanted to put me on lithium, but I decided (with support of my therapist) to hold off a bit and seriously look into going to a partially institutionalized program for women, thinking that my issues gave me mood swings. My mother kept suggesting something Christian but I didn't think anything churchy would help.

12. I read info on Pleasant Valley and thought I might as well try. Without reading any of the material, I signed up and took the course.

13. By the end of the week, I was healed of fibromyalgia, cyclothymia, and by that next Monday was off all medications. Upon returning home, I immediately got a job at a local café where I developed some close friendships with the girls there and walked out into a new medicine-free lifestyle. Within three months I began a full-time Ph.D., and within six months after that I was still off all medications, had close male friendships, was having no severe mood swings, and was leading a balanced lifestyle for the first time in my life!

K.K., Cincinnati, OH USA

### Healed of Tuberous Sclerosis

My wife and I want to give a special thank you to all the staff at Pleasant Valley Church, for all the work they do in saving souls and restoring godly order in not only our lives personally, but for everyone they come in contact with. Our trip to GA was a real blessing—the most wonderful blessing God has ever bestowed upon us as a family. Not only has He healed our daughter of Tuberous Sclerosis, but He has created a new "creature" in both my wife and me through His Holy Spirit.

About 5–6 weeks before we went to GA, my daughter ended up in the emergency room at the hospital because she was having multiple seizures. Being only 21 months old, it is quite disturbing to see her having seizures. As it turned out, they increased her anti-seizure medication because the medicine was low according to her blood level. Recently, her neurologist called once again to have it increased.

He was informed NO, we need to start a slow decrease in her medication. Her recent blood level was checked again, and it was lower than when she was in the emergency room with seizures. She is doing fine. A slight seizure here and there, but she is on her way to total recovery. With all the many denominations out there, we always hear about these curses being passed along to the 3rd and 4th generations. Never do we hear a way around these curses. It is like, "Well sit back and enjoy the ride because there is nothing we can do to change it." Thank you, Henry Wright, for sharing with us the gift God has bestowed upon you. We cannot feel, see, taste, hear or smell God, but experiencing this creative miracle in our daughter makes God all of a sudden seem to us so very real. We feel such a close relationship with God as a result of this healing.

R.S.

## Rashes Healed

I was dealing with a rash and had just made an appointment with my dermatologist. BINGO…you hit the nail on the head with "Is Someone or Something Getting under Your Skin?" God's timing is always perfect!! I have been going through a severe hurt in a friendship that threw me into a tizzy. What was at the root of this was self-condemnation, fear of man/failure/rejection. I have been going through a series of healings in this area, and this "hit" devastated me. It was a repeat of a repeat of painful memories incurred as a child, except I'm no longer a child. Thank you, Lord, though the Pleasant Valley Church ministry, that I was able to face the enemy head on. The "creep" still tries to attack in this area…the relationship problem has not been resolved as of yet…but I know what the sick feelings and rash are all about.

K.M.

## Many Healings!

Things God has healed me of through Pleasant Valley Church:

1. MCS/EI - multiple chemical sensitivities

2. Food allergies

3. Migraines - since age 5, diagnosed and treated unsuccessfully

4. Chronic lower back pain and spasms - since age 12, had tried chiropractic, acupuncture, physical therapies unsuccessfully

5. Arthritis - shown in X-ray

6. Fibromyalgia

7. Neck pain

8. Face pain

9. Interstitial cystitis, sensitive bladder

10. Depression

11. Suicidal Ideation

12. Anxiety Disorder, panic attacks - 15 years of psychotherapy and psychmeds, all unsuccessful

13. Pain in pancreas

14. Chronic constipation

15. Chronic cough

16. Chronic stuffy nose; chronic sinusitis

17. Candidiasis - overgrowth of candida in eyes and mouth

18. Adult acne

19. Eczema

20. Sound sensitivity

21. Exaggerated startle response

22. Blocked hearing

23. Face ground disability

24. Joint pain in hips at night

25. Sensitivity to cold and hot temperatures

R.L., Boston, MA USA

## Healed of Crohn's Disease

Back around 1998/99 I heard some of your tapes of a seminar from Houston, TX, and because of things I heard you say, I was healed of Crohn's disease. Currently I am stationed at a camp in Kuwait about 10 miles south of the Iraqi border. I am not a pastor, but I do some teaching at our post chapel under the supervision of a pastor and the post chaplain.

Anyway, I have told many people of my testimony and of your ministry. I have also told many people what your Web site address is. I would like to thank you for your ministry. Your ministry has not only helped me, but many other people on their way up to Iraq and people staying in Kuwait!

R.K., Kuwait

## Wonderful Childbirth Experience

After the conception of our first child, I began preparing my heart for the labor and delivery process. Honestly, the idea was frightening to me due to the TV documentaries I had seen and also the myriad of discouraging accounts I had heard throughout my life. However, at my church and from other friends, I had begun to hear testimonies that really gave me encouragement. In my heart it was my hope that the Lord had a better way for birthing, and I wanted it for my own experience.

Even while pregnant, I could not bear to see pictures in the birthing book that my husband and I were reading and therefore decided that I was not ready to continue reading. The pictures looked so painful and only seemed to back up the negative experiences I knew many other women were having. My fears were being stirred up. I knew I had to work through those fears of birthing, which had compiled along the years.

My husband led the way for our family to have a wonderful birthing experience. He read the birthing books and then would explain to me what the process would entail. The education took much mystery out of the childbirth. I felt relieved that though I would be the one giving birth to our son that my husband would be fully aware of what was going on, too. He earned a new place of trust with me, and I relied on him for support during the preparation and the actual delivery.

> **Wives, submit yourselves unto your own husbands, as unto the Lord. For the husband is the head of the wife, even as Christ is the head of the church: and he is the saviour of the body. Therefore as the church is subject unto Christ, so let the wives be to their own husbands in every thing.** [*even childbirth—my emphasis added*] **Ephesians 5:22**

> **The wife hath not power of her own body, but the husband: and likewise also the husband hath not power of his own body, but the wife. 1 Corinthians 7:4**

These Scriptures say that husbands have a special covering over their wives unto which the wives can submit. Also, I understood, that even in birthing, the power of my body belonged unto my husband, and he had authority over it.

The Lord led me through a gentle process of recognizing my fears related to birthing, and one by one I repented and asked forgiveness for being in agreement with a spirit of fear.

> **For God hath not given us the spirit of fear; but of power, and of love, and of a sound mind. 2 Timothy 1:7**

Many times in the Word, God has said, "Fear not." When I am in fear, I am not trusting in God and therefore am being disobedient to His commands. As I renounced my fears it gave a place for God to bring a blessing into my life in those areas.

I came to understand that it was not really God's intent for women to have awful birthing experiences as a result of the fall of man in Genesis.

> **Unto the woman he said, I will greatly multiply thy sorrow and thy conception; in sorrow thou shalt bring forth children; Genesis 3:16**

I spent time with my pastor's wife who has had 6 natural childbirths. Her positive experiences and understanding of the Word of God gave me insight into what God intends for us today.

Jesus Christ took all of our sins, iniquities, punishment, and curses on Himself at the cross.

> **Christ hath redeemed us from the curse of the law, being made a curse for us: for it is written, Cursed is every one that hangeth on a tree: Galatians 3:13**

Why then do we still have curses in our lives and in this particular dilemma, why are many women still having very difficult childbirths? It is because, though Jesus Christ paid for these penalties, we are not appropriating the blessing now made available through the cross. What does appropriating mean? It means I must obey His commands so He can honor His Word in my life. It means I must break any generational curses coming down my family line (Jeremiah 32:18, Deuteronomy 5:9). It means that I must break alliance with any ways of the enemy that I am in agreement with, such as the spirit of fear (2 Timothy 1:7).

God honors his Word, but if I am not living by His Word in my life, then He cannot honor His Word in those circumstances. If I continue to choose to live in fear, one of the practical results is that in the labor process, I will have a physiological response of tensed up muscles, which according to medical research sets up my body for a more difficult labor process.

Understanding this I chose to spiritually labor to enter into rest.

**Let us labor therefore to enter into that rest, Hebrews 4:11**

As often as the self-pity, mistrust of God, and fears such as a fear of pain would come up, I would go to the Father and repent and let Him restore my heart in that area. I broke the power of the words that had been spoken to me such as, "Giving birth is the most awful and painful experience I've ever had." Maybe it had been for them, but that doesn't mean that it was necessarily what God intended. I repented for any possible curses in my family line around the birthing process that might be a setup for problems. I started to hope for a wonderful birth, which I began to really believe God intended for families to have. He had a beautiful plan for birth even before the foundation of the world, before sin and the curse entered in, and I wanted to experience it.

**For we which have believed do enter into rest, as he said... although the works were finished from the foundation of the world. Hebrews 4:3**

**Now faith is the substance of things hoped for, the evidence of things not seen. Hebrews 11:1**

It was time to hope in God and His plan, not to put faith toward the bad report. Did I have hope? Yes, finally! Then that meant I had faith according to Hebrews 11:1.

The weeks before our due date I meditated on Matthew 11:28 and Psalm 23.

**Come unto me, all ye that labour and are heavy laden, and I will give you rest. Matthew 11:28**

While in the delivery room, I wanted to remember from Psalm 23 that the Lord is my Shepherd, that He would be there to comfort me and that surely goodness and mercy would follow me right into that room.

My husband and I asked our pastor's wife to be present with us during the labor and delivery process. We wanted to have her as an experienced resource since this was our first birth, we wanted to have a godly authority with us, and also she helped coach me through the stages of labor. My husband and the pastor's wife held the medical staff at bay so I could just labor. I didn't have to deal with anyone, but let them take care of everything that came up.

A few months in advance, my husband and my pastor's wife told me I was not allowed to be a martyr in the delivery room. If I needed any pain medication down to an epidural then I was to get it. My husband and I desired to have a natural childbirth, but he would not let me idolize it at my expense. Being released from that expectation brought rest to me.

My labor and delivery was short and intense, but not painful or traumatic. I did not even need any pain medication. To my surprise, my body just took over and did it all. My job was to keep my peace, keep my body relaxed and let God have my body do what He created it to do.

I reflect on that time as one of the most incredible experiences I have had as a woman. God was with us. It was a holy time, and I will forever treasure it. I'm not saying it was effortless, but I know it was more in line with what God intended from the foundation of the world. My hope is that giving birth to our daughter in a few months will be even more in line with the blessing of birth that He planned.

A.S., GA USA

## *Back to Normal!*

Well, we're back! After several years of sporadic communication at best, we are finally again fully functioning members of society! SO, here's the update.

The biggest news is the phenomenal healing the Lord is bringing to Martha. He has answered our prayers and broken through, bringing health and strength after suffering for 6 long years with a combination of severe pain, sleep problems, allergies, severe back pain, and digestive challenges. We tried countless methods of natural and medical treatment without success. To make a very long story short, the Lord graciously introduced us to a ministry in Georgia that specializes in identifying the spiritual roots of disease. This ministry is based on a book by Henry Wright, called *A More Excellent Way*™. It turns out that about 80 percent of diseases and conditions people suffer from have spiritual roots. It is fascinating! We had never heard of this approach before, but now, after attending two seminars, we know "all about it!" Anyway, after discerning the spiritual roots of my wife's problems, with lots of answered prayer and persistence and the Father's love and faithfulness, she is walking into freedom! Oh, there are still some battles, but the war is won, and we are so very thankful.

With her huge change, life is quickly returning to "normal." For us, that means lots of activity with church and ministering to the needs of people there. I am teaching about the ***more excellent way,*** equipping the people to minister healing to the city. I am also involved with a group of pastors seeking God for the city. My wife teaches a ladies' Bible study at church and talks to everyone she can about the Father's love and His ministry to her! We are also loving being grandparents to our FIVE grandchildren!

So, there you have it! We are happy, blessed, challenged and thankful. The Father continues to reveal Himself in deeper ways, and we just keep walking a step at a time.

D.B., NE, USA

### Fibromyalgia, Chronic Fatigue, Other Chronic Diseases Healed

> I waited patiently for the LORD; and he inclined unto me, and heard my cry. He brought me up also out of an horrible pit, out of the miry clay, and set my feet upon a rock, *and* established my goings. And he hath put a new song in my mouth, *even* praise unto our God: many shall see *it*, and fear, and shall trust in the LORD. Psalm 40:1–3

I accepted Christ as my savior at a very young age and never wickedly departed from my God.

I tried to be perfect, but kept failing. I know now that no created being can hold up to perfection.

I identified with the verse in Matthew 23:27, "Woe unto you, scribes and Pharisees, hypocrites! For ye are like unto whited sepulchers, which indeed appear beautiful outward, but are within full of dead men's bones and of all uncleanness. Even so ye also outwardly appear righteous unto men but within ye are full of hypocrisy and iniquity."

My desire was to be godly. I did not know why I felt, in my heart, the way I did.

I remember the first time I read the book of James and the verse in 1:8, "A double-minded man is unstable in all his ways." This verse troubled me. Sometimes I felt saved. Sometimes I didn't feel saved. Sometimes I felt like God loved me. Sometimes I didn't feel like God loved me. I tried hard to follow God's ways, but continued to sin and "fall short of the glory of God." I was so distressed because I didn't understand how I could call myself a Christian and commit such sin. I would repetitively repent, but never felt forgiven or peaceful. I did not feel secure in my salvation. I know now that double-mindedness is like having a split personality: one-half of your thoughts are from God and one-half of your thoughts are from Satan.

As a child, I suffered from debilitating asthma, multiple allergies, and consistent nosebleeds. Without any knowledge of spiritual roots, healing began at age 19 when I married and was relieved of the fear of abandonment for a season. At age twenty-one, I began having terrible migraine headaches, which continued until I was healed while at Pleasant Valley in 2000. I was diagnosed with osteoarthritis at age twenty-three and was told that I would eventually have to have surgery when I could no longer tolerate the pain in my back.

In 1986, in what should have been the prime of my life, I was diagnosed with a number of chronic diseases: fibromyalgia, chronic fatigue syndrome, chronic costo chondritis, heart arrhythmias, high blood pressure, depression, anxiety, fibrocystic breast disease and panic attacks. Seven different prescriptions were prescribed initially, and many others were added throughout the years. I had the best doctors that the medical profession had to offer. I also added many other healing modalities along the way. "And the vessel that He made of clay was marred in the hand of the potter" (Jeremiah 18:4).

I was bound with chains of disease, which produced terrible pain and discomfort throughout my body. I was unable to use my arms, and I lost the ability to function in simple daily matters. All during that time, I was intently reading God's Word continually and asking the Holy Spirit to help me to be acceptable to God. I did not understand about evil dwelling within a Christian. I did not know that sin was a being. I did not know how to separate the sin from myself. I thought the sin was me, and how could God love me? I always felt condemned. I kept asking God to "create in me a clean heart and renew a right spirit within me." I knew something was wrong with me, and I didn't know what to do about it.

In my despair, I would read the verse in Matthew 12:20, "A bruised reed shall he not break, and a smoking flax shall he not quench." I would thank Jesus and I would say to Him, as a prayer, Psalm 17:15, "As for me, I will behold thy face in righteousness. I shall be satisfied when I awake with thy likeness." That was my hope until another voice would quote from Matthew 7:23, "I never knew you. Depart from me, ye that work iniquity."

My husband was diagnosed with a rare form of cancer in 1990, which took his life in 1993. I was calling out to God for mercy and healing and grace to sustain me in those dark hours of distress. The only way I was able to overcome, at the moment, the fear that was in my heart, was to cry out to the Lord with a song of praise on my lips, "I love You, Lord, and I lift my voice to worship You, oh my soul, rejoice. Take joy my King in what you hear. Let it be a sweet, sweet, sound in your ear." I'll never forget that song. I began to sing songs of praise and worship more and more to sustain me through weakness as I watched him go through test after test to determine what was happening in his body that had been so strong and able. The singing enabled me to go through many deep valleys of sorrow and suffering with him. You can offer a sacrifice of praise when your spirit is overwhelmed by circumstances. My song became a weapon to war against the enemy as he tried to steal my peace and continue to sow fear in my heart. It was the only way I could defeat him and receive some momentary peace. It was during this time that I was diagnosed with reflex sympathetic dystrophy in my right foot and was in a wheelchair, with excruciating pain, unable to walk for 5 months. When the neurologist told me that I would have to undergo surgery in order to cut the nerve so I would not feel the pain, I told the doctor, "No, my God is able to heal me." I forced myself to bear the pain, and I walked out of his office, never to return. In God's time, healing did begin very slowly. I began to learn about "putting on the garment of praise for the spirit of heaviness" as in Isaiah 61:3.

I continued to suffer with these conditions and in fact, was placed on Social Security disability. Chronic, unbearable, insomnia began in 1999. In December of that year, I read in Isaiah 61: "The Spirit of the Lord GOD is upon me, because the LORD hath anointed me to preach good tidings unto the meek; He hath sent me to bind up the broken hearted, to proclaim liberty to the captives, and the opening of the prison to those who are bound." I cried out to the Lord, "I am in a prison. Please cut the bars," to no avail.

In February 2000, a dear friend encouraged me to attend a week-long seminar led by Henry Wright. By that time, my ability to sleep had plummeted to one hour out of twenty-four. The daily migraines had become so intense that I could not lie down in the bed, but rather had to sit upright, with an ice pack tied to my head. Because of exhaustion, I could only attend portions of the teachings, but my spirit was in agreement with everything I heard and the lights went on. I realized the truth of 2 Timothy 2:26 and I knew that I was in "the snare of the devil who had taken me captive at his will." The last Sunday of the meeting, Henry and I were the last ones to leave the church. While walking up the aisle to the door, Henry looked at me and said, "Come out of the prison house. The body of Christ needs you." I said, "I want to." He said again, "Come out of the prison house. The body of Christ needs you. "I said, "I'm trying. " He said to me the third time, "Come out of the prison house. The body of Christ needs you." With that we parted ways. Little did I know that I would be in Georgia the very next Thursday. My friend did send me, but the details of how it happened are another testimony to the intimate love and care of our Father.

I went to Pleasant Valley Church, a nondenominational ministry in Thomaston, Georgia. I lived there for 5½ months and learned about *A More Excellent Way*™, a teaching on the spiritual roots of disease, led by Henry. I went with the hope of being healed. After being there for about a month and a half, the day came when I looked up into the heavens and said, "Father, I just want my spirit to be healed. The body will be a bonus." I had been treated by a Japanese acupuncturist who told me, "Until your spirit and heart are healed, your body will not be healed." I said, "Oh, Dr., I am a Christian. Second Corinthians 5:17 says, 'Therefore if any man be in Christ, he is a new creature: old things are passed away; behold all things are become new.' My spirit is totally healed." I did not know how sick my spirit was. At Pleasant Valley I learned to separate myself from the part that is not me. I might sin, but I am **not** sin. I might act unrighteous, but I am **not** unrighteous. I learned how to love myself, even with evil in me. I learned that not all of me is polluted. There are parts of my spirit that are perfect.

The real me was buried deep on the inside, entangled with spiritual roots with a wall of protection all around. Upon hearing the constant message from Henry that the Father loved me, and the infusion of love and acceptance that I received through the teachings and those that ministered to me, I began to have the desire to find that favored daughter of the Most High God who was "chosen before the foundation of the world, and who was called out of the darkness into His marvelous light."

Through the teaching *A More Excellent Way*™ by Henry, I came to realize that there are many voices in the world, none without signification. Not only do I hear my own voice and others, but the Spirit of God speaks and the spirit of Satan speaks. I was caught between two kingdoms. I had to decide whose voice I would listen to.

The door was opened for demons to have access to my human spirit through my family tree and personal choices. As the Holy Spirit empowered me, I was able to identify the evil that was within my spirit…evil, such as the spirit of fear, unloving spirits, the spirit of rejection, accusing spirits, spirits of bitterness, spirits of envy and jealousy, the spirit of guilt and the spirit of shame. I repented and I renounced all of the evil. **They were cast out.**

I learned to face what was in me. I faced Satan's kingdom and God. With the help of the Holy Spirit and the ministry team at Pleasant Valley, I was victorious.

I had opposed myself. I had to repent for the evil I had allowed, and I did recover myself out of the "snare of the devil [who took me] captive at his will." I am "working out my salvation daily, with fear and trembling." I am being made whole progressively. My spirit, soul and body did come out of the "prison house." I will be blameless before I get to heaven, and I look forward to hearing Him say, "I love you. I am well pleased with you."

There is victory in Jesus Christ. I was gloriously healed and restored. I love to declare the words from Chuck Girard's song, *The Heart of God*, "God's love for me has set me free and now I am free forever." Not only did He make me free from disease and pain, but He also delivered me from all medication and all of the ungodly sorrow, grief, guilt and the spirit of death that came into me following the death of my husband. I am a new person. I am so excited about life and the opportunity God has given me to express His love to everyone and declare His desire and ability to "set the captives free" in every area of life. He has given me a new life, and He has given it to me abundantly.

God provided a home for me in Florida where He continued to strengthen my spirit, mind and body. As people heard about my testimony, they began to call and inquire about God's provision for healing in my life. They wanted to know how they too might move the hand of God to be free of disease. As I shared what Jesus had done for me and as I heard the pain in their voices, God birthed in me the desire to serve Him by helping His suffering children.

In the midst of my deliverance, I developed MCS/EI along with electromagnetic field sensitivity. I was alone but I knew the spiritual roots of these diseases and continued with Henry Wright's teaching tapes daily. God's word to me and encouragement from my friend in Dallas helped me through a most difficult time. God showed me that although I was following in the path of my Shepherd, the enemy was tracking my every step, waiting for the opportunity to devour any area of my life that was open to fear. God is faithful to His Word, and I walked out of it in 2 and ½ years.

When the Lord showed me I was to return to Dallas, I went back to Georgia and received training in ministry concerning spiritual roots of chronic disease. I am privileged to work with individuals who have chronic diseases, teaching them the possible cause and effect, the spiritual dynamics involved, and the mind-body connection.

I always wanted to do something **for** God. I am truly blessed to be called to work **with** my Father and share *A More Excellent Way*™ with others.

S.A., Dallas, TX USA

## Cholesterol Level Dropped!

In May 2002, I had emergency surgery for gallbladder problems that had impacted my pancreas and liver functions. The bloodwork showed my cholesterol level was 320, and I didn't even think about this because of the other complications involved.

After surgery and during the next several weeks, I read Henry Wright's book *A More Excellent Way*™. I saw many sin issues discussed in the book that were a part of my life. One in particular was self-bitterness, self-hostility and self-anger. I did not really make the high cholesterol connection, but I did recognize my sin. I repented of this, confessing my sin to God and the iniquity of my forefathers that I also clearly saw.

About 5 months passed, and I felt urgency in my spirit to have my cholesterol checked again. (I had the thought then that the cholesterol level was probably "out the roof"!) My doctor was shocked! My cholesterol had come down 90 points without medication, dieting or exercise. He asked me how this could have happened and I told him. He asked me to write out my testimony and give it to him, minus my name, so he could use it in his medical practice. He is a Christian.

C.H., Lakemont, GA USA

## Fibromyalgia Gone

Praise God! In August of 2002, we visited your church for the *For My Life*™ program. About 8 weeks after leaving the ministry program, my wife realized that fibromyalgia had left her. After visiting Pleasant Valley, she is TOTALLY healed. Praise God!

S.M., Charleston, IL USA

## Healed of Seizures

Thank you for the ministry I have received from this church. The Lord healed me of seizures. I am so grateful to the Lord for all He has done for me.

L.C., TX USA

## Healed of Ovarian Cancer

Several months ago I was diagnosed with Ovarian Cancer.

At first, fear tried to come in with having to face death. There is a Scripture that says, "If you try to save your life you will lose it." I had to come to the point of releasing everything to God and take my hands off. The moment I did, I heard God say, almost audibly, "This test has come to pass."

I called Pleasant Valley. Two years ago I attended a seminar there and was healed of life-threatening allergies. Knowing the ministry there and their faith, I felt free to call. A minister prayed with me. Roots were dealt with, and she spoke to my body, basically telling it to come into order.

After this, I kept hearing the word "integrity." I realized there was still some fear, and I wasn't trusting Father God's integrity. I deeply repented, knowing He has life for me, not death; good, not evil; and even His thoughts for me are good, not evil. This word carried me through the test and still carries me daily.

I did have surgery and 99 percent of the cancer was taken out. Knowing God doesn't do a 99 percent work, I knew the last 1 percent was for some other purpose.

My oncologist was a Christian and a wonderful brother in the Lord. I shared my faith easily with him.

I sensed God had touched me outside of the surgery. I asked the doctor what tests I could take to prove if, in fact, I still had remaining cancer. He told me of 3 but the most accurate was the blood test. Meantime, many people were praying and supporting me.

I had my blood drawn, and the doctor called me, saying, "You confuse me." I asked, "How?" He said normal blood count was 35, yours is 23. I thought it would be 200. (23 is very good.) The second blood test, my count was 17.7. The doctor said, "You are clear, come back every few months to keep a check." I told him, "I know in my knower I'm healed." But I will do it.

Later, a minister came here. I shared my testimony, and he prayed for me to be sealed physically and spiritually so the cancer can't return. So, I'm healed and sealed. Hallelujah!!

J.P., Duluth, MN USA

### Healing Is Happening!

I came to Georgia a very desperate woman, driving 4 days. As I got closer to Atlanta, my sinus and chest secretions changed color. Now I'm sneezing less and less congested. I had lost my senses of smell and taste, and yesterday I smelled meat cooking. I was deaf in one ear with loud tinnitus, and now that is less loud. My body is less stiff. My head feels clearer without heaviness. Joy is coming back, and laughter and my appetite has improved. As you see, healing is happening, and I know I will soon write another testimony!

I believe more and more in the connection between sin and disease.

F.S., Ottawa ON Canada

### Sound Teaching!

I asked Jesus in my heart at a church camp when I was 12 years old. That same year, my father went through his 32nd degree initiation with the Freemasons and was in a very serious car accident where his intestines ruptured and he nearly died. A year later, I was in the hospital having about 50 cm. of my intestines removed as a result of Crohn's disease after being seriously ill for two years.

I wanted more than anything to serve God, and so, five years later, after being filled with the Holy Spirit at a Young Life Camp, I left home to join what turned out to be a very destructive religious cult along with my older sister. Of course, I didn't know that it was a cult or that it was destructive at the time, just like my father was not aware of the occultism behind Freemasonry! I was a part of that cult for 8 years, but ended up going from that to a very abusive marriage for 13 more years until I found out about my oldest daughter's abuse by someone in my immediate family. At this point, my world fell apart.

I left God and for the next almost 10 years, went through more than I could've ever imagined as I struggled with anger, bitterness and depression. I was also very suicidal. During that time I tried various things to find healing and peace, including various "New Age" techniques, psychotherapy, Jungian therapy, prescription drugs and more unhealthy relationships.

About 3 years ago, I finally gave up and came back to the Lord, wanting more than ever to put Him first in my life as I knew I had made a mess of it without Him. I heard about Pleasant Valley Church through a missionary friend last August, and knew that I needed to go. I made the decision to take a week off work for the *For My Life*™ retreat, as God provided a sub (I teach) and a dear sister to take care of my 15-year-old son and youngest child. (I'm 3 times a grandma!) In one week of the most sound and helpful teaching I've had since I left the cult, I learned about "The Father's Love," resting in Him and getting off the performance track, generational sins, the absolute need for forgiveness (to myself, God and others) AND the need to be delivered of all the spirits I had allowed to come into my life through the various doorpoints that were described in the teachings. I thank God for making me free and I plan to come back with my son, and to also do the *For Their Life*™ retreat at some point.

Now I have a HOPE to share with my brothers and sisters who were also victims of the cult I was in, as well as my older sister who is still in (and has been for 33 years)! There is also hope for my children and my grandchildren, as I broke off the curses that had been passed down (and which I also allowed) to any future generations!

Praise God! Hallelujah! And thank you, my brothers and sisters at PVC for your faithfulness to live out His truth and to teach it so diligently with much authority, gentleness, humility and love.

In the Father's love and for HIS glory,

T.B., Atlanta, GA USA

## Healed of Tourette's Syndrome, Diabetes and Incontinence

You told me the truth and the truth set ME FREE!

I was at Pleasant Valley and was healed of Tourette's Syndrome. Also, along with that healing, I was delivered of high blood pressure, high cholesterol, diabetes, insomnia and incontinence. PRAISE THE LORD! GOD is GOOD!

Thank God for you, your ministry and your staff. I have high respect and love for you and all who are included in your ministry.

God is still working in other areas of my body, life, soul and spirit. I am believing I am receiving total victory.

I want to be a blessing to others and work out what God has for me. Thank you again for leading me in the right direction. To God be the GLORY!

A.L.

### Healed of MCS/EI

God, in His great mercy, healed me of a medically incurable disease.

For seven long years, I struggled with Environmental Illness, also known as Multiple Chemical Sensitivity. I had pesticide poisoning, and my immune system rapidly declined. Eventually, I became allergic to nearly everything, including cigarette smoke, perfume, cleansers, detergents, lotions, car exhaust, pesticides and anything new. I developed dust, mold and food allergies.

My allergies were so severe it was hard to leave my home. I could not attend church, movies or other events. I could not go into shopping malls, theaters, office buildings, grocery stores or even most people's homes. We had portable air filtering machines in our home, where I was a prisoner. The fear, pain and isolation were unbearable.

Eventually, we sold our beautiful home because we added new insulation and the chemicals emitted from the attic made me sick. We bought another home, and I was never able to move in because the previous owners had saturated every nook and cranny with mothballs, and we were never able to get the chemicals or smell out. We had no choice but to sell this house also.

I finally got my hopes up when I discovered a doctor who specialized in environmental medicine. He felt he could help me and started new treatments. To our horror, this good, caring man's treatments made my allergies even worse. I was desperate. I had no place to live now, so I had to move to my car. My husband took the back seats out of our van so I could at least lie down to sleep at night.

I spent many hours searching for answers. I went to many doctors and experts across the country. Each time I tried something new I would be filled with hope. I always believed I had at last found the answer and could get well, but it never happened. I was in despair. I was preparing to die.

I went to an environmental health center and returned home in even worse condition. I am 5'9" and was down to 99 pounds because my food allergies were so severe. My esophagus closed when I ate. I had an oxygen tank. My circulation would shut down.

I heard about how God could heal illnesses, but I totally rejected it. Then a woman I barely knew gave me a book on the power of praising God and how He heals when you turn to Him. I had never read anything about this. I felt some faith stirring in me, and I wondered if it was true. I realized I had been trying to do this myself. So I had a talk with God: "Okay, God, I'm Yours. I'm either going to die or I'm going to get well. I'm in Your hands. I am through seeking for answers. I'm through worrying about it, struggling and fearing. I just can't do it anymore. I'm putting my life in Your hands and turning everything over to You."

I felt a burden lift from me. I actually felt some hope and joy. I realized that although I had been a church-going Christian all my life, I did not really have a personal relationship with God. I had no teachings about the gifts of the Spirit or how God heals today. I had to step outside my religion to get my healing.

A friend of mine called and insisted that I call a nondenominational church in Georgia. Pleasant Valley Church is led by Henry Wright, an expert on environmental illness and many other diseases. He teaches that there are spiritual roots to many diseases and that there are also many blocks to healing. He feels people are not healed when prayed for because often they have not dealt with the spiritual roots and removed the blocks.

I called. One of the things they told me was to read the Bible every day. I spent many hours each day reading the Word of God, and it filled me with hope and faith to receive my healing. There is healing power in God's Word, like medicine, and I made sure I took my medicine morning, noon and night. The Bible, the holy Word of God, was the most powerful instrument in my healing.

I also prayed for my healing every day. I prayed healing Scriptures and God's promises back to Him daily. I thanked God daily for healing me, even though, in the beginning, there was no strong evidence that He was. Repentance is also a key to healing. I went through my life and repented for anything that I might have done, no matter how small or seemingly insignificant.

My sister held a family gathering one evening, where nine people prayed for me. That evening, I had some dramatic healing and improvement in my back. My sister came by daily for many months, laying hands on me and praying for my healing.

I read a book that really gave me the faith to seek a complete healing. I was so excited as my sister and I learned how to pray for healing. But as years went by and I only got worse, I lost all belief—but God's time is not our time.

In the summer of 1997, I spent a month at Pleasant Valley Church's retreat. I received wonderful teachings on the Word of God and met a number of people whom God had healed and many in the process of healing. They showed me the spiritual roots of my illness and the blocks to healing. Upon returning home, I was finally able to move into a house.

It took over a year from that time to completely heal from this incurable illness, but my allergies are gone. I now go wherever I want, do what I want, eat what I want. I shop at my neighborhood supermarket without worrying if the food is pesticide-free. I have gained my weight back and more. I have flown on an airplane, driven across country, eaten in restaurants and stayed in many motels. I can go anywhere now, no matter how foul or polluted the environment is. More incredible than all of this:  last summer I helped my husband paint our house!

I now belong to a wonderful non-denominational charismatic church that believes in all of the gifts of the Holy Spirit. They also believe strongly that God heals today and have an active healing ministry.

No doctor or alternative medicine or any 12-step program or other works of man could accomplish my healing. But God can do anything.

God is our Healer, our Physician, our Deliverer. Praise God!

M.G., Overland Park, KS USA

## The Apple of His Eye

I realized a few months ago that all my memories of my father (who didn't have a father, worked most of the time, and didn't relate to me much) were of the side of his face. I do not remember him making eye contact with me. I also realized I had put that "earthly father issue" on God, feeling that I only had the side of God's face—with His full attention on the really important things (not me).

This week, as I considered Deuteronomy 32:10, *"he kept him as the apple of his eye,"* I read the literal translation, which is "little man of his eye." When you look at someone's pupils, straight on and closely, you can see yourself reflected sometimes. You do not get that when looking at the side of someone's face.

So I am standing in that truth, that I have God's full face, and I see myself as the "little woman of His eye."

S.W., Garland, TX USA

## Healed of Cancer!

Henry Wright met with a woman from our small church the Monday morning before he left our town (he spent two hours ministering to her, addressing spiritual roots and all). And I wish you could have been in our services Sunday before last. I do not think there was a dry eye after she gave her testimony.

She was diagnosed with a second go-round of cancer before the seminar. The X-rays showed it in her lungs, and her bones were very painful so they told her it was probably already there, too. A bone scan was given.

On the day she was to get the verdict of the scan, she stopped at the Post Office on her way to the doctor's office. A man tapped on her car window and when she rolled it down to speak with him, he handed her a small red book with Scriptures. He said, "God is with you today." She reached down to get some Kleenex as she was crying, and when she looked back up to tell him "thank you," he was gone. He was not in a car, he was not in the PO, he just was not anywhere to be found.

After several tries, she finally got the message the bone scan did not show ANY cancer in her body. Thank you, FATHER.

Our Father heals and He answers prayer. Only believe ALL things are possible.

S.W., TX USA

## Walking Again!

My friend ordered your tapes because she had Chronic Fatigue Syndrome.

She seems to be doing much better! I had never seen her walking before—until this week! I've known her for 16 years!

L.G., Sumter, SC USA

## Healed of Food Allergies and Blood Sugar Problems

I gave my heart and life to Jesus Christ on September 2nd, 1996, during the extended lunch break of your New York seminar. God extended it for that to happen! Praise God!

Since then, all food allergies have disappeared, blood sugar problems have also been healed by Him. I had over 100 food allergies and was binging and using laxatives daily. I had no life except for thinking about my illness, etc.

God bless you all for the work you're doing.

J.W., New York, NY USA

## Healed of Epilepsy!

I am a 22-year-old who had epilepsy for nineteen years, and I was told about this place Pleasant Valley by a good friend. I looked through the brochure and read about the things offered and the insights provided. When it came about time to go, Satan knew something was up and he comes to rob, kill and destroy. I started saying, "I'm not going to go," and that's when the jealousy started rising up. I said to my sister, "You and Daddy will get a closer relationship." But Satan did not win. I give God all the glory. I did go because I was blessed. When I came, my life was changed from the inside out, the anger and bitterness that I had toward the abusers is no longer there. And the jealousy I had of my sister was released. When I released it all, God said that He did something marvelous in my life. It was a miracle.

During the lessons of fear and unloving spirits, I asked God to forgive me once again, for I had held so much inside of me. When God said to me to release it, all of this was released, and they called out epilepsy. I claimed my miracle and was amazed claiming the miracle: I got it! When we returned back to where we were staying, I realized I had gotten my miracle because where I had brain surgery, a portion of the left temporal lobe was removed in 1997, I could put my fist in the area where it was removed. I no longer can do that! God created a new portion of my brain and brain cells!

I give Him all the praise and glory. Thank You, Jesus!

I called my dad last night, who is a non-believer. I'm believing God is going to use this awesome miracle for his salvation.

May God richly bless you all.

M.H.

## Many Healed from TBN Special

Thank you so much for helping make the television special "A Night of Miracles"! At last count 200 people have called to say God has healed them!

P.F., USA

## *My Pilgrimage to Meet God in Georgia*

I flew over two-thirds of the United States, leaving on a cold, snowy night for my appointment with God to meet Him in Georgia. He had had this plan for me forever, but I had to step into it in December of 1998, as Henry Wright had been in Las Vegas a year before, so I could learn about this place called Pleasant Valley. God knew what He was doing when He sent me there. He never does anything halfway. NO, He went all the way.

I'm 65 years old now. I've been an insulin dependent diabetic for over 8 years. During that time, I had asked for prayer from three different ministries for diabetes. Three times the spirit manifested and left. Three times it came back. That became my question to God—why does this spirit have the right to be here? What had we missed? After hearing what he had to say about the roots of diseases and my phone call to him, I knew what we had been missing. The spiritual root of the disease and the serious kingdom of self-hatred, self-rejection, self-abandonment and guilt that had been an active part of me most of my life without me even knowing it or recognizing it for what it was. Yes, His people perish for lack of knowledge. But that was about to change.

Education is the basis for continued success for those who spend time at Pleasant Valley. Education completes the process to make it possible to maintain freedom, along with the actual ministry. It works. The results are phenomenal and lasting!

Because of 16 days at Pleasant Valley, because he overcame his past and followed God's calling, because the staff has a burning desire to be instruments of healing for God and stayed there, because there is a vision that provided a converted school building, a campground, a chapel, and many, many others who knew they were destined to stay and manage it—my life will be forever changed.

Diabetes will never again have its chance to ravage my body, sending my blood sugar up and down, making my eyes blurry, making my body carry extra pounds of fat and water, changing my personality because of drivenness and aggressive irritability and other personality disorders. None of that will ever happen again. It is gone. Healed forever. An incurable disease defeated and sent on its way packing. Henry says, "Book it!"

Pleasant Valley Church has to be a unique place. One of a kind in the whole world. Some people are so sick they hardly have an ounce of energy, but you know they are in the middle of recovery and walking out of some terrible life-threatening disease. Sometimes God just holds them together by a thread, and they are so brave! At one chapel service, everyone had a chance to get up and give their testimonies. A song, a little poetry, a word—I was surrounded by people who were getting up and expressing God's Heart. It was so touching I was just overwhelmed by His love and His presence in the midst of His people.

Biggest victory: One staff member held me in one of her "heavenly" hugs, and self-hatred left. The next morning, I looked in the bathroom mirror, and it just popped out of my mouth without a thought: "I like you." Imagine that!

Being at Pleasant Valley felt like being a part of one big most-of-the-time happy family. There was a lot of laughter on Friday nights, and that had to be good, even for those who could only lie down and listen.

Since being back home, I have continued to heal and overcome lingering symptoms. God even healed my love of food so that area is under control. I have lost 12 pounds and see what my body is like without a terrible disease. My personality is quieter and kinder. The fruit of the spirit of gentleness is now a part of me, and I have even learned with the help of several what I can and cannot talk about!

The first morning back home, I got up and went downstairs and sat in my chair and praised the Lord. Was it my imagination or was there a small heavenly host in my living room quietly applauding?

Thank you, Pleasant Valley Church. Thank You, Father.

UPDATE, several months later: I continue to be totally free of diabetes and when anyone asks me how my diabetes is, I just say, "I do not know; I left it in Georgia!" I'm down 20 pounds now, which is just right for me since I stopped insulin.

J.F., Carson, NV USA

## Lupus and MCS/EI GONE!

We wanted to share our joy with you! Words cannot even begin to express how grateful we are to God for leading us to Pleasant Valley. I am walking out MCS/EI, was borderline lupus, it is gone! We are loving God, ourselves and each other in a deeper way. Our new baby is the fruit of my healing. We are hoping to bring our entire family to Pleasant Valley this year or next year! Thank you so much for obeying God and for your ministry!

R.S.

## Four-Year-Old Boy Healed of Allergy to Dairy Products

When I learned of your ministry, my 4-year-old boy had an extreme allergy to dairy products. The doctor that we took him to could do nothing successful. I started looking at his deeper issues and found several problems. One was a spirit of fear. I applied what information I had from Henry Wright and what the Lord has taught me over the years.

My son is now healed. We still battle the spirit of fear at times, but he is learning to stand against it.

I started working on the rest of my family, and the results have been the same. My 11-year-old daughter has been troubled all her life. The Lord Jesus is doing great things in her life.

My wife has had a spastic colon from childhood. She could not eat red meat among other things. It took awhile to find the issue, but the Lord brought it to the surface. She now eats red meat and anything else she wants and has no problems. This is a dramatic change. No more doubling over with pain after dinner!

It is the Lord Jesus who is doing the work. But I want to say thank you for your ministry.

D.S., Utah USA

## *No More Panic Attacks!*

It is a miracle! I attended a *For My Life*™ conference. My primary problem was severe anxiety disorder and panic attacks. The worst aspect of this problem for me was my inability to write when people were standing near me. I would experience all the classic symptoms of panic attack to the point of almost fainting sometimes. For 15 years I'd developed incredible coping skills (I could have taught a class on this!) just to live day to day going to the grocery, bank, etc., etc., etc. When I registered for the conference, I had to wear a fake brace on my right index finger to be able to fill out the forms. Over the years I'd been on, at various times, Zoloft, Prozac, Paxil and Zanax, even though I knew all along this was not God's way for me.

During the conference, I came to know that I'd come into agreement with a demonic fabricated personality. This had gained entry as the result of a traumatic assault I'd experienced 15 years ago. I told my Saturday wrap-up group that I WAS NOT GOING TO TAKE THIS DEMONIC/INNER CHILD/FALSE PERSONALITY HOME WITH ME. After repenting of coming into agreement with this thing, it was cast out (along with self-pity, self-hatred and fear, among others).

Over the years, this thing had slowly but surely isolated me. I felt most safe and comforted at home with my little collection of stuffed animals among other comfort props! I was reverting back to a small child, becoming more and more dependent on my husband. I even recently bought new editions of my first grade reader series, *Dick and Jane*! By the way, I am 56 years old.

Needless to say, I'd been crying out to the Lord for many years to heal me. I'd had much prayer, but the ROOT HAD NEVER BEEN EXPOSED! I'd heard of *A More Excellent Way*™ and even tried to contact Pleasant Valley Church a couple of years ago. Then in May of 2003, I was driving with a friend to Florida to plan my son's wedding. We stopped for gas on I-65 a little south of Montgomery, AL. Lo and behold there were copies of *A More Excellent Way*™ for sale at the gas station!! My friend bought one for me for a birthday present, and the rest is history!

Three days after returning from the conference, I was in Home Depot with my husband. We were standing in line to check out. Normally I would feel anxious at Home Depot just standing near that dreaded little black box that you have to swipe your card through and then sign. On this day I FELT NO ANXIETY AT ALL. I swiped my own card and signed my name as if I'd never struggled with this!! It's a miracle. I continue to have victory in this area.

The same day as my miracle at Home Depot, I received a phone call from a young adult woman from church, asking me to pray about teaching/facilitating a young adult women's Bible study once a week. After a couple of days I accepted, believing God was giving me a unique opportunity to WALK OUT my healing. These girls want an adult for a leader, not a little child.

Over the last few years I've all but given up flying. Much to my husband's dismay, I've forced him to cancel a vacation in Italy among other trips. I'm flying to France to visit our son!! An ADULT will be flying. Praise be to God!

It's hard to find the words to express my very deep thankfulness to God and the teachers, staff and volunteers at Pleasant Valley Church. I know the walk-out is crucial, and I'm determined to keep walking in victory!

All praise and honor and glory and power and thanks be to God.

> **When I was a child, I spake as a child, I understood as a child, I thought as a child: but when I became a man, I put away childish things. 1 Corinthians 13:11**

B.K., Brentwood, TN USA

### Healed of Glaucoma

I was down to get help with glaucoma. When I came back, I went to see my opthamologist to have my eye pressure tested, and without taking my drops, it was normal. Thanks be to God for His tender mercies.

D.B., Calgary, AB Canada

### A More Excellent Way™: A Testimony of Divine Healing

Before the age of 30, I developed hypoglycemic symptoms and was tired most of the time. After our daughter Jennifer was born, the symptoms intensified. My doctor recommended tranquilizers and counseling. A chiropractor diagnosed hypoglycemia and exhausted adrenal glands. I was treated with natural supplements and experienced much improvement. When Jennifer was 11, I went back to work for another 11 years. I would pretend to feel good during the day at work. Then in the evening at home, I would go to sleep in a chair if I sat down. I would go to bed very early in order to get through another day of work. I thought, if only I could quit work and just rest a month or two, maybe I would get better.

Finally the day came in 1997! My last day of work was on a Friday, and my mother passed away the following Wednesday. Exhausted, I barely made it through the week of the funeral. I started noticing soreness in my right ankle, and within a week, I was sore in many other parts of my body. The Lord gave me peace as only He can, and I was amazed at how well I handled my mother's death.

I then began to develop more symptoms like extreme tiredness, burning and soreness in my feet, neck and back pain, hip pain, sore and weak knees and weight gain. The doctor diagnosed fibromyalgia. I have probably taken a truckload of supplements and have been to chiropractors, a neurologist, an endocrinologist, a podiatrist—even an acupuncturist! I was like the woman in the Bible who spent all she had at the physicians! I had been in every healing line I could find. I knew my only real help had to come from God. I experienced temporary relief of symptoms after prayer a few times. I even received several personal prophetic words where the Lord said my healing was coming and that it was tied to a fear planted in me during my childhood. I never understood that because I always thought I had a wonderful childhood.

For several months I knew I was in the process of receiving my healing because I started noticing that God was revealing things to me. It was like watching a puzzle coming together. In a counseling session, the Lord revealed that the root cause of my insecurities, fears and even self-hatred was abandonment when my father was killed suddenly in an accident when I was three. My mother was such a strong Christian. I only remembered being loved and spoiled by my mother, older brothers and sisters. The counselors felt that my mother was so upset by my father's death that she probably was not really there for me the way I told myself she was.

I called my sister, expecting her to verify that my mother was the strong person I remembered. My sister said that she and my other siblings had to take care of my mother and me at that time. The part she remembered most was my waking up every morning calling for my daddy to come get me up from my bed. Since my mother was just too devastated to deal with that, one of my brothers or sisters would come play with me to get my mind off daddy. They cannot remember if I attended my father's funeral. As a result of nothing being explained to me, I never really grieved his death. This confirmed to me that the counseling I received was a revelation from the Holy Spirit.

Around this same time, a friend gave me the book *A More Excellent Way*™ by Henry Wright. In this book he links every symptom I had to fear, stress and anxiety. Henry Wright's book became a very important part of my healing. When I heard him speak at Life Center on April 5, 2003, the Lord revealed to me that I had experienced abandonment a second time when my mother died. I had always wondered why all the soreness had come so suddenly the week of her death.

Gradually, I had started to notice a marked improvement in my energy level. I no longer needed 9 or 10 hours of sleep. My feet no longer burned, and almost all the soreness had gone from my feet. My knees had greatly improved. Now my hip is only slightly sore at times. I have stopped taking the supplement I have taken for years to help with inflammation in my body. I had never allowed myself to run out of it because the pain would be so bad if I ever skipped it. Today I do not even need it! My chiropractor checked me and said he could see definite differences. In fact he said he had no trouble believing that I was being healed. He said it had been obvious to him for months that we were being favored in so many ways! The Lord has spoken prophetically to my husband and me several times that we are walking in His favor. Our chiropractor doesn't know that, and I do not think he frequently hears the terminology "the favor of the Lord"!

The best thing is that I am starting to think differently. I am starting to believe I can do some things I never before would have considered. I have always been cautious about committing to things. Now I say "Yes" to things I am asked to do, and I am loving it! God is so wonderful, merciful and faithful!

M.J., Atlanta, GA USA

## *Multiple Personalities Gone*

I had been going for Christian counseling for several months when my counselor told me that I had Multiple Personality Disorder (MPD). She said I had three separate beings and that with continued counseling they could be integrated. In other words, I could get these three beings to become happy roommates within. I was devastated.

Then two people on two consecutive days told me to read *A More Excellent Way*™. I did just that and was determined to get to Pleasant Valley Church for their seminar. I was totally set free not only of MPD, but also other chronic illnesses like high blood pressure, rheumatoid arthritis and my blood sugar dropped over 200 points. I went from over a dozen pills a day to 4. I do not have to have prescription pain pills just to manage a day. I still believe God for total healing.

When I returned home, I overheard my mother say, "The light is back in her eyes."

D.D.

## *My God Is an Awesome God*

I just want to share my story with some of you out there who have lost hope and think there is no way out. There is hope and that hope is Jesus! You are not alone. I have been in bondage with Environmental Illness (EI) and have been miraculously healed!

I had lost my life both physically and emotionally. The Lord has given it back to me. Oh what a miracle! I wasn't a strong believer. I heard of many people who were healed of Environmental Illness (EI), but never in a million years would I have thought it would happen to me. I never thought I was worthy of being healed (but no one can be worthy of being healed). The Lord has shown me that He loves me unconditionally and I am a child of God and nothing I do can change that.

My health started to slowly deteriorate in 1989. I was becoming slowly allergic to everything I ate and to every chemical, pollen and dust in the air. My children were five and three years old, and when it all started, I could no longer care for them. They had to live somewhere else. It was horrible! I was diagnosed with malnutrition, malabsorption, allergies, thyroid, Environmental Illness (EI), nervous disorder, hormone imbalance, etc. I didn't know why all this was happening. I had to be fed intravenously for months at a time just to stay alive. I couldn't even tolerate my own home. I was having heart palpitations, and my body was shaking every day. I would have severe panic attacks and would wake up every hour from sleep. I felt nauseous and drugged every day. I almost died several times from too much medicine.

My husband and I went to at least 30 doctors trying to get help. We moved to upstate New York away from New York City in hopes that cleaner air would help my condition. However, I became very ill living upstate. There was so much wood-burning smoke around that I couldn't breathe. I was also losing weight fast and was too weak to even walk.

When I could no longer function, I went to a clinic in Dallas, Texas. I was so thin, weighing 72 lbs., that my rib bones could be seen coming through my chest. I was slowly dying and I didn't care.

In Dallas, I was placed in a special environmental hospital free of all smells and chemicals. I had a special tube put in near my heart to feed me. By this time I was only drinking liquids. I was so depressed that I wanted to die. I cried day and night. I became more allergic to people and was put on oxygen to help me breathe. I stayed in the hospital for two weeks and another two weeks at the clinic. It was a nightmare!

While in Dallas, someone told me about other EI people who had been healed through a church called Pleasant Valley Church. Pleasant Valley uses prayer and the Bible to help EI patients get healed. It was God working through them. I really did not believe that I could be healed, but what did I have to lose? I called PVC from my hospital bed but was too weak to talk longer than a minute.

After being in Dallas for one month, I returned to New York with no place to live because our home was infested with wood-burning odors. I also could not ride in my car any longer. I smelled the gas fumes and couldn't breathe. I needed oxygen even in the car and had to wear a mask all the time.

Fortunately, I stayed with a wonderful caring friend from Connecticut whom I met on the phone while in Dallas. She also had EI. I stayed with her one month until my husband and I rented an apartment in Tarrytown, NY. In our new apartment, I was very housebound. I had four air filters, four fans and an air-conditioner running constantly. With all this, I still needed oxygen to breathe in the apartment. I still could not go outside or be with any other people.

On top of this, my dad died the following month. I was still very sick and had to stay in a separate room at the funeral parlor. What a nightmare life was becoming!

At this time I started calling PVC and spoke on the phone to many wonderful people. I know the Lord sent me to them. Many of them had been sick with this illness for years and were healed. They were an inspiration to me and gave me so much hope and love. They encouraged and strengthened me and ministered to me about the love of God and how much the Lord loves me. They gave me Scripture to read and prayed with me. PVC definitely was sent from heaven. I could never have done it without them. Everyone at PVC is so loving and wonderful and a gift from God!

I wanted to read my Bible and felt so much power and love from the Holy Spirit. It was beginning to change my life forever. For the first time I now had a reason to live.

It didn't happen overnight. Each day I became stronger in the Word and love of God. I was also becoming stronger physically. I was happier and began eating things I had not been able to eat for 10 years. I could be near people and was even able to go into a store. I walked down the street and no longer needed oxygen. I praised and thanked God. I ate my first piece of cake and first sandwich and stuffing in 10 years on Thanksgiving Day, 1995. I was living again. Oh, it was heaven!

I was able to eat cookies, candy and pizza. What a miracle! I went to the movies and a Broadway show. It was wonderful to live again. But the most wonderful part of all is that I was healed in my heart.

Today I no longer live in a bubble. I can go anywhere and eat anything. PRAISE THE LORD! I went to New York City and walked around with thousands of people. I was able to attend a church in Times Square with 2000 people singing and praising God. It was a taste of heaven!

I thank God so much for what He has done in my life. I joined a health club and walk three-and-a-half miles a day. God has healed my heart, and I know that having this illness has changed my life forever. I have met so many wonderful people through this illness. I learned I wasn't alone in my struggles. I know that fear is the biggest part of this illness to overcome through God's love. I am able to get rid of some of the fear related to this horrible illness. As I become stronger in the love of God, the fear becomes less. I know I can depend on the Lord to be with me in trouble. Jesus said: "I will never leave thee nor forsake thee." And He kept His promise. I thank God for letting me have my life again—even better than it was before.

The Bible verse that helped me the most and that I clung to was 2 Timothy 1:7, "For God has not given us the spirit of fear; but of power, and of love, and of a sound mind."

The Lord has really worked a miracle for me. He gets all the glory! He worked a miracle because I am a child of God. God's promises are true. 2 Samuel 22:30 says, "For by thee have I run through a troop: by my God have I leaped over a wall." He can do that same miracle for you. I am so excited to have a reason to live. I just want to share with everyone the power of the love of God! AMEN!

K.B., Tarrytown, NY USA

## MCS/EI Testimony

I am writing to thank you for your commitment to God in your life and to tell you how much I appreciate the time you have willingly given in helping people like me that you do not even know.

God has saved my life through you and I am so grateful. I had MCS for 6 years after working for the local council where their office was a damp, moldy basement that even had frogs in it. I was told the damp had knocked out my immune system, which caused this illness. I lost my job, went to every doctor, and you know this very familiar story—nothing worked and I received no compensation. I prayed, read my Bible and still did not get well. I was very desperate and allergic to anything that had a smell: petrol diesel, plastics and my dog. My then 20-year-old daughter, who lived away from home, had to change her clothes when coming to visit because of the soap powder she had used and she had to wash her hair using perfume-free shampoo. My 15-year-old son could not wear any of the colognes they enjoy at that age and if his friends came around, I would have to sit in the garden. I spent 18 months in the hall because, after having a new three-piece lounge suite delivered, the new smell of it made me ill. I will not bore you with the rest. I knew all this behavior was bondage but had no understanding of the roots and where it was coming from. I lost touch with everyone from the church I had been attending because I stopped going, and they really didn't understand what my problem was. So I felt really isolated and at times very desperate.

One very desperate day, I started playing around on the Internet, and I stumbled upon your book. I ordered the book and the above story is now history. I have literally gotten my life back. I am not 100 percent better, but I consider myself better compared to how I was. I had the classic case of a broken heart even though I had forgiven my dad years earlier. He is an unloving father who abandoned me when I was 5 years old due to an affair (many years later he married this lady). And although I had contact with him, he was cold, controlling and unfeeling, always expecting me to be the top of the class (I was always at the bottom). I suffered very badly as a child from asthma, bronchitis and severe colds, and so missed nearly all my schooling. God healed me of my asthma when I became a Christian 20 years ago.

I never considered myself abandoned because I had a lovely mum, but she had a dreadful time, financially and emotionally dealing with me as a sick child and my 14-year-old sister. Dad was in business with my mum, and she helped him to achieve his success, but he had no problem keeping her very short of money when they split up whilst he lived the good life. Dad has lived most of my life abroad, and I have no bonding with him, but he knew that he always fell out with everyone. If I did not please him, he would not talk to me on the phone or correspond. On one occasion I used his flat and was wrongly accused of leaving his sun bed out. For that sin he did not talk to me for 4 years and told everyone I was not talking to him. There are plenty of stories like that. I would go for holidays to see him, but that was always because I was pressured to go, and his moods were horrid. My dad was and still is a very difficult character but can also be very charming.

Dad came back to England 10 years ago at 80 years of age, and you can guess he decided it would be nice to have a family in his old age. He lived a 30-minute car drive away, the closest I have ever lived to him. His wife died last year after having a dreadful illness and living with him. My sister and myself supported them both at this time. I was so fortunate to have read your book and my healing had begun because I would never have coped with the many issues I had to face with my dad. It did delay my progress, but I am sure God used this at the specific time for His reasons. He only wants contact now with my sister and myself because he does not have his wife to be unkind to. He is verbally abusive to both of us, constantly trying to play one against the other.

My daughter knows I am writing to you and also says thank you; she had various allergy problems with food and is now so much better.

I feel God has told me to write to encourage you even though I know you must have letters all the time telling you of healings. I am so grateful that you have continued the Lord's work despite the many hardships you face.

I have bought an extra copy of your book *A More Excellent Way*™ so I can hand it out to people to read. I did give a copy to the vicar of the church I now go to; he says it is sound teaching. I would just like others to have the help I have had. I will try to continue to pass this book to as many people as possible in order that they too may be helped.

With much love and many thanks to you and the team for giving my family and me a life worth living.

A.J., Dorset, England

## Healed—Multiple Personality Disorder and Many Diseases!

One of the case histories in the book is featured in a TBN prime-time special called "A Night of Miracles," and they've reenacted some of her diseases. They went to San Francisco to the house where she was in the foil-lined room. They've re-enacted her journey, her healing. Before she was saved in 1989 in San Francisco, she lived in a foil-lined room. She's trying to read a book in a specially created glass covered box exhausted to the outside window, putting her hands to turn the pages protected, because she is so allergic to the glue in the binding and the ink on the page. She was down to two foods that she could eat. She was 56 when she came to us. She's been healed now for twelve years. She's an active member of our staff, she looks like she's still in her thirties, and she was healed of seventeen incurable diseases. God used us to get her saved, healed, delivered, and she is actively defeating the kingdom of the devil today. What God has done for one, He'll do for another. Some of the diseases that she had that God healed—these are documented diseases, medically documented diseases—and she doesn't have any of them today; they included:

Multiple chemical sensitivity (universal reactor). She was allergic to all foods and chemicals, causing anaphylactic-type reactions and throat closure. At one time she was naked due to the inability to wear white cotton clothing. She only had one least reactive food, had to live in foil-lined rooms in areas of mountains or near ocean. Oxygen and adrenalin were necessary for survival, and she was in this condition for ten full years. She had electromagnetic field sensitivity. That's being allergic to electricity. Would cause heart attack-type symptoms and faintness. At one point, a 20–watt light bulb couldn't be turned on. Heaters that were electric could not be used in the winter.

She had immune disorders; helper suppressor cells inverted, abnormal elevated complement C-3 was 212 (normal is 70 through 176). Complement total Hem lower than 20 (normal is 70 to 150). Low B cell count, 176. Low T-cell count, 700 (normal is 1000 to 2500). She was diagnosed with moderate to severe atypical organic brain syndrome, mostly right hemisphere affecting the limbic system, hypothalamus and right frontal lobe. Had dyslogia, which is short-term memory loss, aphasias. She had a drop of 25 points in IQ for ten years from over sixty electroshock therapies and a prolonged coma. Her IQ has been totally restored.

She had disequilibrium, loss of balance, falling several times per day. She had hyperparathyroidism, hypothyroidism, primary renal calcium leak (a rare kidney disorder). Secondary estrogen deficiency due to total hysterectomy, multiple fibroid tumors and pre-cancerous cysts in both ovaries, cervical and lumbar osteoarthritis with narrowing of C-5/C-6/L-5 through S-l interspaces requiring braces, traction, Demerol and hospitalization.

She had leukopenia, neutropenia, secondary kidney dysfunction due to previous renal shutdown requiring hemodialysis and was in a coma for one month. There was a chronic high sedrate indicative of inflammation in the body, for ten years. She tested positive in IgE Rast tests for traditional allergies elevated from childhood, perennial allergic rhinitis to dust, molds, trees, animal danders, food, and bee stings.

She was diagnosed with psychiatric disease, schizophrenia, paranoid catatonic episodes, beginning in 1962; manic depressive, circular depressed, beginning in 1976. Multiple personality disorder: she had fourteen multiples from age five. Since childhood (age eight), chronic suicidal ideation and attempts. Anorexia nervosa and bulimia. Had to be hospitalized and tube-fed, beginning in 1964. All of the above included obsessive-compulsive behaviors, free-floating anxiety and panic disorders.

Chronic generalized myositis, diffuse arthralgias, tendonitis and bursitis and chronic severe bladder infections.

And today she is totally healed from all of the above conditions.

A.H., GA USA

## *Virus Growths Gone!*

My husband and I are attending a *Be in Health*™ Sunday night class. I have subscribed to the 7000 project and will probably need forms, etc., because I am beginning to have people ask a lot of questions and for prayer, etc.

There was a rather dramatic thing that happened during the class deliverance on occultism/yoga stuff. During the casting out of evil spirits attached to yoga, something snapped to attention at the base of my spine and rapidly spun and wiggled up and out the base of my skull. It felt like a moving electrical/shocking snake. I just said to myself, "Wow!! OK, this is cool!" The next morning I woke up and realized that for the first time in 35 years I had no lower back pain. Then I remembered that when I was in a new age cult group at that time, I got talked into messing around with Chakras and Kundalini. Well, the bottom line is that I have not had lower back pain since the deliverance ministry done for the whole class on November 9, 2004.

Also, all the growths on the skin of my neck simply disappeared within a week after returning home. Now the growths on my back have either turned gray and dropped off or disappeared. My doctor had told me, prior to my coming to PVC, that I had a virus and nothing could be done to stop the growths. Well...I do not "had" a virus anymore! My immune system is beginning to behave properly.

Early in March I am to have another blood test to see if I can stay off Avandia (diabetic med). My doctor said my cholesterol has improved so much that I may be able to go off Lipitor. Hoping the thyroid medicine will be the next to go. By the way, my hemorrhoids are shrinking...a little graphic...but very important to me...since they have been there for 45 years.

Guess I am a success story in progress. Deepest thank you's to all the staff who so selflessly laid down their own interests on behalf of me and all the others. Every-so-often I hear a voice saying, "Deal with it."

S.B., Tacoma, WA USA

## The Father's Love

*All my life* I served the unloving spirit brought down by parents, etc. I so see the mercy of God upon all my days—HIS great mercy but also faithfulness. I know now that HE really does love  me just the way I am and that I found "Daddy." For the first time in my life, I truly have a Daddy now. I am so grateful to God for bringing me into HIS freedom and out of bondages of serving that spirit of evil. Now I can truly minister "The Father's Love" even though I have before. Now it will be IN HIS fullness. I'm home in HIS love. All my life I looked for HIS love. Now I have it! *Thank you, Jesus*!

J.C., MN, USA

## Healed of Sciatica

I was invited to Pleasant Valley Church by a friend in August 2004. I had never heard of the church and had never read the book *A More Excellent Way*™ by Pastor Henry Wright.

I was suffering with sciatica in my left hip and leg, so much that I could hardly walk. I had been taking Tylenol PM at night for approximately 6 months in order to sleep. I was seeing a chiropractor often. It was not helping. I was getting into alternative health care, nutritional health foods, vitamins and supplements in order to regain and maintain my health. I was becoming more fearful, as I was getting older, of being crippled and sick in my old age.

I also had a hiatal hernia and acid reflux disease and had to sleep propped up on 3 pillows.

On the second day I was at the *For My Life*™ seminar at Pleasant Valley Church, I was healed of sciatica. Since then, one-by-one as I have learned to apply the teachings that I have learned, I have been healed of all of the above diseases also. I have taken back my life.

I am thankful to the Lord for taking me to Pleasant Valley Church.

S.G., Sulphur, LA USA

## Toxic Brain Syndrome and SRA

God led me to GA from my home in CO almost 3 years ago. I became disabled last December as a result of pesticides and toxic mold. I had begun to think Satan had led me here due to my loss of health and cancer and my dog's death (cancer) until I came to this ministry in April. Then I realized that I was led here to be blessed by this ministry with recovery from satanic ritual abuse. I attended *For My Life*™ two weeks in a row last spring. I have more cognitive function. My friends noticed immediately that I could think better (Toxic Brain Syndrome was one of my diagnoses). I noticed an increase in my energy level. It is not an overnight thing, but daily I'm improving. I am grateful for the teachings, ministry and deliverance.

I especially am grateful that the thoughts in my head toward myself are kinder and more loving. Praise God! Also, "my" thoughts toward others are more compassionate. I'm so grateful for y'all's ministry.

L.G., North Branch, MN USA

### Gout, High Blood Pressure and High Cholesterol Gone

My wife came first to Pleasant Valley Church. I have seen many healings in her life since she came in September 2001. I decided to come and work out problems in my life. We came together in the summer of 2002. Also I came back by myself in February 2004 *For My Life*™. I was dealing with high blood pressure, gout, overweight (289 lbs), high cholesterol, superstitions from my childhood, injury of back many years ago.

After working with my doctor, checking my blood pressure and blood over 6 months, I've been healed of high blood pressure. I'm eating right (smarter), and I've lost 70 lbs. (now weigh 219 lbs). I have no more gout or high cholesterol. I've gone from 5 medications down to one (Ibuprofen tabs 800 mg twice a day). I'm ready to work out (walk-out) other things that the Lord shows me.

T.H., Durant, FL USA

### No More Seizures!

I had seizures since age 13 (for 22 years). I was set free at Pleasant Valley. Before coming to Pleasant Valley, I was having 50 seizures a day and was up 24 hours a day. Doctors never had the medication right. At Emory University they wanted to do 3 tests. I wanted to go to Pleasant Valley. I read the book and lots of healings came forth.

I am also a praise and worship leader and found that this was a hindrance to the ministry. Now there are many open doors.

Praise be to God for no sickness.

A.R., Dalton, GA USA

### Walking Out Addictions

I came here knowing I had an addiction. I did know I had other areas of my life that I need to deal with. The sin I've given into for many years is lust, pornography, and masturbation. I'm coming away from this week knowing God loves me. He desires to see me free. He doesn't reject me because of this sin. There is hope to overcome because of His love. As I walk out my freedom and receive God's love, I'll be able to love myself and others. My wife has asked for a divorce. I've been able to release her while here. I'm making a trade with the Lord. My cheap pearls for the genuine article.

K., Monroe, GA USA

### Healed of Septicemia

Thank you so much for all your help!

My husband's cousin was in the hospital, in a coma, dying of Septicemia. The doctors gave up all hope. He is only 24. Within two days of praying what your ministry told me to do and rebuke, he was sitting up and talking. 3 days later he was sent home with a clean bill of health! They told us he would have all these other issues if he came out of this, but he is perfectly healthy!!

PRAISE THE LORD!!! Thank you again sooooo much!!!

G.S.

### Arthritis Healed

I've been healed of arthritis in both knees and my lower back!

C.V., Marietta, GA USA

### Dyslexia, Chronic Infections, ADD Gone

When we came to Pleasant Valley in June (2003), I had Chronic Fatigue Syndrome for 15 years, allergies to chemicals, foods and environment, A.D.D., Dyslexia, sleep disorder, chronic eye, ear and vaginal infections, fear of man, self, life! (You name it, I was afraid of it.) I hated myself—everything about me! I also suffered the effects of many traumas throughout my childhood and adult life.

My healings have been a process over the last year. We came back to P.V. 5 times (total of 5 weeks), and each time the Lord pealed another layer of the "onion" off my life. I truly believe that by the time I came to P.V. the Lord had me primed and ready to receive His Word, truth and healing. For 23 years I had fought to stay alive and get healthy, and we tried everything under the SUN. I always believed that I was not made to walk in sickness that God could and would heal me, but the frustration of trying this modality and that modality was exhausting in itself.

In November 2002, our then 26-year-old daughter came home from completing her Masters in physics in England, and she was very ill. Fibromyalgia, A.D.D., Manic Depression, emotional torment from a rape at 16 years old. By April we were beside ourselves trying again everything the world offers and praying and believing for God to intervene with a miracle. I had bought *A More Excellent Way*™ at a Christian conference but was in the process of moving, so it got put away in a box. In prayer for my daughter, I remembered the book. She read it, called P.V. and in May (2003) came to P.V. sick and came home *healed*—the 1ˢᵗ stage; then came again in September for a week. 2 weeks later and she is today in London working on her Ph.D. in physics—*no medication*, no sickness.

So when we saw in one week what God's Word through the teachings at P.V. had done for our daughter, then I had to come!

Today I am healed from chronic fatigue, A.D.D., dyslexia, fears, infections, all allergies, and through the teaching on Father's Love and Scripture study, I am loving myself—my Creator, my family, and other people. I am *nothing* like the 54-year-old woman who drove here one year ago. I am truly a "*New Creation*" but I know that I am now becoming that new creation God had intended me to be from the foundation of the world!

Plus, I am so very thankful God in His mercy and goodness did not heal me through those 23 years because, if He had, He would have condoned all of my sins that were responsible for my sickness.

Yes, this was hard work, and it is a process; but it was *far* harder walking minute-by-minute in physical, emotional and spiritual torment. God has given us the tools to freedom. He wants all of His children to walk in freedom, and He is no respecter of persons!

Has this changed my life and our families? Each of our 3 children have had healings and are in and/or doing ministry. And as for my husband and me, well, we have given away or sold over 200 books in the past year and seen many of these people head down to GA for their own journey into wellness. We minister and teach wherever we can. How can we not? God has given us *so* much, we *have* to share and serve others so that they will know His love and His freedom!

B.K., Liberty Township, OH USA

## Panic Attacks and Back Pain Healed!

I became a Christian approximately 31 years ago. I had such a miraculous change in my life at the time of my salvation that I saw four of my family members come to know Christ as a result of these changes that were happening with me. I have done my best to follow Christ and to find His plan for my life through the years, but there was always something missing. I could never gain victory in areas of stress and anxiety. I gradually lost the joy of my salvation over the years. I was searching for the truth, and I just couldn't seem to find it. We all know that Satan comes to steal, kill and destroy. He not only stole this from me, but he was stealing my health as well. I had so much fear and stress resulting from a series of events that had happened to me and my family in the 1990s. I had watched my nephew (who was more like a brother), die a horrible death from brain cancer, just to name one. I prayed for God to heal him, and I searched all alternative healing methods to find a cure for him. I made sure that these were Christian people who were practicing these alternative treatments. I thought this was the right thing to do since the traditional medical route wasn't working. I lost my nephew to cancer in 1994, and I just couldn't believe that he wasn't healed. I just knew that God would heal him. I must confess my faith was shaken. I didn't know there were spiritual roots to disease, and I didn't know about blocks to our healing.

I began to have more and more problems with panic disorder and began to withdraw from all the things I loved doing and the people that I had enjoyed being around. I prayed for God to heal me. I prayed for a church that was REAL, and I prayed for the joy of my salvation to be restored and for God to renew a right spirit within me. I continued to spiral downward. I had literally begged God for answers for at least 5 years, when God told my husband and me through a prophecy that he was going to restore all the things that Satan had robbed us of.

Shortly thereafter, a friend of mine from Atlanta called and asked me to tell her about the healing ministry we had in Thomaston. I promptly told her that we didn't have one! She said, "Oh, but I'm reading a book called *A More Excellent Way*™ by a man in Thomaston!" "Thomaston?" I asked. This was my hometown. We had just moved back here a few years ago, and I had no idea that we had a healing ministry here. I told my friend that I would go and check it out. The rest is so awesome. I knew the minute that I set my foot in the door of the sanctuary that this was the church I had prayed for. I knew this was the answer to my prayers.

I went through the *For My Life*™ program and found the truth that I had been missing. Oh, how awesome it was! I have been healed of anxiety attacks and panic disorder, and I no longer take Klonopin! God gave me something during the week that I didn't even ask for. I had been in an auto accident in 1980 and injured my right hip. I was in constant pain. I had physical therapy; I had gone to chiropractors for years; I had many treatments that had not helped at all. The pain was so bad that I couldn't sleep on my right side at night at all. During the week of the *For My Life*™ program, I discovered that my hip wasn't hurting anymore. I couldn't believe it! Could this possibly be true? I have had this pain for 20 years! The pain never returned. I found out firsthand what happens when the spirit and soul line up with the Word of God, THE BODY STARTS HEALING ITSELF THE WAY God intended! This was a wonderful bonus!

My husband and I are so, so grateful to the Lord for the blessings that are coming our way as a result of the teachings that we have heard and applied to our lives since being at Pleasant Valley. This was truly the missing link in my Christian walk. I can truly say that I have experienced freedom from fear for the first time in my life.

M.T., GA USA

### *Healed of ITP!*

In September 2000, with no explanation, I noticed reddish-purple spots on my ankles and feet. After several days of praying, I went to the doctor on Friday to learn that I had almost no platelets in my blood system. As one of the platelet's jobs is to keep the blood in the blood vessels, mine was leaking out and (by gravity) moving to my feet. Had I not gone to the doctor on Friday, I would have had internal bleeding and probably not lived to Monday.

The diagnosis was Immune Thrombocytopenic Purpura (ITP), a chronic autoimmune disorder of the blood platelets with no apparent predisposing cause. The immune system, which was supposed to guard me, was eating the platelets! The medical community knew of no cause, no cure short of removal of the spleen (the offending organ), and informed me that since I had also had Crohn's disease approximately 20 years earlier, I would just get another autoimmune disorder/disease in the future.

I chose to keep my "parts" and, under "house arrest" so as to not be injured, use a high dose of prednisone for 6 weeks (it then took 4 months to fully stop taking the drug), even knowing some of the side effects, rather than have surgery. Having begun to understand the workings of both Crohn's and ITP, I could see that there must be some spiritual reason that I had developed both diseases. I wanted to let God have time to work on me. I guess I had more faith He could heal side effects than replace a missing part.

Before being saved, I had lived with Crohn's for years, on and off medication, even having surgery for an abscess. Not long after I was saved, God in His awesome mercy and grace healed me of Crohn's. (Not any symptoms for decades now!) He showed me that the cause for the Crohn's was that I was in an oppressive situation and that I tried to change myself so as to be loved and not rejected or abused.

During the treatment with Prednisone, God dealt with me that He had, through His mercy, again healed me. The Oncologist/Hematologist released me in 6 months with platelets at a manageable level and, according to his staff, no one with ITP had been released from their office in less than 2 years and surgery. But...they said I would probably get another disease. However, I knew God was greater, and I prayed and asked what had caused all this to happen. Again God showed me that I had been in an oppressive situation (this time a very controlling "Christian" cult), and that I had tried to change myself to fit in with people who were wrong. I repented immediately. The last blood test I had then showed platelets back at normal.

God is so loving and faithful, and knew that there was an even deeper set of reasons and led a friend to tell me about some of Henry Wright's tapes of a seminar. After hearing the tapes, I knew that this was the answer. I then went to see him in Daytona Beach in 2002 at the *Be in Health*™ Seminar. I sat just listening to truth, with tears running down my face, as God began to liberate me from the bondage of the cult I had been in.

My two best friends and I then knew we had to go to Georgia to check this out more. Within the first 24 hours of listening to truth in class, God began to unravel a lifetime and generations of iniquities that held me in bondage. I began to see that self-hatred and self-rejection came through my family where my mother had rheumatoid arthritis (autoimmune) and died as a result of suicide; my father taken by cancer. I was open to the truth and God met me and set me freer than I had ever been. God knew what the roots were, and now, so did I. I took responsibility.

I took back foods to which I had been allergic. My skin color went from pale to pink for the first time I remembered. My hair that had a lot of gray from the illness turned back to ash blond overnight. Returning home late at night, the next morning my 12-year-old son did not recognize me still sleeping. Even my voice changed and, in telephone conversations when family members heard me speak, they asked me what had happened.

Immediately, due to the changes my husband saw in me, we made plans to return as a family for the *For My Life*™ program. Even my sister and her husband came! Then members of his family came as a result of changes they saw in us.

Now, we live in Georgia, helping others to become free, restoring relationships with God, themselves, and others. My two friends—well, their lives have been changed magnificently by this ministry, and they have invested in an inn here to provide a place for people to stay so they may come to Thomaston to restore their relationship with God and their health. We owe our sanity and our lives to God and what He is doing in our lives through this ministry and this loving family of people.

S.G., Port Saint John, FL USA

# BOOK REVIEWS from Amazon.com

## A Simple and Powerful Prescription For Healing

In *A More Excellent Way*™, Henry Wright gives us a clear prescription for healing which is both simple and powerful. The author believes that most diseases have spiritual roots and are the result of separation on three levels. These can be summed up as separation from God, yourself and others.

All spiritual healing begins with the sick person coming back into alignment with God and His Word, accepting himself or herself in right relationship to God and making peace with others. There are many spiritual blocks to healing, and the most important one is unforgiveness.

Henry Wright emphasizes the prevention of disease and appreciates that spirit, mind and body are interconnected in this effort. A large section of this book is devoted to a discussion of individual diseases and their respective spiritual root causes.

P.K., Birmingham, AL USA

## I Was Completely Healed of MCS/EI

I HAD MCS/EI which is a severe allergy to the environment, chemicals, foods, molds, etc. My life was deteriorating daily and no doctors knew what to do with me. Fears and sickness progressed daily. After I cried out to God one evening, the next day my sister found this book on the Internet with someone's testimony.

To make this a short story, I did purchase this book; God provided me the money to go out to Henry Wright's ministry in Thomaston, Georgia, where I spent a week at their *For My Life*™ seminar. There they teach on the spiritual roots of disease through Scripture (what this book IS about) and then every day you're led through repentance of sins like bitterness, unforgiveness, self-hatred, envy, jealousy, addictions, etc., and then through deliverance ministry. By the second day, the mask that I had to wear most of the time was off! I started to take back foods immediately. My body immediately started to heal, and I mean immediately, and now over 4 months later, I am living a normal happy life full of joy, laughter, freedom and a deeper relationship with God, especially God the Father, than I have never known until the seminar.

I highly recommend this book to all—not just Christians. Do not let that stop you from getting set free. His ministry has healed over 400+ illnesses and counting. Anything from varicose veins, hemorrhoids, depression, addictions such as drug and alcohol and food, ADD, multiple personality, EMF sensitivity, chronic fatigue, fibromyalgia, candida, etc. Everyone that lives out there that works in this ministry has been healed of something. Their testimonies are amazing. There are miracles happening out there and I am one of them.

Do not miss out on the blessing. You could be healed of diabetes, asthma, allergies, etc. They have phone ministry also if you can't make it out to one of their seminars. They have tapes that are healing people as well. Someone was healed of fibromyalgia from repenting of fears after hearing the fear tapes. I am not getting paid for this advertisement—just a very happy, healthy and healed individual who wants to give God all the glory! Praise You, Jesus Christ, for bringing me to the Father and healing my life!

Reader, Leesburg, GA USA

### As Seen on TBN, A Night of Miracles

This book on healing and seeking God needs to be in the hands of everybody—doctors, pastors, Christians, New Agers, parents, common folks—everybody! We have read about the mind-body connection, but God sees us as a triune being: We have a body, a mind and a spirit. All three will affect our health and our lives. Thank you Mr. Wright for making the connection.

You will be changed with the truths in this book! The truth alone just may make you free!

Reader, Hoboken, NJ USA

### This is the first book that should be given to cancer patients

I wish I had read this book when I was first diagnosed with cancer, instead of 6 years later. You can do all the medical treatment that is out there, but if you do not deal with the "root" of what caused the cancer (or other disease) in the first place, you might have to walk a much longer, tougher road on the "cancer (disease) journey." Henry Wright's idea of healing through sanctification makes so much sense. This is a very "medical" book and also a very "spiritual" book; the two are blended beautifully, and it really makes sense! It addresses healing in a way the church just doesn't talk about. It brought me a huge measure of HOPE!

K.S., La Canada-Flintridge, CA USA

### Growing in the Spirit

I found this book to be most helpful. It brought home the entrances Satan uses to place sickness, illness, infirmity and disease on our bodies. It gives us a real root to cut in our healing prayers. The Word says, "My people are destroyed for lack of knowledge" (Hosea 4:6). Following the principles in this teaching will bring healing to many who have not understood why their healing has not manifested. Have a teachable heart when you read this book. Ask the Holy Spirit to quicken it to you. It **IS** God's will for you to be healed. This book will show you who to credit with your illness and how to come against it. Be blessed as you read this.

S.F., Clarkesville, GA USA

### Just what the doctor ordered

This book reveals the missing piece of the mind-body puzzle. We do not have to believe the programming of our past...we can WALK OUT of our (emotional, physical, psycho) PRISON and NOT be TORTURED any longer. Sweet freedom!

D.B., Indiana USA

### A More Excellent Way

This book is a lifesaver. Have you tried prayer, healing, laying on of hands and not gotten healed? Have you tried deliverance and not gotten delivered? This book will tell you the blocks to healing and what you need to look at to get out of your yucky stuff and back on your road to healing and deliverance.

B.R., Encinitas, CA USA

### You Can Be Healed

I was bewildered by the fact that sick people at church were not getting healed. Some were, but more were staying sick and even dying. I couldn't understand why prayer, a lot of prayer, did not work. Then I read this book and now I understand. God does want to heal but the sin in our lives keeps us from being healed....The concepts in the book are easy to understand and can change lives. Most people just do not know these concepts. This book...can save so many lives. I would recommend this book over any book I have ever read.

L.C., Chesapeake, VA USA

### Finally Free!

This book changed my life. I've been a believer of Christ, earnestly seeking Him for 20 years, yet I have never understood why today's church is so ineffective. This book explains it—as well as the scriptural reasons we are so physically and emotionally sick!

And the answers are for everyone—believer or not.

Just reading the book set me free from horrendous allergies I've been fighting for 30 years. I've now been free from allergies for 4 months! My husband who has been crippled with rheumatoid arthritis since he was 19 has also found freedom from pain!

A note to Christians who are put off by the "healers" you see on TV: I never believed any of that was real. This book is real. The healing you will find is real. And not a bit of it is Hollywood. You can literally be free from disease by just applying the biblical principles Henry Wright has outlined.

Reader, Fort Lauderdale, FL USA

### A More Excellent Way™

This book has helped me put together the pieces of the puzzle of the Christian life. Every person needs a working knowledge of the things taught here. I personally have been set free from tormenting sin through this ministry. I've come to a place, through these insights from God's Word, where I'm confident that we can appropriate God's healing and deliverance. If healing or deliverance are not obtained after ministry, simply work through the "Blocks to Healing" list. God's will **IS** that we have perfect health, but we must line up with God's Word to appropriate it. I've been convinced of the authority that I've been given through Christ to minister healing and deliverance. This book provides a working reference for ministering to the sick and/or oppressed. I carry it everywhere along with my Bible. It is the best book I've ever read, except for the Bible, of course.

Henry Wright and his staff are ministering to thousands who come from all over the world to be healed and delivered and to learn to do the same for others. They work long hours and live very modestly. My wife and I spent a week with them and I know. The book, the man and the church behind them are all the real deal! I praise God for all of them because His ministry through them to me has been instrumental in bringing the kingdom of God to me and mine.

D., Ft Worth, TX USA

### Read and live—this will save your life

If you have illness and incurable diseases, physical, spiritual or psychological, and you want to get well and live a healthy life, then read this book. It will set you on the right path. Reading and APPLYING the principles in this book transformed my life in every way. I no longer have PMS, I can love and receive love from my husband, I have been healed of herpes simplex, I no longer have chronic pain in my hip, right gluteus and leg, I am no longer allergic to foods I thought I was, and this is just the beginning. It is a must read.

H.B., Bethel Island, CA USA

### This is a Life-Changing Book

I was a bit of a skeptic when I first began reading Henry Wright's book. It sounded a little wacky to hear that the sin in our lives can make us sick. By the end of the book, I was a believer! He demonstrates how the Bible clearly shows that God cannot tolerate unconfessed sin and that there are consequences for our sin, even after we trust Jesus as our Lord and Savior. Sanctification is the goal of Henry Wright's ministry, and it is now my personal goal as well. My husband and I have both been healed through applying the principles of this book to our lives. If you read and apply this book to your life, you will experience the peace, love and joy of God like you never have before!

M.R., Wake Forest, NC, USA

### Life Changing!

I have never read a book as life changing as this one.

I have been a Christian for many years, yet continued to struggle in certain areas of my life both with God and with myself.

The principles in this book have made such a difference! Not only is God healing me of addictions, back pain and insomnia but my mom who has had a crippling fear of heights all her life has been healed and no longer has any fear! This book has enabled me to deepen my relationship with God and with others. There is no way I could describe the fullness of what the knowledge contained in this book has done for me. I thank God and give Him the glory for giving Henry Wright this knowledge.

D.G., Roswell, GA USA

### No Longer Sick

My husband and my two sisters-in-law had years of debilitating chronic illnesses. Through understanding the biblical teachings in this book and applying them to their lives, they are no longer ill and live completely normal lives. This teaching has brought our marriage into wholeness. EXCELLENT!

Reader, GA USA

### Henry Wright's Book Is Awesome!

This is the only book I have ever read that tells me the truth about sickness and what causes it. I need truth because I want to get healed!! I have been prayed for over and over and over, but healing never manifests itself. Henry Wright gives us the truth! I went to their ministry for help. They are sooo very caring and love people!! I have been healed in a many areas, and the rest of the healing will come as I walk out my healing by keeping God's Word in my ears and coming out of my mouth. The wonderful care they give and show each and every person no matter what their problem is! Henry Wright is a man of true love and concern for God's children! He is the only person brave enough to tell us the truth about why we get sick and how to get healed. His book is bathed in Scripture. If we won't own up to our own negative thoughts that turn inward on us and bring sickness in our bodies, then we won't get healed or get free. I was seeking healing and freedom. I got it!! Awesome!! Everyone who wants to be healed and get the whole truth and nothing but the truth—this is a must read book!!

T.M., Prattville, AL USA

### Candida, Food Allergies and Rosacea Gone

A friend called to tell me about the book; she said I had to buy it. I did and it changed my life. I never knew there could be reasons that I was not healed. I love God and had been prayed for many times. For 4 years I have dealt with Candida, food allergies and Rosacea. I have been on a strict diet and tried many ways to be healed. This book has saved my life. I think everyone reading this book will receive something different from it. It will depend on why you are reading it and how honest you can be with yourself. The author just tells you the truth; you can do what you want with it. I did not read it from a theological perspective; I read it as one looking for answers in my own life. I needed help, and I found it from someone honest enough to tell me the truth.

B. S., South Bend, IN USA

### My Life (and yours, too, if you want) Will Never Be the Same!

*A More Excellent Way*™ is just that—*a more excellent way*™ to live your life! This book has been my ticket to freedom: with myself, others and God. No longer do I suffer oppression, depression and brokenheartedness. I also personally know others who have been freed of glaucoma, cancer, MCS/EI, asthma and lupus. This is no game—it's your life. If you are serious about fighting for it, get this book. The ministry of Henry Wright is biblically based and very loving and full of hope. Fight for your life—the devil is!

D.P., Calgary, AB Canada

## *Profound and Gets Results*

Prior to my wife's introduction to Henry Wright, she was homebound with disease that was identified by him as fear-based. In accordance with sound biblical teaching, "perfect love casts out fear," the teaching of *A More Excellent Way*™ became the foundation for my wife's freedom from a disease that was incurable, medically speaking. She was healed within four weeks as his the ministry applied the word of God's love into our lives. She had been housebound for 6 years.

I have seen scores of people who, when they honestly address the spiritual roots of disease mentioned in the book, are released from diseases including diabetes, cancers, arthritis, lupus and so many more. The scriptural references are numerous and are given in context with each teaching in *A More Excellent Way*™.

To me it is impossible to truthfully deny a thorough biblical basis for the teachings set forth. Had I denied it, my wife would be homebound, and we would still be childless. This book revealed that spiritual roots needed to be dealt with before we could carry a child past the first 5–8 weeks of pregnancy. Thanks to the principles revealed in this book, with no medical intervention. My wife is expecting our second child in less than 3 months. We had been childless for the first 15 years of our marriage.

This book is written from the transcript of a seminar in which a close friend of ours was healed and set free from her oxygen, wheelchair and life of isolation in disease.

It works because another lady, while attending the seminar the book is founded on, was healed totally of breast tumors. Not only that, but her brother upon applying the teachings of the tapes she sent was likewise set free of debilitating disease.

This book is on the cutting edge of the healing of disease. The book shows the value of medical and psychiatric practices, but also shows that God has established healing as part of His church. *A More Excellent Way*™ establishes the necessary inter-relationship of pastoral care with the medical and psychological professions. It also documents the superiority of God's healing to man's disease management.

You will enjoy this expose of how God's will to heal and prevent disease can be manifested by a simple, pragmatic application of our hearts to the Word of God. You will read of people, I personally have come to know, who are now healed. It is about the need to be freed from the broken relationships and abuses we have taken into our hearts. *A More Excellent Way*™ shows how bitterness, rejection, fear and other spiritual roots, trip us up in our spiritual dimension, causing associated biological and psychological manifestations. When the medical profession labels a disease "incurable," *A More Excellent Way*™ shows the value of going before God with a disease and going to work to root out the spiritual roots that do not show up in a blood test or under the microscope.

Just buy the book! It could save your life, or the life of a loved one. It gave me happiness, a family and so much more....

T.R., South of Atlanta, GA, USA

### Truly A More Excellent Way

This truly is *A More Excellent Way*™ of dealing with deliverance and healing. I personally have been touched by this book as well as others whom I have come into contact with.

Just a note regarding other comments (no offense meant). But scripturally it is possible for an infant to have a disease. Curses are passed onto future generations. So according to Scripture you could even receive them through the womb. It certainly is good information to know when you come against a disease to know what curse was passed from a prior generation. You can stand in the gap and break that curse from being passed on to future generations. Thank you Lord for sending the information to us. I recommend the book to anyone…caution…be ready for change.

Reader, Washington State, USA

### An Excellent Resource for Biblical Healing

This book is a must for anyone involved in prayer-based healing and deliverance and for those who find themselves victims of persistent and/or incurable diseases. It provides invaluable information about the spiritual roots of many common illnesses. (Some of these spiritual roots are inherited…just as the tendency for the disease is inherited!)

However, I agree with the "caution" below, that the information in this book is not for legalists and novices. It must be used under the guidance of the Holy Spirit. Much harm can come from telling others that their diseases are caused by certain spiritual roots…especially if it's done in a direct, forceful and unloving way. We must use this information as Jesus would. He did not lecture those who came to Him for help about the spiritual roots of their diseases. He forgave their sins (and thus healed the spiritual wounds feeding the problems), rebuked the disease and healed the person…physically and spiritually. They left feeling healed and liberated, not condemned for their faithlessness or sinfulness!

The book has a very strong biblical base, and is also based on much work "in the trenches" of an international healing ministry. One of my favorite parts of the book is the chapter on blocks to healing. It is both convicting and enlightening.

I pray that this book will help many to overcome the harm done by the spiritual forces of evil (Ephesians 6:12), and to resist the enemy who prowls around like a roaring lion looking for someone to devour (1 Peter 5:8).

G.B., Alpharetta, GA USA

### It's All about Relationship and Honesty

I found this book to be a confirmation of much personal experience (both for myself and others). It has challenged me to not become introspective (i.e., naval gazing), but rather, **honestly** examine my full relationship with God. Since I fully believe in the Trinity, I must be in fellowship with Father, Son and Holy Spirit.

We are a culture of pill-poppers. I would wonder what Eastern cultures and Native American cultures would think of this book, since the Western world is so quick to separate the physical from the spiritual. Like the title suggests, there must be *A More Excellent Way*™.

Reader, Los Angeles, CA USA

## Caution

Although I agree with much of what is written in this book, I would like to draw your attention to the author's own warning. This or any other book should not become a method, a science, a formula, or a quick fix to take the place of a relationship with God. Unfortunately, I have already seen what can happen when information like this gets into the hands of the legalist. Legalism results in condemnation and guilt. This is not a book for a novice or new Christian. If you read this book, please rely on God's wisdom in using it. It may be better to lead someone to find a spiritual root for a disease than to point it out to them. It may also be better to mentor someone to yield their life to the lordship of Jesus Christ, and it will be amazing that many of the roots will be exposed by the Holy Spirit. Then you are in a relational position to lead someone in healing, armed with the information you have learned in this book. Please use the information in this book guided by wisdom of Holy Spirit and with the humility of Jesus Christ.

Reader, Red Lion, PA USA

## Finding a Real Jewel!

Reading this book was like finding an expensive, priceless jewel in a jungle after looking for years! Words cannot express the freedom I have from reading in this book and understanding the simplicity of the deep foundational biblical truths. I have read and reread it. I encourage anyone who is hungry for the truth to read it prayerfully and with an open mind and heart. There are so many questions in life and it is not easy to find the answers. Reading this book is as if you are given entrance to the stage door and get to watch the performance from the back—then you are able to understanding how they do it. It is called discernment, and it is only valuable to you if you incorporate it into your daily life. Finally, I understand that sin is not a part of me but separate and that my freedom is in falling out of step with it and out of agreement with it and denying it use of "me" to express itself. This is actually just believing the truth...which is found in the Bible. Although it is written from transcripts of audio tapes, it is totally readable.

Reader, Paoli, IN USA

## One of the Most Significant Works on Healing Available

This book is birthed out of a frustration with the lack of healing taking place in the church today. Even in churches who believe that God is still actively healing today, only a small percentage of people who are prayed for are actually healed.

Henry Wright has done extensive medical and biblical research in order to trace out the spiritual roots of disease. Until these roots are dealt with, healing is unlikely. He addresses a whole range of diseases including environmental illness/allergies, cancer, heart disease, etc.

I have not yet seen the most recent edition, but previous editions are essentially a transcript of a seminar, so it reads a bit differently. However, the value of the material presented easily overcomes any weaknesses in presentation.

M.F., Dallas, TX USA

### The Road to Freedom

I became acquainted with Henry Wright's book through a friend of mine who received her healing because of the scriptural principles found in the book. I am now receiving my freedom from years of emotional torment. The scriptural principles in Henry Wright's book are truths taken directly from Scripture and applied to daily living. This book is all about getting free from the perpetual garbage of sin in our lives. It deals directly with personal and generational sin and teaches us how to recognize sin in our lives and in our generations and then to take responsibility for that sin and repent to God for it. This is the way I am gaining freedom from the destructive patterns in my own life.

I thank God for men like Henry Wright, who care enough about people to do and say the unpopular things.

It's a book for freedom. If freedom is what you're after, I mean freedom from repeating the same destructive things over and over again, or freedom from disease…read this book. You'll be blessed.

Reader, Thomaston, GA USA

### A Book for Everybody!

I recently met a pastor who bought a copy of this book for every single member of his flock. Now, that is a good, caring pastor! For anyone with a *Merck Manual* on their shelves, they must have a copy of *A More Excellent Way*™ as a companion.

What did I learn? Well, I tried for ages to heal myself and couldn't. I went to a thousand doctors and they couldn't do it either. Went to a few thousand more quacks and they didn't do much better. Did they want to help? Of course. Were their hearts in the right place? Mostly yes. But, only God can heal a spiritually rooted disease. Many of us just do not know how to let Him fix us. This book will help YOU let HIM.

This book will help repair the breach between you and your heavenly Father. That alone is worth the price of admission! It's not a quick fix and the ride may get bumpy, but it is definitely worth it. Will some sacred cows get chain-sawed in the process? Perhaps. Will your thinking change? Hopefully. Is it written in love? Definitely!

This book is for everybody. I was not even saved at the time when this gem fell in my lap. But, when we line up with godly principles, He will bless us.

Please bless someone with this book. It's worth sharing!

Reader, Hoboken, NJ, USA

# About the Author & His Ministry

Henry W. Wright is the President and Chief Executive Officer of Be in Health™ in Thomaston, Georgia. He has presented seminars internationally across broad and diverse audiences for a number of years and is recognized for his understanding of diseases from a spiritual perspective.

He believes many human problems are fundamentally spiritual, with associated psychological and biological manifestations. Because of his pre-med background and insights into the medical as well as the spiritual aspects of disease, he brings a unique and fresh perspective to the process of ministering to the sick. He is convinced that many diseases have an often-overlooked spiritual root, which must be identified and dealt with from a biblical perspective. He has applied these principles successfully in bringing healing to people with a great number of diseases, many of which are considered incurable.

These principles can be found in an international best-selling book, *A More Excellent Way*™, detailing spiritual roots to disease, pathways to wholeness and disease prevention.

Wright's parents were ministers. He grew up with the knowledge that God heals, because of his mother's own miraculous healing. She was dying from fibro-sarcoma cancer with a fast-growing and fatal tumor wrapped around her jugular vein just two months after his birth. Paralyzed, wasting away and dying, she was carried to a church service on a stretcher. In that condition, she cried out to God to heal her so she could raise her son. She repented of bitterness and made a Hannah-type covenant that she would raise him in the knowledge of God if He would heal her. In this private moment of prayer, God healed her instantly.

One week later, her doctors were amazed to find no evidence of cancer. No medical treatment had been given. Even more remarkably, her healing broke a pattern, a genetic factor, from her past. As her mother had died of cancer soon after giving birth to her, so she was dying of cancer after giving birth to her own child. *With the cancer defeated*, she lived another 33 years.

In his later years, Wright dedicated his life to God and the study of the Scriptures. The Scriptures seemed to indicate God wanted to heal all of our diseases, yet he observed that only a small percentage of people ever defeated incurable diseases, including those who looked to churches for help. He understood the frustration of psychologist Carl Jung, who observed his minister father seemingly offer no solutions for the diseases of the soul and body.

Today, psychology is the fruit of this frustration as an attempt to manage the diseases of the soul through therapy and drugs. Wright observed that the church, religions, alternative medicine, spiritual groups, allopathic medicine, chiropractic, and eastern mysticism trying to decrease the effects of disease through various methods, but for the most part, and in the end, all he saw was "DISEASE MANAGEMENT."

Over the years, God has shown him many insights into why mankind has disease. It is not that God cannot heal, or that He doesn't want to; the problem is man does not understand disease. We have gone into captivity and are perishing either because of lack of knowledge or just because of no knowledge at all. His investigation over the years from the Scriptures and by practical discernment has unearthed many spiritual roots and blocks to healing. In fact, the basic principles that, when applied, will move the hand of God to heal are the same that, when applied, which will *prevent* disease.

Wright does not advocate a boycott of doctors. On the contrary, he works in cooperation with the medical community. Be in Health™ has a network of doctors, psychologists, pastors and other individuals all over the world who share information about disease and spirituality.

God's perfect will is not to heal you…His perfect will is that you don't get sick. Today, Be in Health™ stands not for "disease management," but for "disease eradication and prevention."

**Beloved, I wish above all things that thou mayest prosper and *be in health*, even as thy soul prospereth. 3 John 2**

- Attended Union College in Kentucky as a pre-med student
- Spent 10 years in radio as an announcer, 5 of which were in Christian radio as an announcer and teacher
- Began ministry in 1986 and is currently the president of Be in Health™ in Thomaston, Georgia
- In 1994, the ministry purchased an existing recreational campground and converted it into a retreat on 43 acres in the beautiful foothills of central Georgia near the famed Callaway Gardens and FDR National Park.
- In 1997, the ministry purchased an existing county school complex. At this location there is a church sanctuary, teaching facilities, and offices supporting Be in Health™ globally.
- President of Be in Health™, a non-profit organization dedicated to the healing, eradication and prevention of all diseases globally. This is accomplished through conferences, networking, collaborating, publishing and ministry.
- Founder of For My Life™, an internationally acclaimed one-week ministry program held in Thomaston, GA. This is a cutting-edge program to help people defeat disease and understand the dynamics causing diseases.
- Founder of For Their Life™, an internationally acclaimed one-week training program held in Thomaston, GA. This program is designed to equip individuals to minister to others.
- Founder of For Our Life™, a program designed to allow churches, ministries, organizations and businesses to care for each other utilizing Be in Health™ principles.
- Founder of The 7000 Project™, an international networking project of churches, ministries, and individuals helping others. "We can do this…together!"
- Spiritual Lifeline™, a global program which will utilize modern methods, such as e-mail, phone or fax, as methods of connecting with those who have questions about spiritual, psychological, or biological issues.
- Who's Who. Honored member of the Heritage Registry of Who's Who™, 2004–2005 edition, in the field of Religion and Health, Healing and Disease Prevention.
- Coming Soon (under development)—"The School of the Ignorant and Unlearned" for those *who would turn the world upside down* (Acts 4:13; 17:6). A four-level school of learning and equipping is being designed to release individuals into ministry and care in the body of Christ.
- Television:
  - *Hour of Healing* with Richard and Lindsay Roberts
  - *Make Your Day Count* with Lindsay Roberts
  - *A Night of Miracles*, the TBN television special, which aired worldwide
  - *It's Supernatural!* with Sid Roth, which airs to 50 stations & internationally
  - *The Promise Land* with Marvin and Margie Rudolph, which can be seen on Sky Angel
  - *It's a New Day*, a frequent guest with Willard and Betty Thiessen of Trinity Television in Canada
  - *The Gravedigger Show* with host Joe Oreskovich on WATC Atlanta
- Radio:
  - *The Jordan Rich Show* with WBZ in Boston, a 50,000 watt station
  - *Sid Roth Live*, a live call-in talk show in 12 major cities in the northeastern United States
  - *Messianic Vision* with Sid Roth, which broadcasts internationally on 149 stations
  - *Health in Nature* with Jill Harrison in Denver, Colorado

# What We Offer

Now that you've finished reading *A More Excellent Way*™, we would like to make you aware of other resources Be in Health™ has to offer.

### For My Life™

For My Life™ is a one-week program held at the Be in Health™ campus in Thomaston, Georgia. This course is designed for people seeking restoration for their physical, emotional and spiritual health.

We believe most diseases result from a separation between God, ourselves and others. These programs will help you identify and deal with the "issues" that may be keeping you from being in health. The For My Life™ program consists of intense teaching and group ministry sessions concluding with individual "wrap-up" ministry.

### For Their Life™

For Their Life™ is a one-week program held at the Be in Health™ campus in Thomaston, Georgia. This course is designed to empower you to minister to others, helping them on their road to recovery and restoration.

We believe you will be well-equipped to identify the issues in the lives of others and be confident enough to disciple them according to biblical principles. Our insights into disease dynamics will be discussed during these sessions. The training will conclude with your participation in actual "hands-on" ministry under the guidance of our trained ministers.

### For My Life™ Children's Program

The For My Life™ children's program is a one-week program held several times per year at the Be in Health™ campus in Thomaston, Georgia. This course is designed to teach children, ages 6–12, the same age-appropriate topics offered in For My Life™. The children will participate in praise and worship and ministry and deliverance with their parents. Parents must attend a For My Life™ program simultaneously in a separate area while their children are in this program.

### For Our Life™

For Our Life™ is a program for churches and businesses. It integrates For My Life™ and For Their Life™ into a single platform where an organization may care for its members spiritually. It is a world-class program in which the body of that organization learns how to minister one to another to produce health, to produce wholeness and to remove disease.

### The 7000 Project™

Elijah thought he was the only one trying to help God. But God spoke to him and said there were 7,000 others in Israel who had not bowed their knees to Baal. He was not alone and—neither are you!

In The 7000 Project™, we are looking for individuals, churches and ministries dedicated to establishing the kingdom of God in the earth today. They must be those who have not compromised by mixing the world's system with Christianity.

If you want to help others, we want to help you. Our resources are available to assist you in identifying the problems of disease and the possible solutions from our perspective.

Features and benefits for our associates include:

1. Monthly journal with current topics, testimonies and new revelations.
2. Teaching and training materials as well as discounts on publications and recordings.
3. Access to our medical research via our Web site.
4. Access to ministry support to assist you in ministering to others.
5. Access to specific training and ministry conferences.
6. The possibility to network with others as well as ministries and churches of like mind.
7. Global interaction open forum on www.beinhealth.com 24/7 and 365 days a year.
8. Exclusive admission to equipping conferences.
9. Exclusive access to a weekly 2–hour telephone conference call.

Register as a 7000 Project™ Associate at www.beinhealth.com.

### Be in Health™ Conferences

Live conferences are available worldwide. These range from one to five days in length. If your group or church is interested in scheduling a conference, please contact Be in Health™ at www.beinhealth.com.

### Spiritual Lifeline™

We have a global program called Spiritual Lifeline™ that utilizes modern global methods such as e-mail, phone or fax as a method of connecting with those who have questions about spiritual, psychological or biological issues. This program is an extension of Be in Health™.

Further information is available at our Web site: www.beinhealth.com.

# Index

## (**bold** page numbers indicate testimonies)